UPPERS,
DOWNERS,
ALL AROUNDERS

Dedicated to
The Staff and Clients of the
Haight-Ashbury Drug Detoxification,
Rehabilitation, and Aftercare Program

and to our Fathers
Flu Hitoshi Inaba 1920 - 1993
Philip Henry Cohen 1911 - 1992

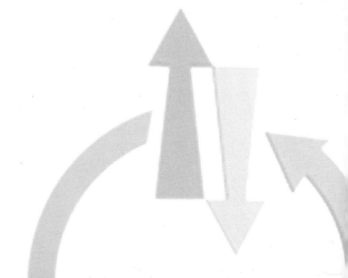

CNS PRODUCTIONS, INC.
Paul J. Steinbroner - Publisher
P.O. Box 96
130 3rd Street
Ashland, OR 97520
Tel: (503) 488-2805   Fax: (503) 482-9252

Second Edition © **1993, William E. Cohen, Darryl S. Inaba**
First Edition © 1989, William E. Cohen, Darryl S. Inaba

Cover/Book Design:

Lee Ann Ranney
Image Grafx, Medford, OR

Illustrations:

Walter Denn, Amy Hosa, Laural Schaubert, Linda Sturgeon

Photos:

Michael Aldrich, Virginia Morgan, Jason Moss, Ed Nelson,
Alan Richardson, George Steinmetz, Paul Waring

Special thanks to:
Michael Aldrich, Ph.D., Drug Historian and Researcher
Michelle Aldrich, Member, S.F. Drug Advisory Board
Greg Hayner, Pharm.D., Chief Pharm., Haight-Ashbury Clinic
Rick Seymour, Ph.D., Drug Educator
David E. Smith, M.D., Founder Haight-Ashbury Clinic

ISBN 0-926544-11-X

Printed in the U.S.A.

UPPERS, DOWNERS, ALL AROUNDERS

PHYSICAL AND MENTAL EFFECTS OF PSYCHOACTIVE DRUGS

by
Darryl S. Inaba, Pharm. D.,
Director, Drug Detoxification, Rehabilitation, and Aftercare
Program of the Haight-Ashbury Free Medical Clinics and
Associate Clinical Professor at the University of California
Medical Center, San Francisco
and
William E. Cohen
Communications Director, Haight-Ashbury Clinic

with
Michael E. Holstein, Ph.D.
Consulting Author and Editor

2nd Edition
CNS Productions

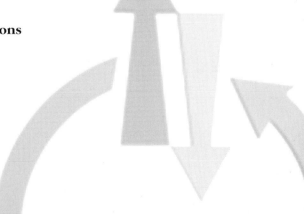

INTRODUCTION

The information and quotations in this book are based on the most current drug-abuse research and particularly on the experiences and clinical expertise of 200 staff members of the Haight-Ashbury Clinics in San Francisco and the 50,000 drug abusers who have been treated over the past quarter century.

The clinic's treatment program has one of the highest caseloads and best success rates in the country due in great measure to our success in drug education. We have found that objective, non-judgmental information about drugs and their effects are important in treatment and crucial in drug abuse prevention.

The Second Edition

The second edition of Uppers, Downers, All Arounders expands the well-illustrated, readable format of the first. It also reflects the changing face of drug abuse in the 1990's: new drugs, new theories, and innovative treatment procedures used to counter drug abuse. As in the first edition, we continue to emphasize the physiological and psychological changes that occur with substance abuse.

The second edition has added 3 new chapters:
    Chapter 9: Drugs and Sports (Chapter 9),
    Chapter 10: Drugs, Love, and Sex,
    Chapter 12: Dual Diagnosis.

In addition, we have expanded information on
    Chapter 1: The history of drug use and abuse
    Chapter 2: Neurochemistry
    Chapter 3: Stimulant abuse treatment and plant stimulants such as khat and tobacco
    Chapter 4: Benzodiazepines
    Chapter 5: Alcohol
    Chapter 6: LSD, MDMA ("ecstasy")
    Chapter 7: Inhalants and "smart" drugs
    Chapter 8: Youth and school, AIDS
    Chapter 11: Treatment

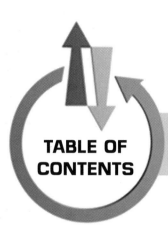

TABLE OF CONTENTS

UPPERS, DOWNERS, ALL AROUNDERS

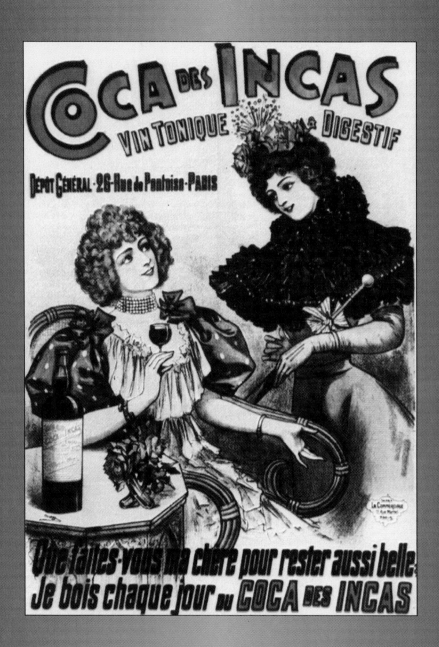

Ad for French tonic wine, made with coca leaf extract. It promised to help the user's digestion and disposition (c. 1896 by Charles Levy - Courtesy of the estate of Timothy C. Ploughman).

CHAPTER 1

HISTORY OF DRUG USE

1921

HARDING'S PEN SPEEDS DRIVE AGAINST DRUGS

President Signs Congress Resolution to Join with Other

1929

HOOVER BACKS U.S. IN DOPE WAR

By Universal Service.

WASHINGTON, Jan. 21.—President Hoover today sent a message to Congress recommending $35,000 be appropriated for American participation in the International Conference on Limitation of the manufacture of narcotic drugs, to be held at Geneva, Switzerland, May 27.

1993

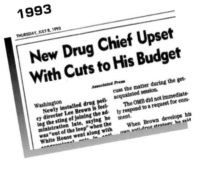

THURSDAY, JULY 8, 1993

New Drug Chief Upset With Cuts to His Budget

Associated Press

Washington
Newly installed drug policy director Lee Brown is feeling the sting of joining the administration late, saying he was "out of the loop" when the White House went along with congressional cuts, he said

cuss the matter during the get-acquainted session.

The OMB did not immediately respond to a request for comment.

When Brown develops his own antidrug strategy, he said

For much of human history, we've searched for ways to alter states of consciousness. Whether it has been to forget our harsh surroundings, come to grips with our mortality, alter a mood, explore feelings, promote social interaction, escape boredom, treat a mental illness, stimulate creativity, improve physical performance, or enhance the senses, we have felt a desire to change our perception of reality.

There are many ways, other than using drugs, to change our perception of reality: we can seek religious experiences; we can drive the body past its physical limits; we can immerse ourselves in work; we can fall in love; we can create works of art or we can read a book, see a movie, or dance until our spines tingle.

But, over the centuries, culture after culture has chosen psychoactive drugs as one of the routes (albeit a shortcut), to an altered consciousness. The physical and mental consequences of using this chemical shortcut are the subject of this book.

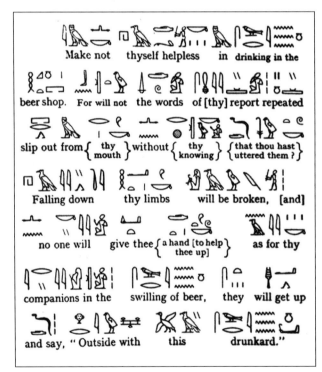

Make not thyself helpless in drinking in the beer shop. For will not the words of [thy] report repeated slip out from { thy mouth } without { thy knowing } { that thou hast uttered them ? } Falling down thy limbs will be broken, [and] no one will give thee { a hand [to help] thee up } as for thy companions in the swilling of beer, they will get up and say, " Outside with this drunkard."

This hieroglyphic from 1500 B.C. advised moderation in drink, as well as avoidance of other compulsive behaviors. Translation from Precepts of Ani, World Health Organization.

ANCIENT CIVILIZATIONS

The history of many countries is partially reflected by their use of drugs and their attitude towards them. In addition, many countries have used drugs for economic gain and political or spiritual control.

Alcohol

Alcohol has been with us since the beginning of civilization. Wherever a forgotten container of fruit or vegetables was left to ferment, some curious passersby tried the resulting alcoholic beverage and liking it, learned how to make some themselves. Many ancient cultures looked on alcohol, particularly wine, as a gift from their gods. In legends, Osiris gave alcohol to the Egyptians, as did Dionysus to the Greeks. The Jewish people have historically used wine as part of their religious celebrations. In ancient Egypt, alcohol was given as a reward to workers building the great pyramids. It also became a social problem.

Opium

More than 6,000 years ago, the Sumerians, living in the area we now call Iran, cultivated the opium poppy. They named it, "the joy plant." The milky white fluid from the dried bulb was boiled to a sticky gum, then chewed, burned, inhaled, or mixed with fermented liquids and drunk. Even then it was used for both its medicinal properties of pain relief or diarrhea control, and its mental properties of cine, wrote about poppy juice and its usefulness as a narcotic painkiller in treatment.

Marijuana

In 2737 B.C., the Chinese emperor Shen-Nung wrote about the medicinal uses of marijuana: for constipation, rheumatism, absent mindedness, female disorders, malaria, and beri-beri. However, other evidence shows that the Chinese were well aware of its stupefying and hallucinogenic properties. In the 5th century B.C., a Taoist priest reported that necromancers (channelers of dead spirits to foretell the future) used it in combination with ginseng root to "set forward time and reveal future events."

In India, almost 1500 years before the birth of Christ, the Vedas (sacred psalms) sang of Cannabis (marijuana) as a divine nectar, able to promote good health, long life, and visions of the gods.

About 500 B.C., the Scythians, whose territory ranged from the Danube to the Volga rivers in Eastern Europe, threw marijuana on hot stones placed in small tents, and inhaled the vapors. The Greek writer Herodotus wrote, "No Grecian vapor bath can surpass the Scythian tent. The Scythians, transported with the vapor, shout for joy." Most often, though, marijuana, or hemp, was prized as a source of fiber, for its edible seeds, as a source of oil, and as a medicine. Archaeologists have found traces of its use in prehistoric times (10,000 years ago) in Asia and Africa.

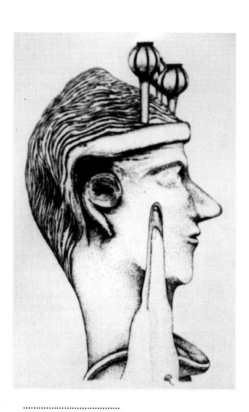

Sumerian crown, decorated with incised opium poppies (c. 3,000 B.C.).

euphoria and sedation. Because it was a potent and therefore a desirable substance, the rulers and holy men tried to limit its use to increase their control over society.

Ancient Egyptian medical texts referred to opium both as a cure for illness and as a poison. Opium was used in many ways. In Egypt it was a remedy for crying babies. The substance, called "shepen," was opium mixed with fly-specks (or more probably opium poppy seeds). In 700 B.C., Homer wrote in the Odyssey about another opium mixture called "nepenthes," given by Helen of Troy to Telemachus "to lull all pain and bring forgetfulness of grief." Even Hippocrates, the father of medi-

Psychedelic Mushrooms

The Indian Vedas also sang of psychedelic drugs. Aryan tribes, in sacred rites, drank an extract of the psychedelic amanita mushroom, also called the fly agaric. In fact, Soma, their name for the hallucinogen, was also the name of one of their most important gods. Over 100 holy hymns from the Rig-Veda are devoted to Soma. (The name Soma has been used in different centuries to represent diverse drugs from a mythical psychedelic in the book <u>Brave New World</u>, to a real prescription muscle relaxant). The intoxication, hallucinations, and delirium produced by the psychedelic have

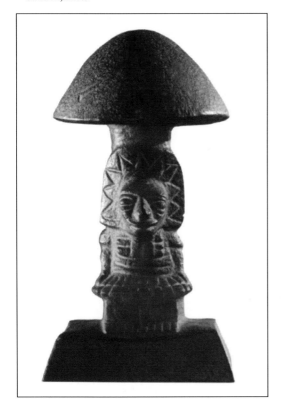

A Mayan stone god, sculpted in the shape of a mushroom (c. 500 A.D.), is one of many sculptures of the psychedelic amanita mushroom. Some date back to 100 A.D. Archives Sandoz, Basel.

been used over the centuries in religious ceremonies by native tribes from India, Siberia, and the Aztec and Mayan cultures in Pre-Columbian Mexico.

MIDDLE AGES

Psychedelic Plants

Other psychedelics used over the centuries are members of the nightshade family: deadly nightshade or belladonna (atropa), henbane (hyoscyamus), and mandrake (mandragora). Though they were most popular with medieval witches and medicine men, henbane has been referred to as early as 1500 B.C. Henbane was used as a poison and a pain-killer, to mimic insanity, produce hallucinations, and generate prophecies. Belladonna, known as "Witch's berry" and "Devil's herb," dilates pupils and inebriates the user. Mandrake, a root occasionally shaped like a human body, was used in ancient Greece as well as medieval times. Its properties, similar to belladonna and henbane, come from atropine, scopolamine, and hyoscyamine, which are all tropane alkaloids.

Psychedelic Mold (ergot)

Another psychedelic which has persisted through the ages is found in ergot, a purple fungus that grows on rye or wheat plants and contains lysergic acid diethylamide, the natural form of the synthetic LSD. The use of this drug (it was called a poison until 1943 when its psychedelic nature was recognized) is referred to in ancient Greek literature. Over the centuries there have been numerous outbreaks of ergot poisoning where whole towns have seemed to go mad and many people have died. One of the outbreaks gave the name "St. Anthony's Fire" to the affliction. Another outbreak is speculated to have been a stimulus for the Salem witch trials in 17th–century America.

Substitutes for Alcohol

After the 7th century throughout the Arab Empire, opium was seen as an acceptable substitute for alcohol which was forbidden by the Koran. The opiate was used to control pain and grief. It was also used recreationally. Extremely strong coffee and tobacco were also used as substitutes for alcohol in order to achieve an altered state of consciousness.

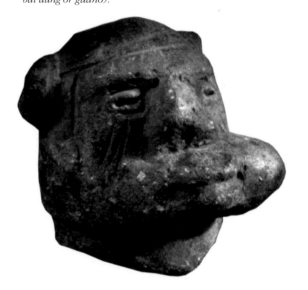

Columbian stone head (c. 1400) depicting user's cheek stuffed with concada (coca leaf mixed with bat dung or guano).

Khat

Another stimulant, Khat, was also permissible in Islamic cultures. The Arab physician Naguib Ad-Din, in 1238 A.D., distributed khat to soldiers to prevent hunger and fatigue. Another Arab King, Sabr Ad-Din, in the 14th century, gave it freely to subjects he had recently conquered to quell their revolutionary tendencies.

Alcohol

In the Middle Ages, the monasteries cultivated wine grapes to assure a supply for their Eucharistic sacrament. As the hordes of invading barbarians, from the Goths to the Huns, swept through Europe, the oft-enslaved peasant found solace in wine. Thus, the Dark Ages were somewhat lightened by hoisting a flagon or goblet.

Cocaine

Almost eight centuries ago in South America, in the Andes Mountains, the Incan Emperor Manco Capac controlled use of the coca leaf, the natural source for cocaine. "The right to chew the coca leaf was prized far above the richest presents of silver and gold." All the nobility carried their precious supply of coca leaves in ornate bags strapped to their wrists. A plentiful supply of the drug, which was considered divine, was buried with the mummified nobility.

Psychedelic Fungi and Plants

To the north of the Incan Empire, about the time Columbus

arrived in the Americas, the Aztec, Huichol, Cora, and Tarahumare Indians of Mexico were digging up the peyotl cactus (which contains mescaline), mushrooms (containing psilocybin), and the ololiuqui vine (containing psylocin), and celebrating their hallucinogenic effects in sacred ceremonies. On the other hand, the Spanish conquistadors and Christian clerics considered peyote and other hallucinogenic drugs as Satanic instruments. In fact, a manual published in 1760 that contained a list of questions to ask potential converts included, "Have you practiced cannibalism or eaten peyote?"

RENAISSANCE AND ENLIGHTENMENT

Tobacco

In 1492, after sailing the ocean blue, Columbus noted that the American Indians smoked tobacco. (He also noted that the Caribbean natives snuffed cohoba which is a potent psychedelic substance). Tobacco was thought to have medicinal qualities (an idea that lost favor after a few hundred years). Soon, the Spaniards in the New World were exporting tobacco to Europe. Tobacco became a large source of revenue for Spain and later for England. It also helped finance much of the U.S. Revolutionary War.

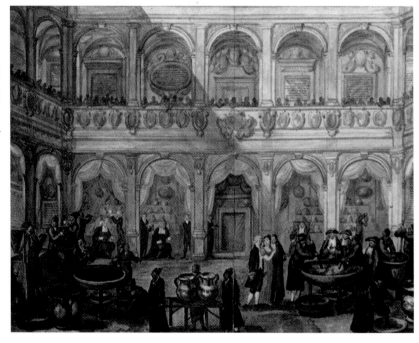

This illustration from Giuseppe Guidicini, Vestiari, usi, costumi di Bologna, in 1818 shows theriac, an opium based cure-all being prepared in batches sufficient for the entire city of Bologna.

Opium

During the Renaissance, the use of opium in medicinal concoctions came back into favor when the works of the 2nd-century physician Galen and the Moorish physician Avicenna became widely used for medical education. Theriac, one of the opium preparations that came into vogue again, was used in the Middle East, in Europe, and even in the New World for almost 2,000 years. It had more than 60 ingredients in it and was prescribed for poisoning, inflammation, and pestilence. Galen compounded it for several Roman Emperors he served. Since opium controls diarrhea, pain, headaches, and anxiety, and produces a certain euphoria, its presence in theriac was thought to be the main reason for the popularity of the drug.

Theophrastus von Hohenheim, in 1524, returned from Constantinople to Europe with the secret of laudanum, a tincture of opium in alcohol, as a panacea or cure-all medication. It was readily available, inexpensive, and soon was widely used (and abused) in all strata of society. To soothe a crying child, laudanum was quite popular. Laudanum, like theriac before it, was advertised as a cure-all for any medical ill. Scrooge drank it in Charles Dicken's <u>A Christmas Carol</u>, and it is still in use today.

Benjamin Franklin, one of America's Founding Fathers, died addicted to opium which he was taking for the gout.

Samuel Taylor Coleridge probably wrote his famous poem "Kubla Khan" while under the influence of opium.

Beware! Beware!
His flashing eyes, his
floating hair

Weave a circle round
him thrice,

and close your eyes with
holy dread,

For he on honey-dew
hath fed,

And drunk the milk of
paradise.

—Samuel Taylor
Coleridge, 1797

Coleridge was a miserable, guilt-ridden addict who drank laudanum daily to control the pain of chronic heart disease. In fact, the excessive use of alcohol along with opium and other drugs has been an occupational hazard for many writers and philosophers throughout the centuries.

Marijuana (hemp)

King George of England sent a proclamation to America in 1750 encouraging the planting of hemp (marijuana). Though the purpose was to establish an American textile and rope industry, the possibilities for smoking were not lost on our forefathers. George Washington grew hemp at his Mount Vernon plantation, but we are not certain whether he also smoked it.

NINETEENTH CENTURY

Nitrous Oxide (inhalant)

Inhaling a gas (as opposed to smoking a drug) became popular in the 1800's with the discovery of nitrous oxide or "laughing gas." Nitrous oxide was first used as an intoxicant and later found to be an anesthetic. Several other gases for anesthesia were also developed in this century, namely chloroform and ether. Nitrous oxide and other sedating drugs were regularly prescribed to women in Victorian times to keep them under control.

This 1830 print from England with its caption, "Living Made Easy," is reminiscent of the 1960's slogan, "Better Living Through Chemistry" (National Library of Medicine, Bethesda).

Opium

The production and distribution of drugs have often had an economic motive. The British government grew opium in India to trade with China for tea. "The Wars for Free Trade" as the British called them, or the "Opium Wars," as the rest of the world called them, were fought from the early to the mid 1800's to enforce the British right to sell opium to the Chinese war lords who in turn sold it to the peasants.

Since opium and its derivative morphine are pain killers as well as euphoriants, their widespread use in the U.S. Civil War to ease the suffering of the wounded rebel and union soldiers created scores of "morphine eaters, drinkers, and shooters." Opiate addiction was

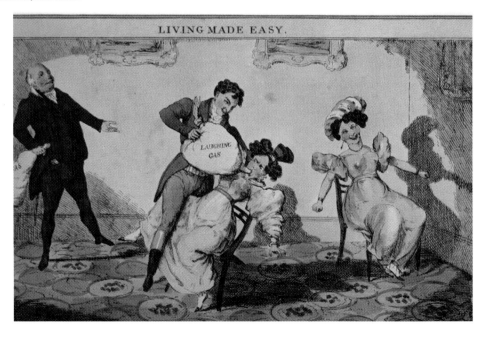

known then as "the soldier's illness." However, in the beginning, opium overuse was considered preferable to alcohol abuse since the user "wasn't as rambunctious or noisy and just sat in a corner dozing off."

Hypodermic Needle

In the 1860's, soon after the hypodermic needle was developed, cocaine was isolated from the leaf of the coca bush, and a few years later, heroin was produced from morphine at St. Mary's Hospital in London. The change from using drugs in their natural forms (i.e. snorting cocaine powder rather than chewing cocoa leaves or using a more potent version of the drug, i.e. shooting heroin rather than smoking opium) accelerated the creation of an ever–growing population of compulsive users and addicts.

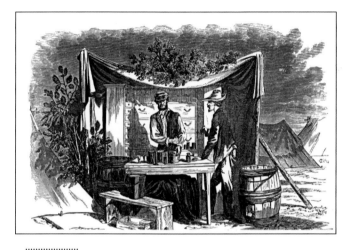

A Civil War pharmacist dispenses drugs (c. 1863).

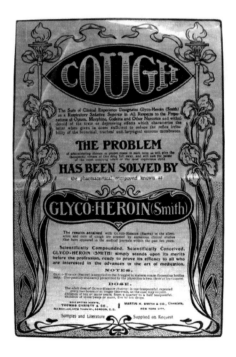

1888 Bayer Pharmaceutical ad promoting heroin for that nasty cough.

Tobacco

One of the changes that propelled tobacco from an occasional indulgence to a health problem was the invention of the automatic cigarette-rolling machine in the late 1800's. Historically, only small amounts of tobacco had been used — a pinch of snuff, a leaf in the cheek, or a gram in a pipe. It wasn't until the 19th century that automation, a more plentiful supply, and advertising promoted the use of cigarettes instead of pipes, chewing tobacco, or snuff.

....

The easy availability of tobacco led to the addiction of millions of Americans. With addiction came untested patent medicines to cure the habit. (William Hefland Collection, New York).

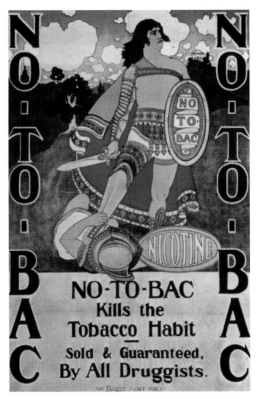

NO-TO-BAC
Kills the
Tobacco Habit
Sold & Guaranteed,
By All Druggists.

TWENTIETH CENTURY

Tonics and Patent Medicines

Vin Mariani, a fine Bordeaux wine laced with coca leaf extracts, became quite popular beginning in the 1890's, spurred on by the first celebrity endorsements from such luminaries as Thomas Alva Edison and President William McKinley.

Other over-the-counter medicines sold at the turn of the century had imaginative names such as Mrs. Winslow's Soothing Syrup and McMunn's Elixir of Opium, all loaded with opium, heroin, cocaine, and usually alcohol. Needless to say, patent medicines were very popular in all strata of society and were used to cure any illness from lumbago to depression, much like theriac and laudanum before them.

Regulation

Heroin/cocaine kits were advertised in newspapers and sold in the best stores. Our ambivalence toward drug use reached its zenith at the start of the 20th century. The age of the average user at this point in our history was 42.

By 1914, the Pure Food and Drug Act, the Opium Exclusion Act, and the Harrison Narcotic Act eliminated the over-the-counter availability of opiates and cocaine. Unfortunately, the tight control of all supplies encouraged the development of the illicit drug trade.

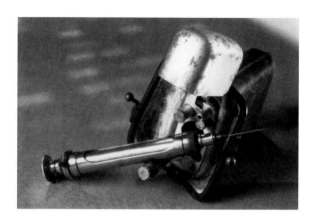

....

Kit on sale at Macy's (c. 1902) included vials of cocaine, heroin, and a reusable syringe (Fitz Hugh Ludlow Memorial Library).

Alcohol Prohibition

In 1920, it took thirteen months to ratify the Eighteenth Amendment prohibiting the manufacture and sale of liquor. Thirteen years later it only took ten months to repeal that same amendment. Americans hadn't changed their feelings about the benefits or liabilities of alcohol. They had simply found out that Prohibition didn't work.

Unfortunately, by that time, a new coalition of smugglers, strong-arm thieves, mafia members, corrupt politicians, and crooked police

1933

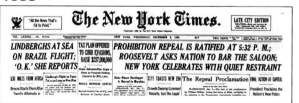

....

Headlines of the time seemed to be happy about the end of prohibition.

gave rise to a multi-billion dollar drug business which continues to promote drug use and therefore makes drugs the leading cause of crime and corruption in the world.

With the end of prohibition, alcoholism became more of a problem than ever. It forced the creation of an organization to help alcoholics recover. Alcoholic's Anonymous, a spiritual program that teaches alcoholics 12 steps to recovery, was founded by two alcoholics, Bill Wilson and Doctor Bob Smith. Over the years, AA and its off-shoots such as Narcotics Anonymous have proved themselves to be the most successful drug treatment programs in history.

Marijuana

In 1937, certain plants of the Cannabis family (marijuana) were banned despite their use in numerous medicines for over 5,000 years. The only Cannabis plants that were legal were those used for growing bird seed and for making hemp. The banning of the medicinal uses of marijuana was inconsistant since opiate-based medications, which are stronger than marijuana, were never banned, only controlled through prescription because of their medicinal value.

Amphetamine

In an attempt to improve physical performance of soldiers during World War II, American, British, German, and Japanese army doctors routinely prescribed amphetamine (speed) to fight fatigue, heighten endurance, and "elevate the fighting spirit."

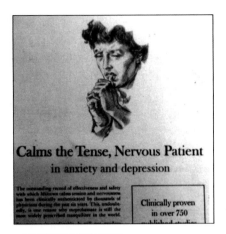

Calms the Tense, Nervous Patient
in anxiety and depression

The outstanding record of effectiveness and safety with which Miltown calms tension and nervousness has been clinically authenticated by thousands of physicians during the past six years. This, undoubtedly, is one reason why meprobamate is still the most widely prescribed tranquilizer in the world.

Clinically proven
in over 750

Miltown ad, targeted for doctors to help them convince their patients of the drug's value (c. 1955).

Sedative-Hypnotics

Barbiturates, first used at the turn of the century, came into their own in the 50's. The indiscriminate prescribing of those drugs, their widespread misuse, plus the development of Miltown and other "milder" tranquilizers, document an era of downer abuse during the 40's and 50's.

LSD

Dr. Timothy Leary encouraged the children of the 60's to "Turn on, tune in, and drop out." The guru of LSD spoke out for drug experimentation to "alter the mind." Psychedelics and stimulants (LSD, marijuana, and speed) were the most popular. Better communication, faster travel, a "do-your-own-thing" attitude, along with criminal organizations engaged in drug trafficking, helped spread the use of psychoactive drugs other than alcohol and tobacco. A flood of new synthetic psychedelic drugs like DOB, DMT, 2CB, CBR, and others, combined with the new experimental attitude of the times, made many believe in the slogan, "Better living through chemistry."

The increase in drug use was met with attempts to address the problem of addiction and crime brought on by drugs. The three methods tried were treatment, interdiction, and prevention.

Under treatment, alcoholism and other addictions were slowly being recognized as illnesses, and the treatment of compulsive use became a social science. Some of the treatment protocols tried were therapeutic communities, treatment hospitals, free clinics, and methadone maintenance.

Methadone and Heroin

Methadone maintenance programs that substituted a legalized narcotic for heroin were developed in the 60's in New York. They spread throughout the country. This was an attempt to bring the heroin addict population under control. The idea was that if they didn't have to steal for their drug, crime would go down. It was an early example of "harm reduction" for society rather than a drug-free treatment goal for the addict. Methadone maintenance continues today as the medical treatment model for addiction.

In the 70's, an unpopular war in Vietnam, along with a flood of opium from the Golden Triangle (Burma, Laos, and Thailand), encouraged the use of downers such as heroin. A whole new group of heroin addicts was created during the years of America's involvement in the war. This new junkie population was composed principally of younger, more educated and affluent heroin addicts than ever before. Only a very few Vietnam Veterans continued their heroin use after the war. The new junkies were those who had remained home to protest the war and question society's direction.

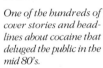

One of the hundreds of cover stories and headlines about cocaine that deluged the public in the mid 80's.

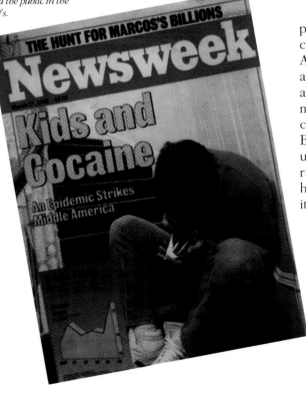

Stimulants (cocaine and amphetamines)

During the 1980's, a decade of stimulant abuse, cocaine took the country by storm. The traditional method for using cocaine, snorting, gave way to smokable cocaine, known most commonly as freebase "crack," or "rock." The "crack epidemic" was partially fueled by the media's heavy-handed news coverage, but mostly by the cheapness of a hit, the addictive properties of cocaine, and its spread from the suburbs to the inner city. At the beginning of the 90's crack was firmly entrenched in the drug culture.

In the late 80's a new and more powerful smokable amphetamine called "ice," came to the fore. Also called "LA glass," "shabu," and "rose quartz," it was stronger and lasted longer than regular methamphetamines. The initial center of "ice" abuse was Hawaii. By the beginning of the 90's, its use hadn't spread nearly as rapidly as had been feared, perhaps because of the greater severity of its toxic effects.

TODAY AND TOMORROW

At the beginning of the 1990's cocaine remains in widespread use, whether by itself (snorted, smoked or injected), or in combination with other drugs such as amphetamine ("super crank"), PCP ("space base" or "whack"), LSD ("sheet rock"), tar heroin ("hot rocks"), and marijuana ("hubba").

Psychedelics

There has also been a resurgence in the use of psychedelics, particularly LSD, MDMA, and high potency marijuana. LSD is sold in lower dosages than in the 60's and 70's and acts more like a stimulant than a psychedelic. A new, chemical variation called LSD-49, or "illusion," created in the 1990's, produces more visual distortions, much like the stronger doses of LSD-25 sold in the 1960's. It is one of the drugs used in "rave" clubs, a 90's version of the psychedelic rock clubs of the 60's. At these parties, sometimes held in legitimate clubs, sometimes in hastily rented warehouses, dancing, partying, and drug use are the rule of the day. "Ecstasy," LSD, amphetamines, alcohol and "smart" drinks used individually or in combination with each other are the most common substances taken at "raves."

MDMA, also known as "ecstasy," "X," "Adam," and "rave," is a stimulatory psychedelic. It is becoming widely used in the 90's much as MDA, a similar drug, was in the 60's. Users claim it is mellower than its chemical kin, MDA or amphetamines. MDMA users claim that it promotes closeness and empathy.

Inhalants

Another disturbing trend is the use of spray-can solvents and their propellants as inhalants. Younger and younger students are inhaling ("huffing") anything from fabric stain-proofers to ethyl chloride. They use it on their own or at "huffing parties." Up to 1,200 deaths from inhalant abuse are reported annually in the United States.

Heroin

Despite all these changes, indications seem to be that the 90's will become an era where downer drugs are back in vogue. Heroin use will see a resurgence in the 90's. Not only is there the traditional "China white" from the Golden Triangle in Asia and the "Mexican brown," there are also Mexican tar heroin, Persian brown, "Afghani," "Columbian," "African brown," and even an American domestic opium in limited quantities. Since the illegal heroin trade can be so lucrative, many of the Columbian drug lords have added it to their cocaine trade to diversify their business. Because of the money involved and the growing number of users, Chinese tongs (criminal societies) have tried to wrest control of the heroin trade in the United States from the Mafia. Indeed, federal reports, for the first time, now list the Golden Triangle in Asia as the primary source of street heroin sold in the U.S., instead of Turkey and Mexico.

Marijuana

One of the drugs that has never been out of favor and is still popular in the 90's is marijuana. The biggest change in this drug is the increase in potency (4 to 7 times as strong) and the increase in price which has gone up 10- to -30-fold since the early 70's.

Alcohol

The other drug that has never been out of favor is alcohol. Heading towards the 20th century, it is still widely used in every age group and in every country (except the Muslim nations). Used separately or in combination with other psychoactive drugs, alcohol

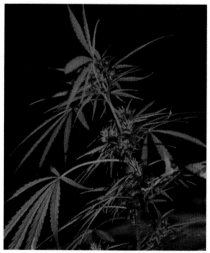

Ripe female marijuana plant (Cannabis sativa) almost ready for harvest. The sinsemilla growing method produces a higher THC concentration which is bringing more marijuana users with bad experiences into emergency rooms and drug clinics in the 90's.

kills over 130,000 persons a year in the United States, compared to 6 to 8 thousand killed by all other illicit psychoactive drugs combined, except tobacco.

Tobacco

From the peak smoking years of 1962, tobacco use in America has been gradually declining. This decline is due to the U.S. Surgeon General's Report on the dangers of smoking in 1965, anti-smoking information campaigns, warnings printed on packaging and advertising, legislation prohibiting smoking on aircraft or in public places, an acceptance by the public of the dangers of smoking, and legal suits against tobacco companies. Between 1962 and 1992 per capita tobacco use has declined by 30%.

The tobacco companies have responded by developing generic brands, cutting prices, developing foreign markets, as well as targeting females, minorities, and younger potential smokers. In certain urban centers it has been noted that "Joe Camel" is more recognizable than Mickey Mouse.

The basic reasons for wanting to alter one's perception of reality and consciousness will stay the same in succeeding generations, and psychoactive drugs will, unfortunately, always be one way that people will choose to try to bring about that change. It is therefore crucial to understand psychoactive drugs because they will affect us directly (physically and mentally) or indirectly (economically and socially) for the rest of our lives.

REVIEW

HISTORY

1. Historically, drugs have been used as a shortcut to an altered state of consciousness.

2. Alcohol and opium, then marijuana and psychedelic mushrooms, were the earliest psychoactive drugs used by various civilizations.

3. Four uses of opium throughout history have been to stop pain, to control diarrhea, to bring on sedation, and to produce euphoria.

4. Two of the psychoactive drugs used in ancient Egypt were alcohol (as a reward for pyramid builders) and opium (as a remedy for crying babies, etc.).

5. Two of the drugs used in Ancient India were marijuana (as a medicine and vision-inducing drug), and amanita mushrooms (called Soma and used for visions and sacred ceremonies).

6. The amanita mushroom and cocaine were used in the Americas in pre-Columbian times.

7. Control of psychoactive drugs was one way political and religious leaders kept control of their people.

8. Six psychedelic plants that have been used in religious, magic, or social ceremonies throughout history have been psychedelic mushrooms, belladonna, henbane, peyote, marijuana, and coca leaves.

9. Tobacco was introduced to Europe from the Americas in the 1500's. Tobacco helped finance the American revolution.

10. Opium was used as a "cure-all" throughout history: theriac, made of opium and 60 other ingredients, was used for 1800 years; laudanum, made of opium and alcohol, was used for 400 years.

11. In the 18th and 19th centuries, nitrous oxide (laughing gas) was used as an anesthetic and intoxicant. Other anesthetics developed were chloroform and ether.

12. The China-England Opium Wars were fought for economic reasons: one was the right of England to sell opium to China.

13. Opium and morphine were used as pain killers during the U.S. Civil War. Thousands of morphine addicts were created, ("Soldier's illness").

14. The invention of the hypodermic needle and the extraction of the active ingredients of opium and coca leaf encouraged abuse of drugs.

15. The invention of the cigarette rolling machine vastly expanded the excessive use of cigarettes.

16. Patent medicines at the turn of the century contained opium and cocaine.

17. The Pure Food and Drug Act was passed in 1914 controlling opiates and cocaine. Marijuana was banned in 1937.

18. The alcohol Prohibition Amendment lasted from 1920 to 1933. In the process it created the multi-billion dollar illegal drug business. The abuse of alcohol encouraged the creation of Alcoholics Anonymous, the most successful drug program in history.

19. An upper-downer cycle has been occurring in the U.S.: the downer alcohol in the 30's, stimulants like amphetamines in the 40's, sedative-downers like Miltown in the 50's, amphetamine-uppers in the 60's, heroin and Valium-downers in the 70's, cocaine (including crack) and amphetamine (including "ice") uppers in the 80's, and heroin or sedative-downers in the 90's.

20. Psychedelics like LSD and marijuana became popular in the 60's. MDA and MDMA (ecstasy) were also used. In the 90's, LSD and MDMA are making a comeback. Marijuana use has remained fairly constant. Alcohol remains the number one drug problem in most of the world.

QUESTIONS

1. What are three reasons that psychoactive drugs are used?

2. Name three ancient civilizations, a psychoactive drug they used, and how they used it.

3. What are some effects produced by psychedelic mushrooms?

4. Describe ergot and some historical consequences of ergot poisoning.

5. What two ways has alcohol been used historically?

6. Name three plants that were sacred to Central American Indian tribes in the 15th century?

7. What was theriac and how was it used?

8. What were the commercial uses of hemp in Colonial America?

9. Name three inhalants and their uses during the 19th century.

10. How did the hypodermic needle and extraction techniques lead to greater drug abuse?

11. How was opium used during and just after the U.S. Civil War?

12. What invention led to greater addiction to tobacco during the 19th century?

13. What were the psychoactive drug ingredients in patent medicines at the end of the 19th century in the United States?

14. How many years did prohibition last in the U.S. and why was it ended?

15. Give some examples of the upper-downer cycle in the United States.

16. What are three drugs making a comeback in the 90's?

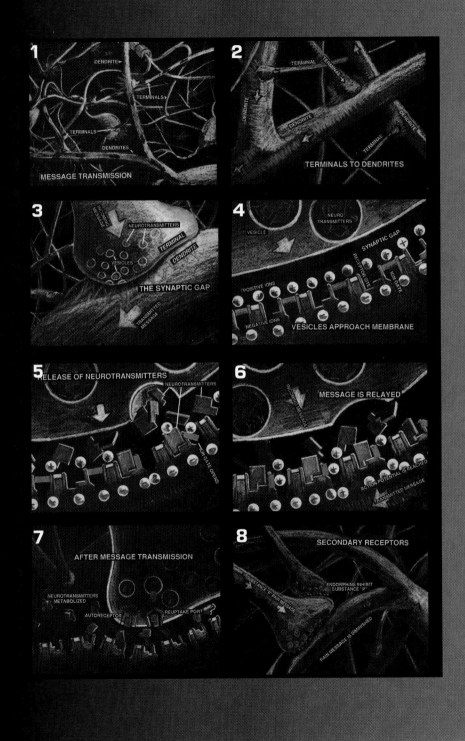

These drawings, by Amy Hosa of San Francisco, are representations of the process of message transmission in the central nervous system at the level of the nerve synapse.

THE PHYSIOLOGY of PSYCHOACTIVE DRUGS

CHAPTER 2

1923

MARIHUANA MAKES FIENDS OF BOYS IN 30 DAYS; HASHEESH GOADS USERS TO BLOOD-LUST

Physicians Called On to Urge Harding Bid
All Nations Meet to Throttle Dope At Its
Source; United States Laws Too Lenient

"The Federal Government, operating under the Harrison Act, and
co-operating fraternally. The state laws always can be appropriately
made and amended upon. The country is divided into thirteen districts,
in each of which is placed a woefully light brigade." —Sidney Howard

By ANNIE LAURIE
ARTICLE 1

1986

A Study Indicates Cocaine May Lead to Heart Attacks

By PETE THOMAS, *Times Staff Writer*

The recent sudden death of Len Bias, former
University of Maryland basketball star, and the
possibility that cocaine was a contributor, has put the
spotlight on the relationship between cocaine and its
effects on the heart.

1893

MANIA FOR MORPHINE.

Grave Charges That Have
Been Made Against Phy-
sicians of Paris.

A SPECIALISTS OPINIONS.

Fifty Thousand Persons in the
Capital Use the Drug

CLASSIFICATION OF PSYCHOACTIVE DRUGS

The question is, what is a psychoactive drug? An easy answer is that it is any drug that distorts the operations of the central nervous system. But, life is not always this easy. Ask people who have used drugs or are involved in drug abuse prevention, and you will get widely different answers.

"Sinsemilla is the number one strength, Thai sticks are second, and Columbian is the worst. Then there's always home-grown, backyard weed that everybody grows." 16-year-old marijuana smoker

"I like nitrous oxide a lot better than the other two thing: isobutyl or amyl nitrite. You shouldn't stand up or walk around when you do them." 26-year-old inhalant user (huffer)

"I started drinking gin and tonic. And then after a while, about a month, I started drinking gin over ice. And then I switched to brandy." 35-year-old woman

"Acid, in our heyday, was a lot stronger. One hit then was the equivalent of 5 or 6 hits today." 38-year-old LSD user

"This doctor I went to started out giving me Nembutal, Darvon, a little phenobarbital, Valium, and Compazine. The drugstore delivered all at one time. My health insurance paid for them. I mean, luxury, right there." Valium user

"I'd been using China White heroin, about 95% pure, for a year and a half. We ran out. I don't remember anything that happened for about 4 days. I do remember trying to drink alcohol to alleviate the pain." Heroin user

"If it's real pure, you get a real intense vibration, like waves of energy. Lots of times there's too much baking soda left in the rock." Crack-cocaine smoker

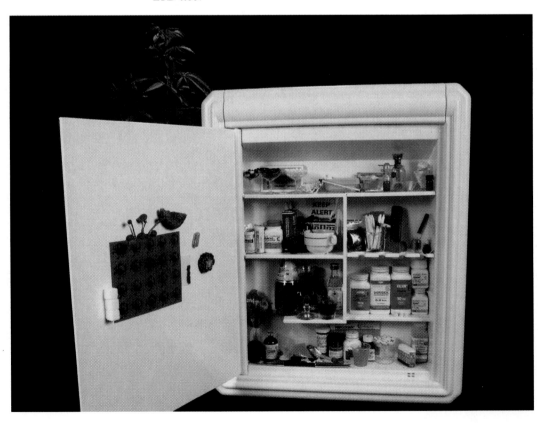

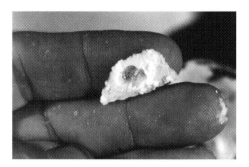

This piece of "crack" cocaine can be called "rock," "boulya," "hubba," or a dozen other street names.

The reason for the wide variety of answers has to do with the differences in the user's personality, the discrepancy in dosages, the settings in which the drugs are used, and the expectations about the effects.

A law enforcement officer might define a psychoactive drug as a schedule I, II, III, or IV substance whose illegal use carries legal penalties.

A doctor in a hospital emergency room treating a drug overdose might define a psychoactive drug as any substance whose excessive use can lead to life-threatening consequences.

A counselor working at a drug treatment center might define a psychoactive drug as any substance whose compulsive use keeps the user from functioning in a normal manner.

To compound the difficulty, drugs have chemical names, trade names, and street names. These street names like "illusion," "rave," "ice," "snot," "flip flop," "crack," "junk," "angel dust," "loads," "crank," "base," "window pane," "Adam," "hubba," "rock," "horse," "ecstasy," and "U4Euh" continue to evolve almost daily among drug users. Each commonly used and abused substance may have ten or more labels. Just as confusing is the continued synthesis of new psychoactive drugs with chemical names such as methylenedioxyamphetamine and alpha-methyl-fentanyl. Trade names such as Prozac instead of its chemical name fluoxetine or Xanax instead of alprazolam further confuses the issue of how to classify psychoactive drugs. Attempts at classifying psychoactive drugs based upon their street or chemical names have been as bewildering as the drugs themselves. Even lawmakers have to be careful when outlawing a drug since they must describe its exact chemical formula.

A more practical way of classifying these substances is to distinguish them by their overall effects. Thus, the terms "Uppers," "Downers," and "All Arounders" have been chosen to describe the most commonly abused psychoactive drugs. Then there are other drugs such as inhalants, steroids, psychotropic medications and a few others which don't fit one of these categories.

When we talk about the effects of drugs, we mean the average effects of a moderate dose on an average person. Since effects can vary radically from person to person and even from dose to dose, our information about the action of drugs on the body should be used as a general guideline and not as an absolute.

UPPERS

Uppers are central nervous system stimulants: cocaine (freebase, crack), amphetamines ("speed," "crank," "ice"), khat, diet pills, "psychic energizers," "look alikes," nicotine, and caffeine.

Physical effects: The usual effect of a small to moderate dose is over-stimulation of the nervous system creating energized muscles, increased heart rate, increased blood pressure, and decreased appetite. A stimulant can cause heart, blood vessel, and seizure problems, particularly if large amounts are used or the user is extra sensitive.

Mental effects: A moderate dose of the stronger stimulants can make one feel more confident, outgoing, eager to perform, and excited. It can also cause a certain euphoria depending on the physiology of the user and the specific drug. Larger doses or prolonged use of the stronger stimulants can cause anxiety, paranoia, and mental confusion.

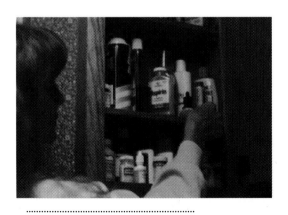

The home dispensary—prescription downers at one's fingertips.

DOWNERS

Downers are central nervous system depressants. The three main categories are:

Opiates & opioids:

Opium, heroin, codeine, Percodan, methadone, Dilaudid, Demerol, Darvon, etc.

Sedative-hypnotics:

Barbiturates, benzodiozepines (Valium, Librium, Xanax), Quaalude, Doriden, Miltown, Soma, etc.

Alcohol:

Beer (and lite beer), wine (and wine coolers), hard liquors (and mixed drinks).

Other drugs used as downers: antihistamines, skeletal muscle relaxants, and bromides.

Physical effects: Small doses slow heart rate and respiration, decrease muscular coordination and energy, and dull the senses. Downers, opiates in particular, can also cause constipation, nausea, and sexual dysfunction.

Mental effects: Initially, small doses can act like stimulants because they lower inhibitions, but as more is taken, the overall depressant effect begins to dominate, dulling the mind and slowing the body. Certain downers can also induce euphoria, or a sense of well being.

ALL AROUNDERS

All Arounders or psychedelics are substances which can distort perceptions to induce delusions or hallucinations: LSD, PCP, psilocybin mushrooms, peyote, mescaline, MDA, MDMA ("ecstasy"), marijuana, 2CB, methylpemoline ("U4Euh"), etc.

Physical effects: Most hallucinogenic plants, particularly cacti and sometimes mushrooms, cause nausea and dizziness. Marijuana increases appetite and makes the eyes bloodshot. LSD raises the blood pressure and causes sweating. MDA, MDMA, and even LSD act like stimulants, but generally, except for PCP which acts as an anesthetic, the physical effects are not as important as the mental effects.

Mental effects: Most often, psychedelics overload or distort messages to and from the brain stem, the sensory switchboard for the mind, so that many physical stimuli, particularly visual ones, are intensified or distorted. Imaginary messages can also be created by the brain, (i.e., hallucinations).

INHALANTS

Inhalants are gaseous or liquid substances, inhaled and absorbed through the lungs: organic solvents such as glue, gasoline, metallic paints, household sprays; volatile nitrites such as amyl or butyl nitrite sold as Bolt, Rush, etc., and nitrous oxide (laughing gas).

Physical effects: Most often there is central nervous system depression. Dizziness, slurred speech, unsteady gait, and drowsiness are seen early on. The solvents in particular can be quite toxic to lung, brain, liver, and kidney tissues. Some inhalants lower the blood pressure, causing the user to faint or lose balance.

Mental effects: With small amounts, impulsiveness, excitement, and irritability are common. Eventually, delirium with confusion, some hallucinations, drowsiness, and stupor can be found in inhalant abusers.

Other drugs which don't fit into these 4 categories will be discussed in later chapters; miscellaneous drugs (Chapter 7), steroids and sports drugs (Chapter 9), and psychotropic medications such as antipsychotics, lithium, and antidepressants (Chapter 12).

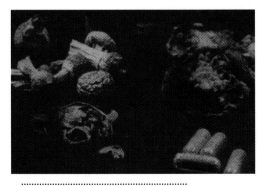

Dried psilocybin mushrooms and capsules of street psilocybin.

DESIRED EFFECTS VS. SIDE EFFECTS

People take psychoactive drugs for a number of reasons, some physical, some psychological.

Confidence

"I felt I wasn't a whole person without it. I needed the drug to become myself, especially dealing with my peers. I was more of an introvert when I was off the drug. When I had the drug, I'd be really outgoing."
Ex-crack cocaine user

Energy

"Very high energy, as though I could walk for miles. I would clean my apartment; use brillo on the floor; just lots of energy. It also made me feel very euphoric."
Amphetamine user

Pain relief

"I'm always in pain. I have bad shoulders, arthritis, and all these things, so it was my excuse cause I knew this stuff would get me high so I would take it. I would say, 'Oh, I'm just killing my pain.'" *Heroin user*

Anxiety control

"It relieved certain anxieties. It alleviated depression which I had. Lots of depression. You tell the doctor, 'I'm depressed.' 'Okay, take some Valium.' Now they try to give you antidepressant medications prescribed by the doctor. I'll take the Valium."
Valium user

Social confidence

"Somebody walks in the room and what do you do, you offer them a drink. It's cordial. That's how you break the ice. You ask, 'Would you like a drink?' And I frankly don't know anyone who says, 'No.' I like to drink. Drink is good. It makes me happy. It makes everybody else I know happy. It's a social event."
Alcohol user

Boredom relief

"It makes time go by fast, sometimes slow, depending on if you're watching the clock and if you're bored. If you're really enjoying yourself, it makes the time go by lots faster." *Marijuana user*

Altered consciousness

"I was really into the literature of the time — The Politics of Ecstasy, *or something like that, by Timothy Leary, High Priest of the LSD movement. It was more like an adventure, looking for things in it. I think people doing it at the time were trying to find out what it was like to have some sort of spiritual experience."*
LSD user

Oblivion or Escape

"I was walking by St. Boniface church and there's this wino. He takes this little bottle of gasoline or paint thinner out and he pours it in this rag and he goes snort, snort, snort. He looked real bad, like death on a soda cracker." *Inhalant user*

Competitive Edge

"I was 125 pounds. Not big enough for the team. I started taking steroids I got from a weight-lifter friend so I could bulk up." Steroid using - high school football player

If drugs did only what people wanted them to, then drugs wouldn't be much of a problem. But drugs not only generate desired emotional and physical effects, they also trigger unwanted, even dangerous side effects.

This competition between the emotional effects that users want, and the physical/emotional effects they don't want is the main danger from psychoactive drugs.

For example, a psychoactive drug such as codeine (an opiate/downer), is prescribed by a physician to relieve pain, to suppress a cough, or to treat a bad case of diarrhea. It also acts as a sedative, gives a feeling of well being, and induces numbness and relaxation. So a user who self-prescribes codeine just for the feeling of well being will also block pain, stop the cough, and become constipated. With moderate use, the user will also be subject to:

- Nausea and occasional vomiting because the drug acts on the nausea center in the brain;

- Pinpoint pupils because opiates affect the muscles which control muscle size;

- Slowed respiration and pulse because the drug affects the part of the nervous system that controls those functions;

- Dry skin and itching;

- Slowed speech and movement.

If users then take large quantities of a drug to get a desired emotional effect, they could

- Suppress breathing to dangerous levels;

- Become lethargic and have drastically slowed reflexes;

- Slow the heart rate, lower the blood pressure, and become unconscious.

And if users wanted those emotional effects over a long period of time, they could

- Become severely constipated;

- Lose sexual desire;

- Become dependent on the drug;

- Cause addiction in a fetus.

So, users have to learn how to use enough to get the emotional effects desired without damaging or mortally injuring the body and spirit. Unfortunately, each drug has certain properties which affect this emotional/physical balance making it difficult to self-prescribe any drug. Factors such as disruption of the nervous system, tolerance, tissue dependence, and withdrawal have to be taken into account.

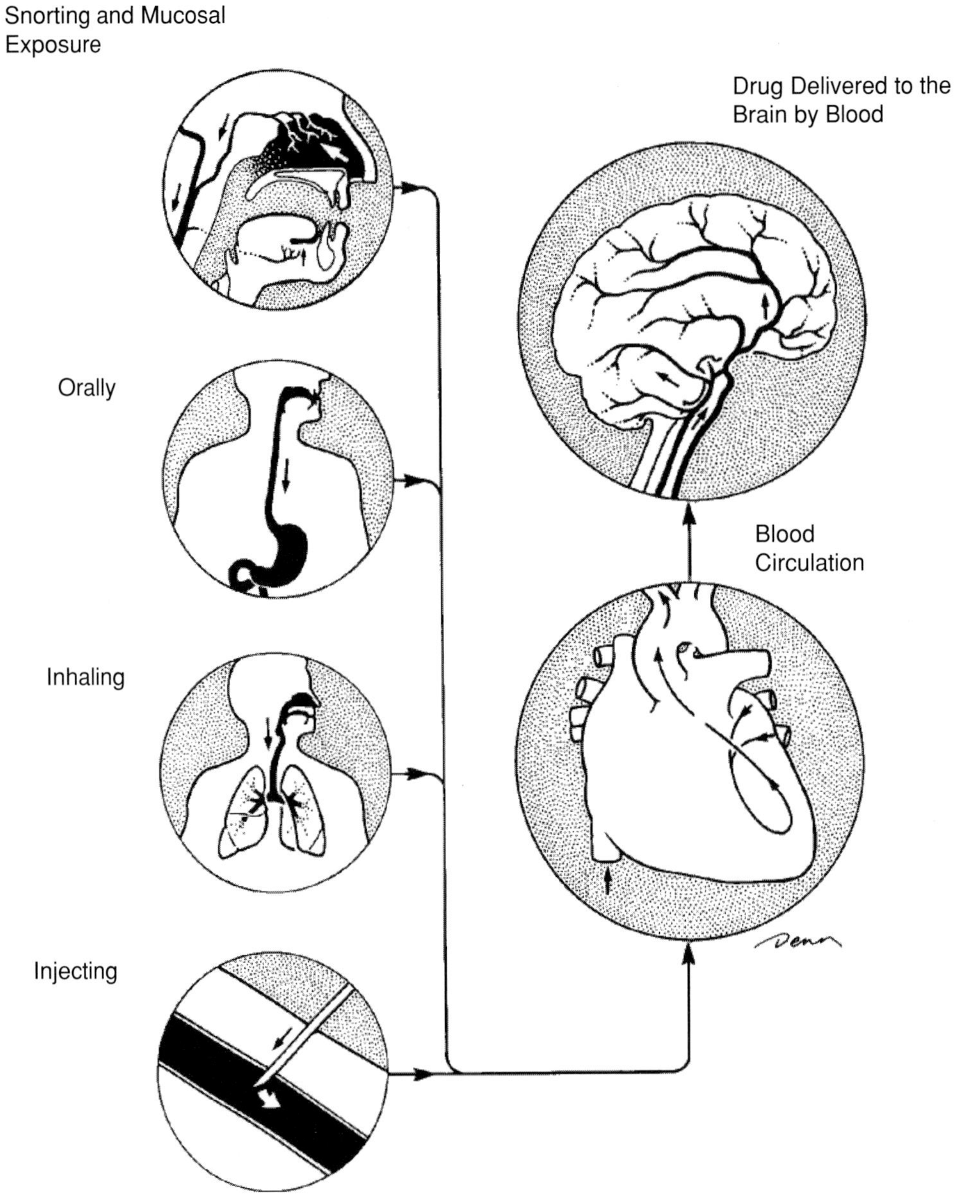

Snorting and Mucosal
Exposure

Drug Delivered to the
Brain by Blood

Orally

Blood
Circulation

Inhaling

Injecting

Fig. 2-1 *Whether taken nasally, by mouth, by inhaling, or
by injection, the drug enters the blood stream and is then
pumped to the central nervous system. It continues to circulate until it is eliminated from the body.*

HOW DRUGS GET TO THE BRAIN

ROUTES OF ADMINISTRATION

There are five common ways that drugs may enter the body:

Orally

When someone swallows a codeine tablet, or drinks a beer, the drug passes through the esophagus and stomach to the small intestine where it is absorbed into the tiny blood vessels (capillaries) lining the walls. Drugs taken this way have to pass through mouth enzymes and stomach acids before they can get to the brain, so the effects are delayed (20 to 30 minutes lag time before effects are felt).

Inhaling

When an individual smokes a joint or inhales freebase cocaine, the vaporized drug enters the lungs and is rapidly absorbed through the tiny blood vessels lining the air sacs of the bronchi. From the lungs, the drug-laden blood is pumped back to the heart and then directly to the body and brain, thus acting more quickly than any of the other methods (only 7 to 10 seconds lag time before effects are felt).

Injecting

Substances such as heroin, cocaine, and speed can be put directly into the body with a needle. Drugs may be injected into the bloodstream intravenously (I.V. or "slamming"), into a muscle mass (I.M. or "muscling"), or under the skin (subcutaneous or "skin popping"). Injection is a quick and potent way to absorb a drug (15 to 30 seconds lag time in a vein, 3 to 5 minutes in a muscle or under the skin). It is also the most dangerous method, exposing the body to many potential health problems such as hepatitis, abscesses, septicemia, or AIDS.

Snorting and Mucosal Exposure

Cocaine and heroin are often snorted into the nose and absorbed by the tiny blood vessels enmeshed in the mucous membranes lining the nasal passages. The effects are usually more intense and occur more quickly than with the oral route. Crushed coca leaves (mixed with ash) placed on the gums are absorbed through the mucous membranes (3 to 5 minutes lag time).

Contact

Liquid LSD has been dropped into the eye where it is rapidly absorbed into the brain (3-5 minutes lag time). Drugs to treat addiction such as nicotine or clonodine are applied to the skin in saturated adhesive patches where they release measured quantities of the drug over a long period of time up to 7 days (1 to 2 days lag time). In hospices for terminally ill patients, morphine suppositories are used for patients too weak for an injection or oral dose of a painkiller (10-15 minutes lag time).

DRUG CIRCULATION

No matter how a drug enters the body, it eventually ends up in the bloodstream. The molecules of the drug then circulate and travel to and through every organ, fluid, and tissue in the body where they will either be ignored, absorbed, or transformed.

In the bloodstream, the drug may be carried inside the blood cells, or in the plasma outside the cells, or it might hitch a ride on protein molecules.

The distribution of a drug within the body depends on the characteristics of the drug as well as on blood volume. As body size decreases, the blood volume decreases, so a small child of 12 might only have 3 to 4 quarts of blood to dilute the drug instead of the 6 to 8 quarts in an adult circulatory system.

The effect of a drug on a specific organ or tissue is also dependent on the number of blood vessels reaching that site. For example, veins and arteries saturate the heart muscles, and since all drugs pass through these vessels, they can have a direct effect on heart function. Bones and muscles have fewer blood vessels, so most drugs will have less effect at these sites.

Most importantly, within only 10 to 15 seconds after entering the bloodstream, the drug reaches the gateway to the central nervous system, the blood-brain barrier. It's on the other side of the barrier that the drug will have its greatest effects.

Fig. 2-2   *This drawing shows only a fraction of the blood vessels of the human body. Miles of capillaries deliver blood to the tissues including the nerve cells of the central nervous system.*

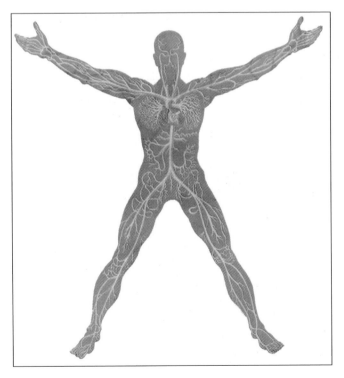

THE BLOOD-BRAIN BARRIER

The drug-laden blood flows through the internal carotid arteries toward the central nervous system also called the CNS (the brain and spinal cord,). The walls of the capillaries surrounding the nerve cells, which make up the CNS, are made up of tightly sealed cells, so that only certain substances can penetrate and affect the functioning of the nervous system. Normally, substances such as toxins, viruses, neurotransmitters, and bacteria can't cross this barrier. One class of drugs which can infiltrate this "blood-brain barrier" is psychoactive drugs (uppers, downers, all arounders, inhalants). Psychiatric drugs such as antipsychotics or antidepressants, and steroids will also cross this barrier. One reason many psychoactive drugs, including cocaine, nicotine, alcohol and the like, can cross this barrier is that they are fat-soluble, so they get to the nerve cells of the brain quickly. The brain and blood-brain barrier, being essentially fatty, keep watery substances out and let fatty substances in. For example, morphine is only partly fat soluble, so it takes longer to cross the barrier. Users who are anxious for an effect prefer heroin because it crosses this barrier 100 times faster. Crack cocaine is more fat soluble than cocaine hydrochloride, so it too crosses the barrier more quickly and gives the user a faster and more powerful reaction.

Note, however, that the brain is the most protected organ of the body, so that drugs which can penetrate its protective barrier inherently possess the ability to penetrate and affect all other organs of the body.

Fig. 2-3 *The inset shows the wall of a capillary in the brain which acts as a barrier to most substances.*

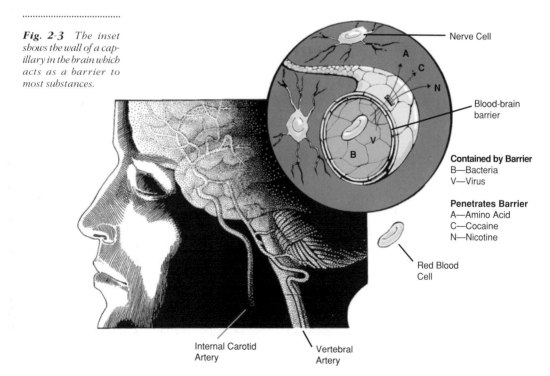

Nerve Cell

Blood-brain barrier

Contained by Barrier
B—Bacteria
V—Virus

Penetrates Barrier
A—Amino Acid
C—Cocaine
N—Nicotine

Red Blood Cell

Internal Carotid Artery

Vertebral Artery

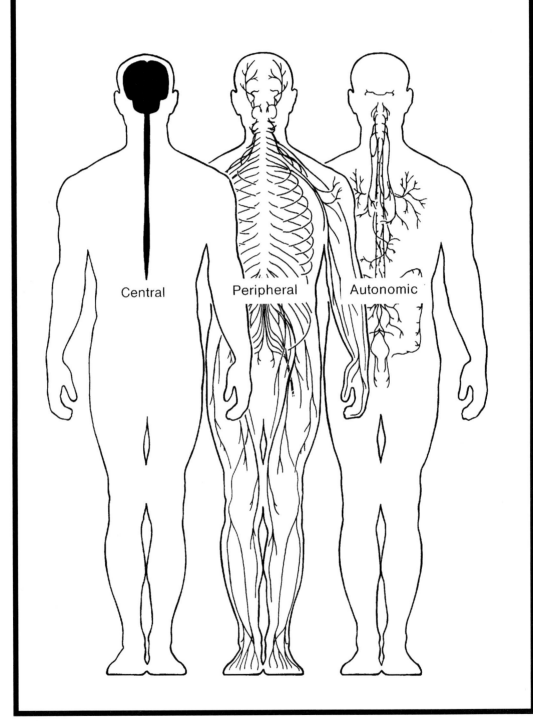

Fig. 2-4 *The three parts of the complete nervous system.*

Central   Peripheral   Autonomic

NEUROANATOMY

NERVOUS SYSTEM

Since the principal target of psychoactive drugs is the central nervous system (the brain and spinal cord), it is important to understand how this network of 100 billion nerve cells functions. The central nervous system is one third of the complete nervous system. The other two parts are the peripheral nervous system and the autonomic nervous system.

The autonomic nervous system, which is made up to the sympathetic and parasympathetic nervous systems, controls involuntary functions such as circulation, digestion, respiration and reproduction. It automatically helps us breathe, pump blood, sweat, etc., to preserve a stable internal environment.

The peripheral nervous system transmits sensory messages between the central nervous system and our environment. (Our senses interpret the environment for the central nervous system.) The peripheral nervous system transmits instructions back to muscles and other organs or tissues from the central nervous system allowing us to react to that environment.

The central nervous system acts as a combination switchboard and computer, receiving messages from the peripheral and autonomic nervous systems, analyzing those messages, and then sending a response to the appropriate system of the body: muscular, skeletal, circulatory, nervous, respiratory, digestive, excretory, endocrine, and reproductive. It also enables us to reason and make judgments.

The complete nervous system helps us distinguish sensations such as light and dark, loud and soft, sweet and sour, pleasure and pain. It governs our emotions such as love, fear, and hate; it controls our physical movements such as walking, flinching, or kissing; it regulates our bodily functions; it lets us think.

A psychoactive drug, being a powerful external agent, alters information sent to our brain and disrupts messages sent back to the various parts of the body. It disrupts our ability to think and reason. A psychoactive drug not only affects the nervous system, it affects the other eight systems of the body as well. It affects them directly while passing through the tissue or indirectly by manipulating the nerves of the central nervous system.

NERVE CELLS

Understanding the precise way messages are sent by the nerves is crucial to understanding how psychoactive drugs affect us.

For example, if a dentist extracts a lower left molar, the damaged mandibular nerve endings (Fig. 2-5 insert) send minute electrical pain signals towards the brain with a frequency of up to 1000 pulses a second and at speeds up to 200 miles per hour. The message is routed from one neuron to the next until it reaches its target in the brain.

At that point, the brain consults millions of other nerve cells, then reacts to the message and sends the appropriate signals back to that part of the body that needs to react. The brain might tell the patient's jaw to bite the dentist's finger.

....

Fig. 2-5 (Following page) Greatly magnified view of the junction of two nerve cells (neurons). The message that travels along this network must chemically jump the gap to continue its journey to the brain and eventually back to muscles and organs throughout the body.

The building blocks of the nervous system, the nerve cells, called neurons (Fig. 2-6), have four essential parts: dendrites which receive signals from other nerve cells; the cell body which nourishes the organism and keeps it alive; the axon which carries the message from the dendrites and cell body to the terminals which then relay the message to the dendrites or cell body of the next nerve cell.

The length of a neuron is determined by the length of the axon which varies from a fraction of a millimeter between brain cells, to a foot between the tooth and brain, to several feet between the spinal cord and toe.

But here's the crucial part. Terminals of one nerve cell do not touch dendrites of the adjoining nerve cell because a microscopic gap (called a synapse) exists between them.

The message jumps this synaptic gap, from the presynaptic terminal to the post-synaptic dendrite, not as an electrical signal but as microscopic bits of neurochemicals stored in vesicles of the nerve cell. This biochemical signal completes the circuit. So, electrical and chemical signals alternate until the message reaches the appropriate section of the brain.

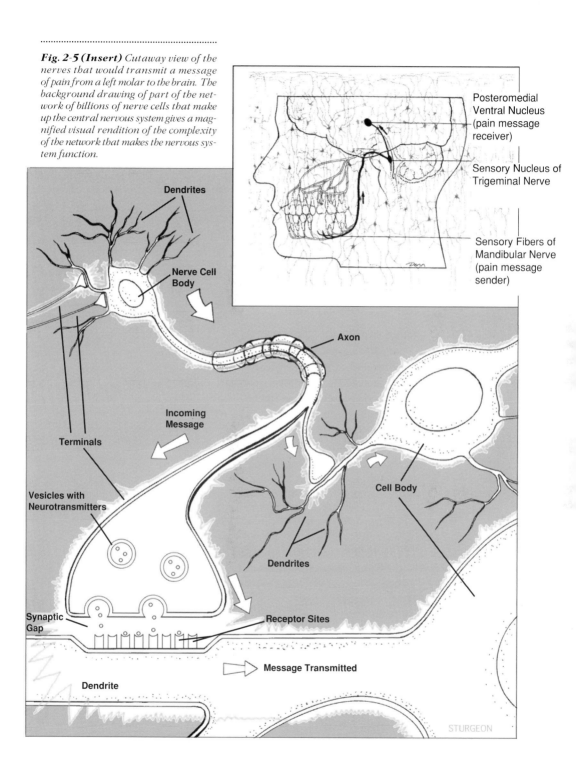

Fig. 2-5 (Insert) *Cutaway view of the nerves that would transmit a message of pain from a left molar to the brain. The background drawing of part of the network of billions of nerve cells that make up the central nervous system gives a magnified visual rendition of the complexity of the network that makes the nervous system function.*

Posteromedial Ventral Nucleus (pain message receiver)

Sensory Nucleus of Trigeminal Nerve

Sensory Fibers of Mandibular Nerve (pain message sender)

Dendrites

Nerve Cell Body

Axon

Incoming Message

Terminals

Vesicles with Neurotransmitters

Cell Body

Dendrites

Synaptic Gap

Receptor Sites

Message Transmitted

Dendrite

STURGEON

NEUROTRANSMITTERS

The biochemicals that transmit messages across the nerve synapses are called neurotransmitters because they transmit information from one neuron to another. The names of some of these compounds are dopamine, endorphin, enkephalin, serotonin, epinephrine, substance "P," acetylcholine, and at least 50 more. A single electrical message might release several types of neurotransmitters from several neurons. A pain message will release substance "P" at one synapse and enkephalin at another (Fig. 2-6).

Normally, the electrical message will cause neurotransmitters to be released from tiny holding sacs (vesicles) and sent across the gap (magnified here 10,000 times). On the other side of the synaptic gap, the neurotransmitters will slot into precise and complex receptor sites, retriggering or inhibiting the electrical message (Fig. 2-7).

Psychoactive drugs disrupt the normal functioning of the neurotransmitters. Sometimes the disruption is useful, sometimes desirable, and sometimes it is extremely dangerous.

For example, an upper such as cocaine will force the release of large amounts of epinephrine and dopamine (without an electrical stimulus) thereby creating, stimulating, and exaggerating messages to and from the central nervous system (Fig. 2-8).

A downer such as heroin, will inhibit the release of substance "P" by attaching itself to the sending nerve cell so the pain signal is dulled, dampened, and weakened. This is a useful effect. It will also attach itself to certain receptor sites in the emotional center of the brain inducing a sensation of pleasure or reward. This is a desired effect. It will also attach itself to the breathing center thereby depressing respiration. This is a dangerous effect. Normally, the inhibition of substance "P" is caused by the release of endorphins, the body's natural pain reliever, by a secondary terminal (Fig. 2.9).

An all arounder such as LSD might stimulate neurotransmitters, but mostly it will confuse them, exaggerating some messages, distorting others, and even creating imaginary ones, particularly visual and auditory images (Fig. 2-10).

In figures 2-6 to 2-10, we showed a simplified version of the synaptic gap and its biochemical activity. Fig.2-11 shows a more complex version of this crucial interface and also shows what happens after the message has been transmitted. Even this version of the synapse is vastly simplified. We show it to give you a feeling of the incredible complexity of biocellular activity in the brain.

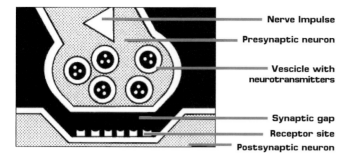

Nerve Impulse

Presynaptic neuron

Vescicle with
neurotransmitters

Synaptic gap
Receptor site
Postsynaptic neuron

Fig. 2-6 *This is a simplified version of the synapse between nerve cells. The electrical message (nerve impulse) arrives at the junction of two nerve cells, the synapse.*

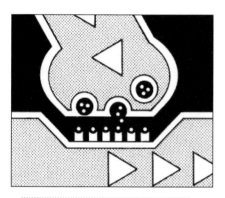

Fig. 2-7 *The electrical message is retriggered in the postsynaptic neuron by neurotransmitters slotting into specialized receptors.*

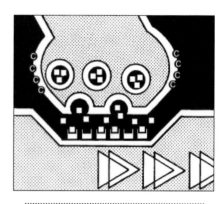

Fig. 2-8 *Cocaine forces the release of extra neurotransmitters, increasing the rapidity of electrical release, thus exaggerating the strength of the electrical signal in the postsynaptic neuron.*

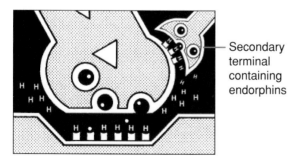

Secondary
terminal
containing
endorphins

Fig. 2-9 *Heroin inhibits the release of substance "P" and also helps block most of the neurotransmitters that do get through. So, the electrical signal is greatly weakened in the postsynaptic neuron.*

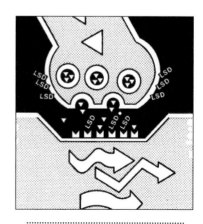

Fig. 2-10 *LSD distorts transmitted messages, creates its own messages, or makes messages jump to the wrong nerve cell. For example, a sound or a taste will become visual.*

In the diagram the precursor (1), an amino acid such as tryptophan or tyrosine which stimulates neurotransmitter production, enters the nervous system; the nerve cell absorbs the precursor (2); the absorbed precursor is used to synthesize the neurotransmitter (3); the neurotransmitters are stored in vesicles (4); when needed, the vesicles move to the surface of the presynaptic neuron (5) and release the tiny bits of neurotransmitter; the neurotransmitters can slot into receptor sites (6) to activate an electrical signal in the post-synaptic neuron; the released neurotransmitters can also be reabsorbed by the re-uptake port (7) in the pre-synaptic neuron, or be degraded biochemically (8), or be flushed from the system (9), or slot on to an autoreceptor (10) in order to signal the cell to make fewer neurotransmitters.

The discovery of naturally occurring neurochemicals (neurotransmitters) with opiate-like activity (endorphins and enkephalins) was the most significant development in the understanding of how drugs work in the body and how they can cause addiction. For the first time, reaction and addiction to psychoactive drugs could be described in terms of the physical

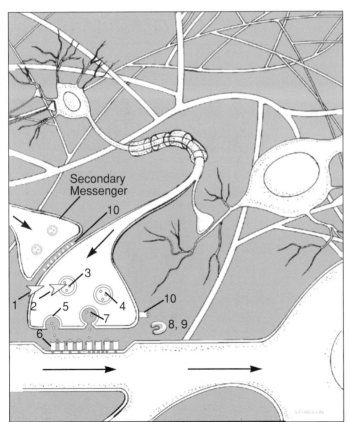

Fig. 2-11 Neurotransmitter dynamics. This drawing shows a more complex version of the synapse. It also shows what happens to the neurotransmitters after they transmit the signal. (Even this version is vastly simplified.)

Fig. 2-12 Psychoactive Drug/ Neurotransmitter Relationships

Drug	Neurotransmitter
Alcohol	Met-enkephalin, gama amine butyric acid (GABA), serotonin
Benzodiazepines	GABA, glycine
Marijuana	Acetylcholine
Heroin	Endorphin, enkephalin, dopamine
LSD	Acetylcholine, dopamine, serotonin
Nicotine	Adrenalin, endorphin, acetylcholine
Cocaine/ Amphetamines	Adrenalin (epinephrine), & noradrenalin (norepinephrine), serotonin, dopamine, acetylcholine
MDA, MDMA	Serotonin, dopamine, adrenalin
PCP	Dopamine, acetylcholine, alpha-endopsychosin

and genetic makeup of a person. As with other diseases like diabetes (a dysfunction of the insulin producing pancreas) or thyroid deficiencies, addiction to opiates was matched to a true biocellular and neurochemical disturbance.

Those who are born with low endorphin/enkephalin capacity have a genetic propensity for opiate and alcohol addiction. Even those born with normal capacities could disrupt and impair their ability to make those neurotransmitters through continuous excessive exposure to opiate drugs. This also means that like other illnesses, addictions are treatable and their progression can be arrested.

Once opiate-like neurotransmitters were discovered, the search for other natural neurochemicals which also mimic psychoactive drugs began in earnest. Although most psychoactive substances affect a number of neurotransmitters simultaneously, current investigations suggest a strong correlation between specific neurotransmitters and specific drugs (Fig. 2-12)

Besides more than 60 known substances such as neurotransmitters and neuromodulators, it is estimated that eventually some 300 brain chemicals will be identified.

THE NATURE OF DRUGS

Microscopic in size, neurotransmitters nevertheless exert powerful control over our actions, feelings, and behavior. A small quantity of a psychoactive drug can affect these neurotransmitters and modify or disrupt every system of our body.

One example might give a sense of proportion about the effects of psychoactive drugs on neurotransmitters. A drug called carfentanyl, a synthetic opiate/downer, is 25,000 times more powerful than heroin, so powerful that a quantity of the drug the size of a grain of salt would be enough to kill 150 people. By contrast, it might take 2 quarts of chug-a-lugged whiskey to kill just one person.

A variety of factors besides strength of the drug—i.e., purity, quantity, how, when, and where the drug is taken, physical and mental makeup of the user, how long the drug has been used, interaction among drugs, exaggerated reaction to a drug, and even age and sex—must be considered when judging the effect a drug will have.

Strength of drug

"Every time I took it, I was experimenting. 'Will I enjoy this or am I going to freak out?'" LSD user

Physical makeup of user

"Sometimes you feel jumpy, ready to go; sometimes not. You just feel like sitting around relaxing, not doing a whole lot. Sometimes, you're running around and playing soccer." Marijuana smoker

Tolerance

"When I first started, I remember having a huge reaction to a small amount of it. Inside of a year, I could shoot a spoon of 'speed' easily, which is a pretty fair amount, and it finally got to a point where I couldn't even sleep unless I'd done some." Recovering 'speed' user

Interaction among drugs

"I went to a party and I started drinking and using codeine, and I became drunk very fast. I didn't realize that mixing the two could cause an overdose." Recovering codeine user

Exaggerated reaction

"When I took cocaine, there was a heavy beating, tachycardia, a sense of not being able to get my breath. There was also the sensation of everything moving very quickly and intensely." Recovering cocaine user

Various aspects of adaptability to the drug reflected by such phenomena as tolerance, tissue dependence, withdrawal, and metabolism are also crucial to understanding how drugs affect us.

TOLERANCE

The body regards any drug it takes as a poison. Various organs, especially the liver and kidney, try to eliminate the chemical before it does too much damage. But drug use over a long period of time forces the body to change and adapt.

For example, the body adapts to a barbiturate in order to minimize the depressant effect on various systems including respiration and heart rate, so the drug appears to weaken with each succeeding dose. More has to be taken just to achieve the same effect.

One tablet of Seconal on the first day, three on the 100th day, and nine on the 300th day might be needed to give the same sedation (Fig. 2-13). One amphetamine tablet in the beginning will energize a user as much as 20 pills on day 100. A glass of whiskey on day one might give the same buzz as a quart on day 200.

Fig. 2-13 This graph shows the gradually increasing amounts of Seconal (depressant) needed to produce sleep or euphoria over time.

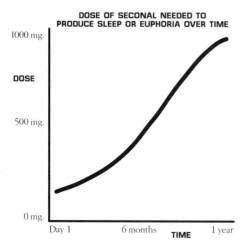

DOSE OF SECONAL NEEDED TO
PRODUCE SLEEP OR EUPHORIA OVER TIME

Dispositional tolerance

The body speeds up the breakdown or metabolism of the drug in order to dispose of or eliminate it. This is particularly the case with barbiturates and alcohol where liver cells produce more metabolizing enzymes as one continues to take the drugs.

Inverse tolerance
("kindling" and tachyphylaxis)

The person becomes more sensitive to the effects of the drug as the brain chemistry changes. A marijuana or cocaine user, after months of getting a minimal effect from the drug, will all of a sudden get an intense reaction.

"Man, at first I could smoke a monster joint and snort half a bindle without feeling a thing. I was wasting my money. Then boom, all of sudden I could get high on just a few hits and a couple of lines." Recovering polydrug user

Pharmacodynamic tolerance

The nerve cells become less sensitive to the effects of the drug and even produce an antidote or an tagonist to the drug. With opiates, the brain will grow more opiate receptor sites and produce its own antagonist, cholecystokinin.

Behavioral tolerance

The brain learns to compensate for the effects of the drug by using parts of the brain not affected. An alcoholic will pass a sobriety test but a few minutes later will be staggering again.

Reverse tolerance

Initially, one becomes less sensitive to the drug, but as it destroys certain tissues and/or as one grows older, the trend is suddenly reversed and the user becomes more sensitive. This is particularly true in alcoholics when, as the liver is destroyed, it loses the ability to metabolize the drug. A wino with cirrhosis of the liver can stay drunk all day long on a pint of wine because the raw alcohol is passing through the body, time and again, unchanged.

> "At first, I could drink a lot, for about 8 or 9 years. They'd say I finished 2 bottles in the bar, but I'd never get drunk. I'd be pretty high, but I wouldn't fall, never passed out. Now, if I drink over about 4 drinks, I go into a blackout."
> Alcohol user

Fig. 2-14 Dose of Seconal needed to produce sleep or euphoria versus the amount needed to overdose.

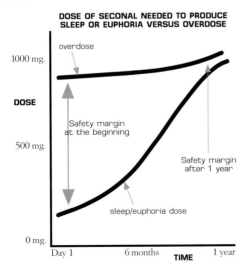

DOSE OF SECONAL NEEDED TO PRODUCE
SLEEP OR EUPHORIA VERSUS OVERDOSE

overdose

1000 mg.

DOSE

Safety margin
at the beginning

500 mg.

Safety margin
after 1 year

sleep/euphoria dose

0 mg.

Day 1   6 months   **TIME**   1 year

Acute tolerance

In these cases, the body begins to adapt almost instantly to the damaging effects of the drug. With tobacco, for example, tolerance and adaptation begin to develop with the first puff. Someone who tries suicide with barbiturates can develop an instant tolerance and survive the attempt with twice the lethal dose in his or her system.

> "When I came to, in the hospital, the doctor said my blood level of seconal was still high enough to kill three people or a horse."
> Barbiturate abuser

Select tolerance

If increased quantities of a drug are taken to overcome this tolerance and to achieve a certain high, it's easy to forget that tolerance to the physical side effects also continues to escalate but not at the same rate, so the dose needed to achieve an emotional high comes closer and closer to the lethal physical dose of that drug (Fig. 2-14).

> "As many pills as I had, I would take. I didn't really care about overdose which I did many times." Former barbiturate user

As more of the drug is used over longer periods of time, the greater are the alterations in the brain chemistry and the more likely that person is to become a compulsive drug user or addict.

TISSUE DEPENDENCE AND WITHDRAWAL

The biological adaptation of the body due to prolonged use of drugs is quite extensive, particularly with downers. In fact, the body can change so much that the tissues and organs come to depend on the drug just to stay normal.

"I would start to feel very abnormal after 2 or 3 hours, and it was like trying to maintain until I could begin to feel normal. And that was the only kind of normal that I knew, Darvon-induced normality." Darvon user

....

Fig. 2-15 *The withdrawal effects are usually the opposite of the direct effects of the drug.*

Heroin Effects	Withdrawal Symptoms
Numbness	becomes pain
Euphoria	becomes anxiety
Dryness of mouth	becomes sweating, running nose
Constipation	becomes diarrhea
Slow pulse	becomes rapid pulse
Low blood pressure	becomes high blood pressure
Shallow breathing	becomes coughing
Pinpoint pupil	becomes dilated pupil
Sluggish muscle response	becomes severe hyper-reflexing & muscle cramps.

An example of biological adaptation can be seen with alcohol. It disrupts the release of certain neurotransmitters in the brain. It also increases the amount of cytocells and mitochondria in the liver that are available to neutralize the drug. The tissues have come to depend on the alcohol to maintain this new balance.

However, when the user stops taking the drug, the body is left with an altered chemistry. There might be an overabundance of one kind of enzyme and a lack of certain neurotransmitters. All of a sudden, the body tries to restore its balance. Usually, all the things the body was kept from doing while taking the drug, it does to excess while in withdrawal.

For example, consider how the desired effects of a drug quickly are transformed into unpleasant withdrawal symptoms once a long-time user stops taking a drug like heroin (Fig. 2-15).

In fact, with many compulsive users, the fear of withdrawal is one reason they keep using. They don't want to go through the aches, pains, insomnia, vomiting, cramps, and occasional convulsions that accompany withdrawal.

"The rush I would get from shooting up again was: all of a sudden my body would not be sick anymore from withdrawal. That was the high." Heroin user

Because the withdrawal as well as the fear of withdrawal can be so severe, many treatment programs use mild drugs to temper these symptoms.

Withdrawal from opiates, alcohol, many sedatives and even nicotine seems to be triggered by an area of the brain stem, known as the locus cereleus. Drugs like Clonidine, Vasopressin, and Baclofen, which act at this part of the brain, block out the withdrawal symptoms of these drugs.

There are three distinct types of withdrawal symptoms: non-purposive, purposive, and protracted.

Non-purposive withdrawal

Non-purposive withdrawal consists of objective physical signs that are directly observable upon cessation of drug use by an addict. These are seizures, sweating, goose bumps, vomiting, diarrhea, tremors, etc. These signs are a direct result of the tissue dependence that has developed.

> *"When I ran out, it was severe. I mean, body convulsions, long memory lapses, cramps that were just enough to—you couldn't stand them. And, it lasted for about 5 days; the actual convulsions, the cramps, and the pain and stuff. And then, it took another couple of weeks before I ever felt anywhere near normal."*
> *Recovering heroin user*

Purposive withdrawal

Purposive withdrawal results from either addict manipulation (hence "purposive" or "with pur-

pose") or from a psychic conversion reaction from the expectation of the withdrawal process. For example, a common behavior of most addicts is manipulative behavior. In an effort to secure more drugs, sympathy, or money, addicts may claim to have withdrawal symptoms that are very diverse and difficult to verify, i.e., "My nerves are in an uproar, so you've got to give me something, Doc!" It is dangerous to the user for the physician to respond to such manipulations.

> *"It takes a doctor 30 minutes to say no, but it only takes him 5 minutes to say yes. We used to share doctors that we could scam. We called them 'croakers.'"*
> *Recovering heroin user*

Within the past few decades, the protrayal of drug addiction by the media, books, movies, and television has resulted in another kind of purposive withdrawal. Younger, addiction-naive drug users expect to suffer withdrawal symptoms similar to those portrayed in the media, when they run out of drug. This expectation results in a neurotic condition whereby they experience a wide range of reactions even though tissue dependence has not truly developed. There is much danger in overreacting to these symptoms.

Protracted withdrawal (environmental trigger & cues)

A major danger to both maintaining recovery and preventing a drug overdose during relapse is protracted withdrawal. This is a flashback or recurrence of the addiction withdrawal symptoms and heavy craving for the drug long after one has detoxified. The cause of this reaction is most likely a post-traumatic stress phenomenon, where some sensory input (odor, sight, noise, etc.) stimulates the stressful memories experienced during drug withdrawal and evokes a re-experiencing of those symptoms and desire for the drug by the addict. For instance, the odor of burnt matches or burning metal (smells that occur when cooking heroin), may cause a heroin addict to suffer withdrawal several months after detoxification. Any white powder may cause the same reaction in a cocaine addict; the odor of hemp burning may do it for a compulsive marijuana smoker; a blue pill may do it to for Valium addict; a crowded bar, for an alcoholic.

"After I've gone through withdrawal and I pass by areas where I used to hang out, and I see other people nodding, in my mind, I start feeling like I'm sick again." Recovering heroin user

Protracted withdrawal often causes users to try their drug again, possibly leading to a full relapse. Unfortunately, these slips are associated with a greater chance of drug overdose since users are prone to use the same dose they were using when they quit. They forget that their last dose was a high one that they could handle because the body had changed and had developed a tolerance. They forget that their abstinence returned their body to a less tolerant state, unable to handle a high-dose.

"We cleaned up because we didn't have any connections when we moved. We had about 15 clonidine to help us through and I was drinking. Then we each did one bag, one $20 dollar bag of cut, and both of us were on the floor." Heroin user

METABOLISM

Metabolism is defined as the body's mechanism for processing, using, and eventually eliminating foreign substances such as food or drugs. So, as a drug exerts its influence upon the body, it is gradually neutralized, usually by the liver or kidneys. It can also be metabolized by the blood, the lymph fluid, or almost any body tissue that recognizes the drug as a foreign substance.

The liver, in particular, has the ability to break down or alter the chemical structure of drugs, making them less active or inert. The kidneys, on the other hand, filter the blood continuously and excrete toxic substances into the urine. Drugs can also be excreted out of the body by the lungs, in sweat, or in feces.

Metabolic processes generally decrease but occasionally increase the effects of psychoactive drugs. Think of the liver, for instance, as a series of tiny chemical factories filled with active body chemicals called enzymes which cause chemical changes. For example, these enzymes help convert alcohol to water, oxygen, and carbon dioxide which are then excreted from the body through the kidneys, sweat glands, and lungs. Valium,

Fig. 2-16   The liver deactivates a portion of the drug with each recirculation through the circulatory system.

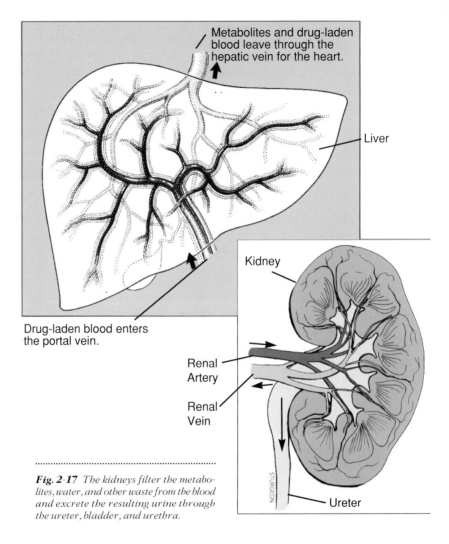

Metabolites and drug-laden blood leave through the hepatic vein for the heart.

Liver

Drug-laden blood enters the portal vein.

Kidney

Renal Artery

Renal Vein

Ureter

Fig. 2-17 The kidneys filter the metabolites, water, and other waste from the blood and excrete the resulting urine through the ureter, bladder, and urethra.

on the other hand, is transformed by the liver's enzymes into three or four compounds which are more active than the original drug.

If a drug is eliminated slowly, as with amphetamines or Valium, it can affect the body for hours, even days. If it is eliminated quickly, as with smokable cocaine or nitrous oxide, the major reactions might last just a few minutes, though other subtle side effects last for days, weeks, or even longer.

The following are some other factors which affect the metabolism of drugs.

Age

After the age of 30 and with each subsequent year, the body produces fewer and fewer liver enzymes capable of metabolizing certain drugs so, the older the patient, the greater the effect. This is especially true with drugs like Valium and other benzodiazepines.

Race

Different ethnic groups have different levels of enzymes. Most Asians break down alcohol more slowly than do Caucasians. They generally suffer more side effects such as nausea and redness of the face. They will, in fact, get drunk on less alcohol.

Heredity

Individuals pass certain traits to their offspring that affect the metabolism of drugs. They might have a low level of enzymes that metabolize the drug; they might have more body fat which will store certain drugs like Valium or PCP; or they might have a high metabolic rate which will usually eliminate drugs more quickly from the body.

Sex

Males and females have a different body chemistry. Drugs such as barbiturates, which are protein bound, generally have greater effects in women than in men.

Health

Certain medical conditions affect metabolism. Alcohol in a drinker with severe liver damage (cirrhosis) causes more problems than in a drinker with a healthy liver.

Emotional State

The emotional state of the drug user also has a major effect on the drug's action. LSD in someone with paranoia can be very dangerous because it can further disrupt the chemical balance of the brain.

Other Drugs

The presence of another drug can keep the body so busy that metabolism of a new drug is delayed. For example, the presence of alcohol keeps the liver so busy that a Xanax or Seconal will remain in the body two or three times longer than normal.

In addition, such factors as weight of the user, the level of tolerance, and even the weather or time of day can affect the metabolism of a psychoactive drug.

THE PHYSIOLOGY OF PSYCHOACTIVE DRUGS

1. The major classes of psychoactive drugs are uppers (stimulants), downers (depressants), all arounders (psychedelics), and inhalants.

2. Drugs can enter the body through eating/drinking, inhaling (smoking), injecting, contact, and snorting.

3. Drugs travel in the bloodstream to reach the central nervous system (CNS). They must cross the blood-brain barrier to reach the nerve cells of the CNS.

4. Drugs which reach the cells of the central nervous system are called psychoactive drugs. These drugs affect the rest of the body either directly or by acting on the nerves of the central nervous system.

5. The central nervous system controls all body functions, thought processes, and emotions, so drugs that affect these nerve cells affect every system in the body.

6. Neurotransmitters are biochemicals found in all nerve cells. It is these biochemicals which are actually responsible for the transmission of nerve impulses.

7. Psychoactive drugs inhibit, stimulate, or distort the release of these chemicals. They can also stimulate or inhibit the actions of neurotransmitters.

8. The magnitude of the effects depends on the quantity and quality of the drug taken and how it is metabolized by the body. The liver is the principal organ for neutralizing drugs. The kidneys are the principal organs for filtering drugs from the blood.

9. The major problem with psychoactive drugs is that when people take them, they focus on the desired mental and emotional effects and ignore the potentially damaging physical and mental side effects that can occur.

10. When a person takes certain drugs over a period of time, particularly depressants, the body becomes used to their effects so more is needed to achieve the same high. The user develops a tolerance to the drug.

11. The body tries to adapt to the increased quantities of drugs taken, and so tissue dependence develops (in particular with downers). The user has to keep taking the drug just to stay in balance.

12. When a user stops taking a drug after tissue dependence has developed (mostly with opiates, alcohol, and sedative-hypnotics), the body experiences many of the sensations and physical changes it was kept from feeling while taking the drug. This backlash is known as withdrawal.

QUESTIONS

1. Name the four major classes of psychoactive drugs and list three drugs in each category.

2. Describe a physical and an emotional effect of heroin.

3. Describe the five ways a drug can be taken and how it reaches the bloodstream. List the five routes in order of speed of action.

4. Describe the route a drug takes when swallowed, from the mouth to the blood-brain barrier.

5. What is the function of the blood-brain barrier?

6. What are the three different parts of the complete nervous system and what are their functions?

7. What are the two parts of the central nervous system?

8. What is a synapse?

9. What are neurotransmitters?

10. How do the different classes of psychoactive drugs (uppers, downers, all arounders) affect neurotransmitters?

11. Name three different neurotransmitters.

12. What is tolerance?

13. What is tissue dependence?

14. Name five effects of codeine and their equivalent withdrawal rebound effects?

15. What organs of the body metabolize and/or filter out psychoactive drugs?

16. Name five factors such as age which govern the metabolism of a psychoactive drug.

The cocaine shot into Duncan Andrew's antecubital vein in a concentrated bolus after having been propelled by the plunger of a syringe. Chemical alarms sounded immediately. A number of the blood cells and plasma enzymes recognized the cocaine molecules as being part of a family of compounds called alkaloids, which are manufactured by plants and include such physiologically active substances as caffeine, morphine, strychnine, and nicotine.

In a desperate but vain attempt to protect the body from this sudden invasion plasma enzymes called cholesterases attacked the cocaine, splitting some of the foreign molecules into physiologically inert fragments. But the cocaine dose was overwhelming. Within seconds the cocaine was streaking through the right side of the heart, spreading through the lungs, and then heading out into Duncan's body.

The pharmacologic effects of the drug begin almost instantly. Some of the cocaine molecules tumbled into the coronary arteries and began constricting them and reducing blood flow to the heart.

Simultaneously the cocaine molecules fanned out throughout the brain, having coursed up into the skull through the carotid arteries. Like knives through butter, the cocaine penetrated the blood brain barrier. Once inside the brain, the cocaine bathed the defenseless brain cells pooling in spaces called synapses across which the nerve cells communicated.

Within the synapses the cocaine began to exert its most perverse effects. It became an impersonator. By an ironic twist of chemical fate, an outer portion of the cocaine molecule was erroneously recognized by the nerve cells as a neurotransmitter, either epinephrine, norepinephrine, or dopamine. Like skeleton keys, the cocaine molecules insinuated themselves into the molecular pumps responsible for absorbing these neurotransmitters, locking them, and bringing the pumps to a sudden halt.

The result was predictable. Since the reabsorption of the neurotransmitters was blocked, the neurotransmitters' stimulative effect was preserved. And the stimulation caused the release of more neurotransmitters in an upward spiral of self-fulfilling excitation. Nerve cells that would have normally reverted to quiescence and serenity began to fire frantically.

The brain progressively brimmed with activity, particularly the pleasure centers deeply embedded below the cerebral cortex. Here dopamine was the principal neurotransmitter. With a perverse predilection the cocaine blocked the dopamine pumps, and the dopamine concentration soared. Circuits of nerve cells divinely wired to ensure the survival of the species rang with excitement and filled afferent pathways running up to the cortex with ecstatic messages.

But the pleasure centers were not the only areas of Duncan's brain to be affected, just some of the first. Soon the darker side of the cocaine invasion began to exert its effect. Phylogenetically older, more caudal centers of the brain involving functions like muscle coordination and the regulation of breathing began to be affected. Even the thermoregulatory area began to be stimulated, as well as the part of the brain responsible for vomiting.

Thus all was not well. In the middle of the rush of pleasurable impulses, an ominous condition was in the making. A dark cloud was forming on the horizon, auguring a horrible neurological storm. The cocaine was about to reveal its true deceitful self: a minion of death disguised in an aura of beguiling pleasure . . .

Just before the EMT's arrived, Duncan finally stopped convulsing and died.

Putnam Publishing Group from <u>Blindsight</u> by Robin Cook, Copyright (c) 1992 by Robin Cook
Coca bush in background.

CHAPTER 3

UPPERS

1897

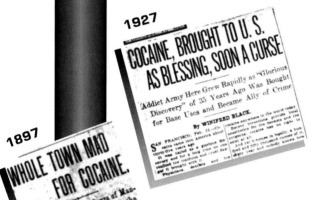

1927

1986

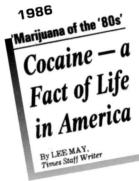

GENERAL CLASSIFICATION

In the United States in 1992 almost 3 million Americans used amphetamines ("speed") for non-medical reasons; over 2 million used cocaine, at least occasionally; 47 million smoked cigarettes; 100 million drank coffee; and almost as many took an over-the-counter medication containing caffeine. From a powerful stimulant such as crack cocaine to a mild one like a cola soft drink, uppers are a regular part of life for most Americans.

Stimulants can be natural, i.e., coca leaf, tobacco leaf, khat leaf, coffee bean; or they can be refined forms of the plant, i.e., cocaine, nicotine, caffeine; or they can be synthetic, i.e., amphetamines, diet pills, and lookalikes.

Fig. 3-1 STIMULANTS

DRUG NAME	TRADE NAME	STREET NAME
COCAINE (from coca leaf)		
Cocaine HCL (hydrochloride)	None	Coke, blow, toot, snow, flake, girl, lady
Freebase cocaine	None	Crack, base, rock, basay boulya, pasta, hubba, bazooko, pestillos
AMPHETAMINES (synthetic) — CRANK, SPEED, ICE, SHABU		
d,l amphetamine	Benzedrine, Obetrol, Biphetamine	Crosstops, black beauties, whites, bennies, cartwheels
Methamphetamine	Methadrine, Desoxyn,	Crank, meth, crystal
Dextroamphetamine	Dexedrine, Eskatrol	Dexies, Christmas trees, beans
Dextromethamphetamine base	None	Ice, glass, batu, shabu, yellow rock
Levo amphetamine	Vick's Inhaler	
Freebase methamphetamine		Snot
AMPHETAMINE CONGENERS (diet pills)		
Methylphenidate	Ritalin	Pellets
Phenmetrazine	Preludin	Pink hearts
Pemoline	Cylert	Popcorn coke
Phentermine HCL	Fastin, Adipex,	Robin's eggs, black and whites
Phentermine resin	Phenazine, Bontril, Plegine, Trimtabs, Melfiat, Pendiet, Statobex	
Diethylpropion	Tenuate, Tepanil	
Methcathinone	None	Cat, khat, chat, miraa
LOOKALIKES		
Alone or combination of two or more of phenylpropanolamine, ephedrine or caffeine	Dexadiet, Dexatrim, Super Toot, etc.	Legal stimulants, legal speed, robin's eggs, black beauties, pink hearts

OTHER PLANT STIMULANTS

Khat (cathinone, cathine)		Qat, chat, miraa, jaad, Abyssinian tea, etc.
Betel nut (arecoline)		
Yohimbe (yohimbine)		
Ephedra		Marwath

CAFFEINE

Over-the-counter stimulants	No Doz, Alert, Vivarin,	
Coffee	Columbian, French roast, etc.	Java, Joe, mud
Colas (from cola nut)	Coca Cola, Pepsi, etc.	Coke
Tea	Lipton, Stash	
Chocolate (cocoa beans)	Hershey, Nestle, etc.	

NICOTINE

Cigarettes, cigars	Marlboro, Kents, etc.	Cancer stick, smoke, butts, toke
Pipe tobacco	Sir Walter Raleigh, etc.	
Snuff	Copenhagen, etc.	Dip
Chewing tobacco	Day's Work, etc.	Chaw

THE EFFECTS

Uppers are central nervous system stimulants. All of these substances act by increasing the neurotransmitter and electrical activity in the central nervous system. This results in the user becoming more alert, awake, active, anxious, and restless: more stimulation than normally experienced.

Day in and day out the body produces a certain amount of energy chemicals, particularly adrenalin (epinephrine) and noradrenalin (norepinephrine). More of these chemicals might circulate at high noon while we are at work than at midnight when we are fast asleep, but the daily output is fairly constant. These energy chemicals can increase heart rate, energize muscles, keep us alert, and help us function normally. In time they are metabolized and excreted from the body.

Sometimes, though, the body needs extra energy: when we exercise, are scared, have to fight, or are making love. At these moments, the nervous system releases extra amounts of adrenalin and other chemicals. Remember the surge of energy the body receives when frightened? The extra adrenalin is soon passed from the body or reabsorbed by certain nerve tissues.

The normal progression of events is

- The body demands extra energy;

- Cells release energy chemicals.

Stimulants reverse the process:

- Stimulants are eaten, smoked, injected, or snorted, forcing the release of energy chemicals;

- These excess neurochemicals then give the body energy and stimulation it doesn't need.

Stronger stimulants such as crack cocaine or methamphetamine keep the chemicals circulating by blocking their reabsorption, so the effects are exaggerated. If this is continued for hours or even days, the body is infused with all this extra energy which has no place to go except by increased muscular activity, hard work, hard partying, talkativeness, restlessness, combativeness, and irritability.

The stimulant cocaine gets the headlines, but the stimulant nicotine is used daily by 54 million Americans.

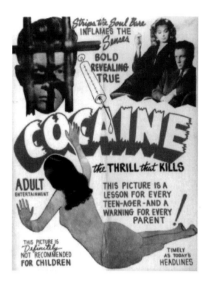

"The Horrors of Cocaine." A movie poster from the late 1930's.

"I would stay up 3 to 5 days, sleep for a day and do it again; 3 to 5 days, sleep for a day, do it again."
Methamphetamine user

If we take stimulants occasionally, the body has time to recover. But if we take stimulants over a long period of time or take large quantities, the energy supply becomes depleted, and the body is left without reserves. We've squeezed it dry. Most systems must shut down in an attempt to replenish the body's energy supply.

It is important to remember that the energy we receive from stimulants is not a free gift. It is a loan from the rest of the body and must be repaid.

With stronger stimulants, this crash and subsequent withdrawal and depression can last for days, weeks, even months, depending on the length of use, the strength of the drug, and the extent of biochemical disruption.

In addition, many stimulants constrict blood vessels, thus decreasing blood flow to tissues, particularly the skin and extremities. At the same time they increase blood pressure so with stronger stimulants, a ruptured vessel (a stroke if it's in the brain) is possible.

The disruption of the body's neurotransmitters also disturbs mental balance. Generally, stimulants increase confidence, create a certain euphoria, and make users feel they can do anything. When they are overstimulated, or continually stimulated, these feelings can quickly turn to irritability, talkativeness, suspiciousness, restlessness, insomnia and even violence.

"It's almost like there's a veneer over the nerves, and it takes off that veneer, that coating, and you are just like a live wire. You'll be on a crowded bus, and you might go into a rage very spontaneously without any real cause."
Amphetamine user

Everything seems exaggerated under the influence of a stimulant: our problems; suspicions, irritability, existing neuroses, and feelings of loneliness. Users need to do something, anything, to use up this extra stimulation.

While cocaine and amphetamines are the strongest stimulants, tobacco is the deadliest, perhaps because it is legal.

COCAINE

Cocaine is extracted from the coca plant which grows on the slopes of the Andes Mountains in South America, in certain parts of the Amazon Jungle, and on the Island of Java in Indonesia.

Incan mask of coca leaf chewer with cheeks puffed out from coca leaf wads (c. 1750).

METHODS OF USE

The history of cocaine can be viewed in terms of the various changes in the methods of use that have been developed.

Native cultures have used coca leaves for thousands of years for social and religious occasions, to fight off fatigue, lessen hunger, and increase endurance. The South American Indians, the Incas in particular, either chewed the leaf for the juice or chopped it up and spooned it under the tongue so the active ingredients could be absorbed by the tiny blood vessels in the gums.

In 1860, cocaine was isolated from the other chemicals in the coca leaf and extracted as a chemical salt, cocaine hydrochloride. Because this extraction from the coca leaf produces pure cocaine, it is much more powerful than just chewing the leaf. Since it readily dissolves in water, users were able to inject it, in solution, directly into the veins, dissolve it in soft drinks like Coca Cola or wine such as Vin Mariani, or use it in patent medicines.

Injecting cocaine results in an intense rush within 15 to 30 seconds, while drinking it results in a milder yet longer-lasting stimulation 30 to 45 minutes after ingestion. Both methods popularized the use of cocaine in the United States by the turn of the century.

Lithograph ad for a French tonic wine spiced with cocaine extract; by Alphonse Mucha, Paris, 1899 (Courtesy of Sasha Runa, Chicago and the estate of Timothy C. Ploughman).

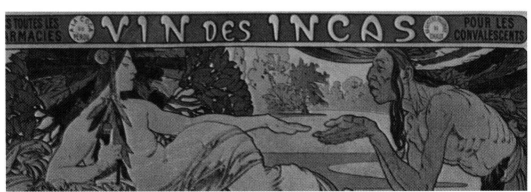

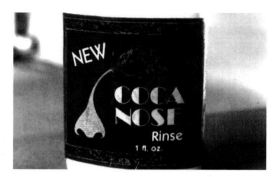

A bottle of rinse to soothe and clean the nasal passages irritated by cocaine snorting.

Around 1914, a pharmaceutical company introduced cocaine cigarettes in America, but the high temperature (198° C) needed to convert cocaine hydrochloride to smoke, resulted in destruction of much of the chemical, and so the cigarettes never became very popular. Instead, the ban on cocaine limited its supply. The 1920's gave rise to a popular new form of cocaine use, snorting of the chemical into the nostrils. Called "tooting," "blowing," or "horning," this method gets the drug to the nasal mucosa, not the lungs, allowing for absorption into the brain within 3 to 5 minutes.

Chewing, drinking, injecting, and snorting cocaine remained the principal routes of use until the mid 1970's. At that time, street chemists converted cocaine hydrochloride to cocaine free base in an effort to purify the street drug from its many cuts or diluents. Unlike the cocaine hydrochloride cigarettes introduced in 1914, "free base" cocaine can be smoked without destroying the psychoactive properties.

Through the lungs, cocaine reaches the brain within only 5 to 8 seconds compared to the 15 to 30 seconds it takes when injected through the veins.

New forms of cocaine like "pasta," "hubba," "primo," and "basay;" a new plant source, the Erythroxylum coca variant ipadu plant; methods for making new forms of free base cocaine like boulya; and different combinations of drugs such as cocaine and marijuana ("champagne"), all indicate a continuing evolution and abuse of this drug for many more years.

PHYSICAL AND MENTAL EFFECTS

Cocaine is not only a stimulant, it is also the only naturally occurring local anesthetic. It is used to numb the nasal passages when inserting breathing tubes in a patient, to numb the eye during surgery, and to deaden the pain of chronic sores. (This topical anesthetic effect numbs the nasal passages when the drug is snorted.) Cocaine will also stimulate the heart muscles directly before it reaches the central nervous system.

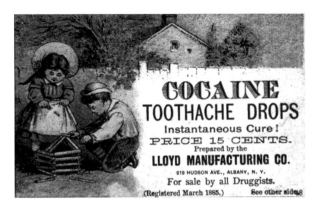

COCAINE
TOOTHACHE DROPS
Instantaneous Cure!
PRICE 15 CENTS.
Prepared by the
LLOYD MANUFACTURING CO.
219 HUDSON AVE., ALBANY, N. Y.
For sale by all Druggists.
(Registered March 1885.)   See other sides

The anesthetic effects of cocaine made the drug a favorite of dentists long before novocaine was synthesized.

"At first, when you put it in your nose, it starts a numbness and you can feel a little drip going down your throat. And then you get hyperactive in 20 minutes. When you smoke it, it's an instantaneous rush."
Cocaine user

Most of the effects, however, occur when the drug disrupts the neurotransmitter balance in the central nervous system. Initially, this disruption and over stimulation of the body's chemical balance seem extremely pleasurable: increased confidence, a willingness to work (sometimes endlessly), a diminishing of life's problems, a euphoric rush.

"I felt real ecstatic, very euphoric; it felt...my mind had a great deal of pleasure. I felt like a somebody. I felt like a super person. I could do anything." Cocaine user

The problem, of course, is that cocaine is not selective about which neurotransmitters it stimulates and how much it disrupts their natural balance.

For example, the greatly increased release of epinephrine (adrenalin) raises the blood pressure, increases the heart rate, causes rapid breathing, tenses muscles, and causes the jitters. It forces the release of excess amounts of these energy chemicals, ultimately depleting the supplies. But initially, the stimulation is intense.

"It exaggerated almost everything that was going on for me. Initially, it exaggerated excitement or happiness or euphoria. It seemed positive. As it became negative, it became extremely negative. Everything seemed out of proportion to everything else." Recovering cocaine user

Besides epinephrine (adrenalin), other disrupted neurotransmitters can cause additional problems. Over stimulation of the brain's fright center by dopamine is the physical cause of most paranoia experienced by stimulant abusers. A shadow, movement or loud voice may suddenly seem threatening. A user reacts in much the same way a deer in the woods reacts to the crack of a twig.

"A person I know does a shot every 15 to 20 minutes. He fights sleep. He'll go days without sleeping and he'll collapse. He looks for people hiding under mattresses, behind door hinges, and in books. He asks why you're smiling." Intravenous cocaine user

Unbalanced acetylcholine, another common neurotransmitter, causes muscle tremors, memory lapses, mental confusion, and even hallucinations.

"My perception of everything was such that I no longer had any clear picture of what was going on. The complete inability to really have any awareness of what was actually happening and having to live in a world where I could only feel what seemed to be happening was the most horrifying thing I ever experienced."
Recovering cocaine snorter

Serotonin helps us sleep and stabilizes our moods, but if it is depleted by excessive cocaine use, insomnia, agitation, and severe emotional depression result. The lack of epinephrine, norepineph-rine, serotonin, and dopamine also causes severe depression and extreme lethargy.

"I realized that I hadn't been outside of my house for a couple of days and hadn't called anybody. I didn't answer my mail for months at a time." *Cocaine snorter*

All these physical effects are very similar to the effects of other stimulants, e.g., amphetamines and Ritalin. The major differences with cocaine are the intensity of the initial rush (stronger), the price (about $100 a gram — on a per dose basis, that's about 5 to 10 times as much as amphetamines), and the speed with which it is metabolized by the body (about 40 minutes compared to several hours for amphetamines).

"After doing it for a while, you just don't want to stop until everything is gone, until all the money's gone, until you have no choice but to stop." *Crack cocaine smoker*

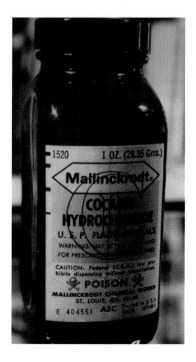

When sold legally in the U.S., one ounce, or 28 grams, costs about $80. In Columbia, one ounce of illicit cocaine would cost about $600 and on the streets of New York or Miami, about $3,000.

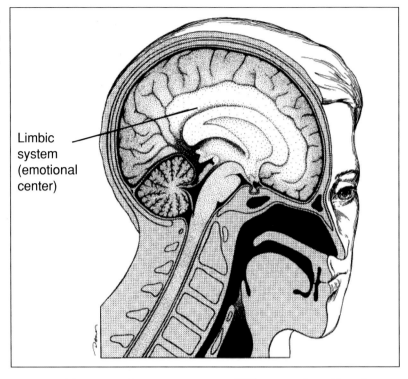

Fig.3-2 The limbic system contains the reward pleasure center which is stimulated by cocaine.

Limbic system (emotional center)

Reward / Pleasure Center

Cocaine disrupts our balance in one other important way. It stimulates our reward/pleasure center, that portion of the brain that tells us when we've done something good. For example, normally, this center gives us a surge of satisfaction when we've satisfied hunger, thirst, or sexual desire. When a drug such as cocaine stimulates this center, it fools us. It signals our brain that we're not hungry, though we've not eaten; that we're not thirsty though we've not drunk; that we're being sexually satisfied though we haven't had sex. This stimulation is perceived as an overall rush, an overall feeling of well being and pleasure. This rush diminishes over time, but the memory lingers on.

"When crack is offered to me, the idea flashes through my head, 'Wow, how nice it was the first time. Maybe this time I can recapture that same experience I had the first time.' But it doesn't happen." Recovering cocaine user

PROBLEMS WITH COCAINE USE

The Crash

The initial euphoria, the feeling of confidence, the sense of omnipotence , and the satisfied feeling disappear as suddenly as the mental and physical rush appeared, so the crash after using cocaine can be particularly depressing. It can be as debilitating as the feeling we would have if we had just run a marathon or if a loved one had died. This depression can last a few hours, several days, or even weeks. It depends on how much we have used, how badly we have depleted our energy supplies, and how severely we've disrupted our neurotransmitter balance.

"I really did want to die, and I remember that as being way out of proportion to the actual events of my life although it seemed like my life was over." Recovering cocaine user

Withdrawal

Contrary to notions held until the 1980's there are true withdrawal phenomena when cocaine is used. Though similar to the crash, withdrawal effects can last months, even years depending on dosage, frequency, and length of use. The major symptoms are anhedonia or the lack of ability to feel pleasure; anergia or a total lack of energy, motivation, or initiative; and intense craving for the drug. These symptoms are also usual for amphetamine withdrawal. It is these symptoms, the last one in particular, which generally cause the compulsive user to relapse.

The time frame for a compulsive cocaine or amphetamine user is as follows: immediately after a cocaine binge, usually lasting several days, the user crashes, sleeping all day long, trying to put energy back into the body, and swearing off the drug forever. A few days later the user starts to feel better and resolves to go into treatment. However, about a week to 10 days after quitting, the craving starts to build, the energy level drops, and he feels very little plea-

sure from any of his surroundings or friends. So, 2 to 4 weeks after vowing to abstain, users feel the craving build to a fever pitch and unless the user is in intensive treatment, he or she will relapse.

Polydrug Use

One of the problems with cocaine is that the stimulation can be so intense that the user needs a downer to take the edge off or to get to sleep. The most common drugs taken are alcohol, Valium, and heroin, though any downer will do in a pinch. Sometimes, the second drug can be more of a problem than the cocaine.

"After the coke would be gone, you'd be all wired up and you couldn't sleep, so I'd always have a little bit of heroin on the side and it'd bring me down. And I wouldn't be all jittery all night and grinding my teeth." Cocaine snorter

Adulteration

Adulteration of cocaine involves dilution with such diverse products as baby laxatives, aspirin, sugar, tetracaine or procaine (both are topical anesthetics), even talcum powder. And as with the intravenous use of any drug, contaminated needles can spread hepatitis, blood and heart infections, and AIDS.

Overdose

An overdose of cocaine can be caused by as little as 1/50th of a gram or as much as 1.2 grams. The "caine reaction" is very intense and generally short in duration. Most often, it's not fatal. It only feels like impending death. However, in a small number of cases, death can occur within 40 minutes to 5 hours after exposure. Death usually results from either the initial stimulatory phase of toxicity (seizures, hypertension, and tachycardia) or the later depression phase terminating in extreme respiratory depression and coma.

"I did too much; my knees buckled; I fell on the toilet stool; I was shaking. If my buddy hadn't grabbed me and put me in the shower, I don't know what would have happened." Crack cocaine smoker

"I have seen a friend go through overdose. His skin was grey green. His eyes rolled back, his heart stopped, and there was a gargling sound which is right at death. And I had to bring him back, and that's enough to put the fear of God in anybody." Intravenous cocaine user

First-time users and even those who have used cocaine before can get an exaggerated reaction, far beyond what might normally occur or beyond what they have experienced in the past. This is partially due to the phenomenon known as inverse tolerance or kindling. As people use cocaine, they get more sensitive to its toxic effects rather than less sensitive as one would expect. With large doses, cocaine can injure heart muscles and blood vessels, making permanent damage to those tissues more likely.

Long-Term Use

The elevations and drops in blood pressure caused by cocaine, plus some toxic effects to the vessels themselves, weaken blood capillaries, resulting in a greater risk of stroke. Strokes occur when a weakened blood vessel bursts, causing internal bleeding in the brain. Chronic cocaine use also causes a disorganization in the usual formation of heart muscles resulting in constriction bands on the heart. This makes chronic users more likely to suffer a cocaine-induced heart attack.

COMPULSION

Considering all the problems with cocaine—the expense, the dilution, the adulteration, the possibility of overdose, the illegality, the physical and psychological dangers—two questions come to mind. "Why do people use cocaine?" and "Why do they use it so compulsively?"

Why do people use cocaine and amphetamines?

Some people are drawn to cocaine and other stimulants because they mimic natural body functions: the adrenal energy rush, the confidence, the euphoria, the increased sensitivity, the stimulation of the reward/pleasure center. It is sometimes easier to get a chemical high instantly

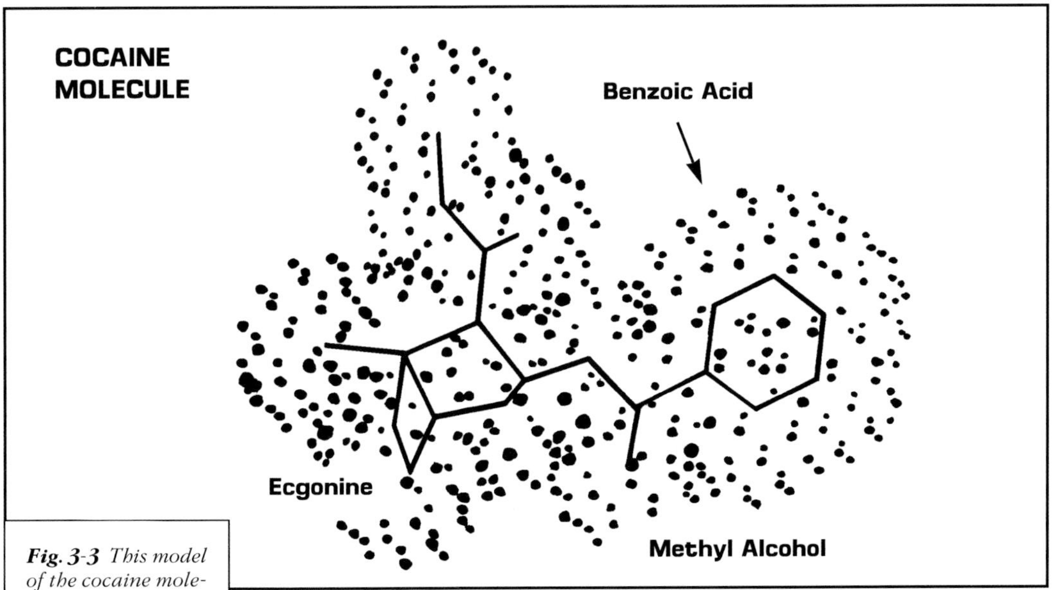

COCAINE MOLECULE

Benzoic Acid

Ecgonine

Methyl Alcohol

Fig. 3-3 This model of the cocaine molecule shows the components of cocaine: benzoic acid, ecgonine, methyl-alcohol.

than a natural high over a period of time. A natural high is a stimulation of our energy supplies or our reward/pleasure center that comes from real deeds, i.e., the completion of a difficult physical or mental task, communion with God, or an emotionally fulfilling relationship. People also use because of peer pressure, curiosity, or availability.

Why are cocaine and amphetamines used so compulsively?

• To recapture the initial rush which is extremely intense. Most find that it can't be done, but that doesn't stop them from trying.

• To avoid the crash that is inevitable after the intense high. In many cases, a user will shoot up or smoke every 20, or in some cases, 10 minutes.

• To avoid life's problems such as difficult relationships, lack of confidence, traumatic events, a hated job, or loneliness.

• To respond to the environmental cues that remind users of their drug use. Many seemingly innocuous sensory cues in our environment will trigger that memory of smoking, snorting or shooting, and create a severe desire to use again. The cues can be seeing white powder, holding the freebase pipe, or having money in one's pocket.

• To answer the demands of cocaine. In and of itself, the chemical will cause a user to keep shooting, snorting, or smoking until every last microgram is gone, until the user passes out, or until he or she overdoses.

• In response to one's hereditary predisposition to use. That is, certain people's natural neurotransmitter balance makes them react more intensely to a drug. They get more pleasure from it. They are in essence pre-sensitized to the drug.

Of the millions of Americans who have experimented with cocaine, 15% use it at least once a month and have had episodes where they find it hard to function. One to two million have severe problems with the drug.

SMOKABLE COCAINE
(freebase, crack, rock, boulya, etc.)

The words "crack cocaine" appeared on the streets and in the media in 1985, tentatively at first, as if society were trying out a new nickname. By 1986, there seemed to be a "crack" epidemic that crossed all social and economic barriers. By the 90's it was ingrained in the American psyche as one of the main causes of society's ills: gang violence, "crack babies," AIDS, crime, and addiction.

The question, however, is, "Was the spread of the so-called rich man's drug to the office, factory, school yard, ghetto, and barrio generated by media attention or by the actual properties of the substance?

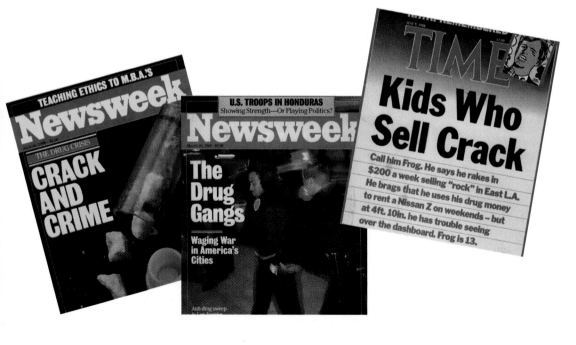

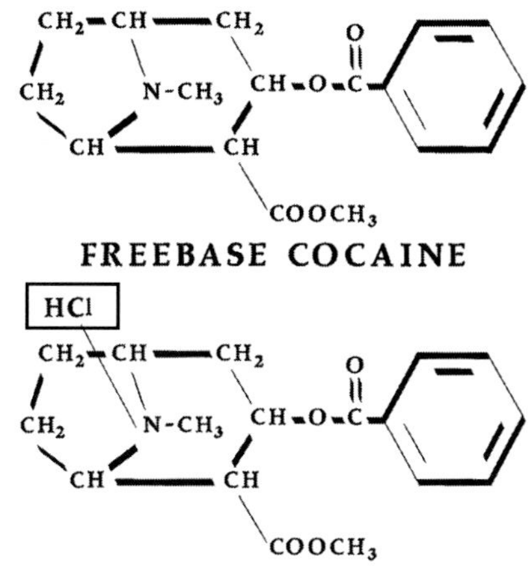

FREEBASE COCAINE

HCl

SNORTING/IV COCAINE

Fig: 3-4 A comparison of the molecular structure of freebase cocaine and snorted cocaine shows the only difference is the HCL or hydrochloride molecule which is also called a "base," hence the name freebase when the hydrochloride molecule is chemically removed.

An important clue to the answer is that "crack" is not an entirely new drug. It is freebase cocaine, and freebase is simply a chemically altered form of regular cocaine, cocaine hydrochloride. Freebase was developed in the mid seventies to make cocaine smokable. Freebase cocaine, also known as smokable cocaine, has been called "base," "basay," "rock," "hubba," "gravel," "Roxanne," "girl," "fry," "boulya," and "crack." Perhaps next month another nickname will appear.

For example, in South America, "pasta" smoking is popular. "Pasta," a form of freebase nicknamed "bazooko" when mixed with marijuana, is an intermediate product of the cocaine refinement process. Being an intermediate product, it contains toxic chemicals such as kerosene and leaded gasoline.

Whatever the name, freebase is still cocaine and when smoked,

causes all the reactions expected from shooting, or snorting the drug, the differences being in the extra speed of delivery to the brain and the greater intensity of the effects.

PHARMACOLOGY OF SMOKABLE COCAINE

There are two basic ways to make cocaine suitable for smoking.

The first method, developed about 1976, uses highly flammable or toxic chemicals such as ether, to convert cocaine hydrochloride, the refined form of the drug, to crystals of freebase cocaine. This creates a purer form of the drug since any additives are filtered out by the process. This method is also called "basing" or "baseballing."

The other technique, developed in the early 80's, sometimes called "cheap basing" or "dirty basing," involves baking soda and heat. This simpler method does not remove as many impurities or residues as the basing technique. Residues such as talcum powder and, particularly, baking soda remain.

The converted freebase cocaine, made by either the basing method or the "crack" method, has two chemical properties sought by users. First, it has a lower melting point than the powdered form so it can be heated easily in a glass pipe and vaporized to form smoke at a lower temperature. Too high a temperature destroys most of the psychoactive properties of the drug. Second, since it enters the system directly through the lungs, smokable cocaine reaches the brain faster than when cocaine is snorted.

Fig. 3-5 The graph shows the intensity of the high and the rapidity of the rush with smokable cocaine versus snorted cocaine. Although I.V. use also produces a rush almost as rapidly as smoking, it also carries with it the dangers of infection associated with needle use.

Freebase cocaine is more fat soluble than cocaine that is snorted (cocaine hydrochloride) and so is more readily absorbed by the fatty brain tissue causing a more intense reaction. Users are also able to get a much higher dose of cocaine in their system at one time because the very large surface area in the lungs (about the size of a football field) can absorb the drug instantaneously.

Crack and freebase cocaine unbalance the brain chemicals more quickly than snorted cocaine, leaving the brain hormonal balance in disarray. Users react in their own way to the drug depending on how much is used, the purity of the drug, and how long they have been using.

"You get heat energy, heat flashes that go all through your body. You get these pins and needles, depending on the cut of course." Crack cocaine smoker

SIDE EFFECTS

Since smoking cocaine causes more intense reactions than snorting, it makes sense that the side effects would also be more intense.

"Physically you feel like you're dying, real depressed, exhausted and wasted, burned out, you know? Like you need to do some more even to function, even to do anything at all."
Crack smoker

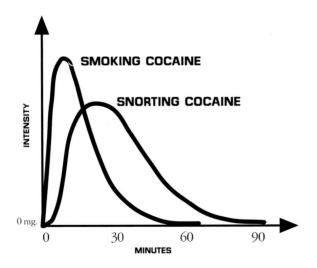

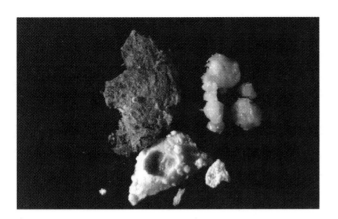

Collection of rocks of freebase cocaine (crack). Each is made in a slightly different manner. The various colors come from the impurities left after heating the mixture.

Because a user inhales an extremely harsh substance, smoking cocaine can also cause breathing problems.

> *"I had a lot of coughing after using it and shortness of breath. I didn't really notice it at the time, but if I went out to ride my bike or lift weights I would really have a hard time."*
> Recovering 16-year-old boy

> *"A friend was freebasing heavily, and he started going into convulsions and throwing up blood. It was real awful. I was really scared, and I thought he was going to die. Me and my other friend, we just kept freebasing...and then when he came out of it, he started freebasing again."*
> Recovering 16-year-old girl

Neonatal Effects

Smoked, snorted, or injected, cocaine is of particular danger to the fetus of a pregnant woman. When a pregnant woman smokes crack, within seconds her baby will also be exposed to the drug. The chances of miscarriage, stroke, and sudden infant death are greatly increased.

> *"I'd been smoking crack for a couple of years, and I had a baby who was born testing positive for coke. Child Protective Services came and placed her in foster care. It took me 2 years to get my baby back."* 17-year-old recovering crack user

Overdose

The most frequent type of overdose that people experience when smoking cocaine is on the mild side: very rapid heartbeat and hyperventilation. However, these reactions are often accompanied by a feeling of impending death. Although most people survive and only get very sweaty and clammy and feel that they are going to die, several thousand, in fact, are killed by cocaine overdose every year.

Polydrug Abuse

As with snorted and injected cocaine, the intensive use of freebase increases the potential for the abuse of other drugs especially alcohol, heroin, and sedative-hypnotics. Some smokers combine freebase and marijuana in a combination called "champagne," "caviar," or "gremmies." In addition, users are even mixing PCP with crack in a nasty mixture called "space basing" or "whack." Further, there is the addition of freebase cocaine to smokable tar heroin to make a smokable speedball called "hot rocks." Finally, "crack" or regular cocaine is being used with wine coolers for an oral speedball known as "crack coolers." When "crack" is not available, users have switched to shooting and even smoking methamphetamine (speed). A mixture of "crank" with "crack" smoked together has also appeared recently and is called "super crank."

REASONS FOR COMPULSIVE USE OF CRACK

Besides the reasons already mentioned for compulsive use of

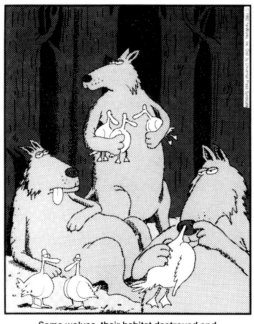

THE FAR SIDE   By GARY LARSON

Some wolves, their habitat destroyed and overwhelmed by human pressures, turn to snorting quack.

cocaine such as the search for the first intense rush, or avoidance of the down side, there are several other reasons for the compulsion associated with smoking cocaine.

First, smoking a drug is more socially acceptable than injecting or snorting it because cigarette, pipe, and cigar smoking are part of our culture (and legal).

Next, smoking is not as dangerous as using a contaminated needle. (While avoiding needles would remove one source of infection, the lowered inhibitions, the overwhelming desire to use at any cost including bartering sex for drugs, and the stimulation provided by cocaine causes users to be more careless about high-risk sexual activities leading to high rates of sexually transmitted diseases, most ominously AIDS.)

The economics of crack cocaine have expanded the potential number of users, especially among teenagers. The reason is in the packaging. Crack is not cheaper than snorting cocaine; it is just sold in smaller units. A gram was the standard amount, going for about a hundred dollars. Now, a twentieth of a gram that has been converted to crack or rock can be bought for 10 to 20 dollars, a manageable sum for teenagers and incidentally, about twice the price of snorted cocaine when figured on a per gram basis.

The economics of crack cocaine have created more dealers, and these people have a vested interest in keeping users using. Many housing projects in the inner city have become a haven for crack houses and dealers. Fifteen-year-old dealers are buying new cars, and drug-gang homicides are expanding at an alarming rate. Gangs from other countries, such as Jamaica and Columbia, have expanded to a number of American cities.

Unfortunately, this burgeoning drug market is making use of the best sales strategies of a free enterprise system: reduce the prices to increase sales; increase the size of the sales force to cover the territory more efficiently; encourage free trade to avoid tariffs and impounding; and create appealing packaging to make the product attractive to a wider segment of the population.

The original question in this section was "Is it the media coverage or the actual properties of a drug that lead to an epidemic?" One conclusion is that the media can hype a drug all it wants, but if the drug doesn't have inherently addicting qualities, then no amount of hype will lead to a sustained epidemic. Smokable cocaine has properties that lead to compulsive use. Those same properties will keep it around for decades to come. In fact, the majority of drug arrests in major cities is for cocaine possession and dealing.

AMPHETAMINES
(speed, meth, crank, crystal, ice, etc.)

CLASSIFICATION

Amphetamines, known variously as "speed," "meth," "methamphetamines," "crank," "crystal," "ice," "shabu," and "glass," are a class of powerful, synthetic stimulants, with effects very similar to cocaine but much longer lasting and cheaper to use. Amphetamines can be taken orally, but shooting, snorting, and most recently smoking have gained in popularity.

There are several different types of amphetamines: amphetamine, methamphetamine, dextroamphetamine, and dextromethamphetamine. Their effects are almost indistinguishable from each other, the major differences being the method of manufacture (methamphetamine being the easiest) and the strength.

Currently, there has been an explosion of methamphetamine use in its various forms and a drastic increase in the number of "meth labs" raided by the authorities, particularly in Oregon, Texas, and

1992

'POOR MAN'S COCAINE'
Methamphetamine Use on the Rise

By Erin Hallissy
Chronicle East Bay Bureau

Once popular mainly with "speed freaks" and motorcycle gangs, methamphetamine is rapidly becoming the drug of choice among partygoers at all-night "raves" and growing

production boom, with chemicals smuggled over the border from Mexico and "cooked" into the drug by a widening array of outlaws.

Recent crime statistics show that manufacturers are moving into suburban areas where they

workers, has been especially hard-hit by the latest boom. In the past two years, drug agents have seized methamphetamine labs across the street from a church in Danville, in a trailer buried near the Concord Police Academy, in quiet neighbor-

California. Illicit methamphetamine manufacture is a risky business. The fumes can be toxic, and explosions can occur if the chemicals are handled improperly. Much of the street dealing in methamphetamines has been taken over by biker gangs because of the money involved and the partiality of bikers to the drug.

HISTORY OF USE

Amphetamines were discovered in the late 1800's, but their medical applications weren't recognized until the 1930's when Benzedrine was marketed as a stimulant to counter low blood pressure. It was also used to dilate constricted bronchial passages, to help asthmatics breathe. Later on, other amphetamines were used to treat narcolepsy, to treat a form of epilepsy, and as a possible cure for depression. At the same time, the stimulant effects came to be appreciated by students cramming for exams, truckers on long hauls, any worker with extra long hours, and soldiers or pilots trying to stay awake for 48 straight hours.

Diet Pills

Pharmaceutical companies in the 50's and 60's promoted the hunger-suppressing and mood-elevating qualities of amphetamines. This led to huge quantities of amphetamines such as Dexedrine, Methedrine, Dexamyl, and Benzedrine flooding the market. Unfortunately, weight watchers found that because of the rapid development of tolerance to this class of drugs, the appetite suppressing effects diminished after a few months forcing the user to take ever increasing quantities to lose weight. Dangerous side effects started to counter the benefits.

*"Well, I almost never ate.
And when I ate, I ate sugar;
colas, cakes; and that was all
I ate. I mean, once in a while
I'd go to a steak house and
treat myself to a fabulous
dollar-fifty-nine steak
dinner. I weighed probably
90 pounds, and I was anemic
and weak, but I always felt
up and energized because I
was always shooting speed."
Speed user*

Many different forms of amphetamines displayed at a Drug Enforcement Administration (DEA) laboratory in San Francisco.

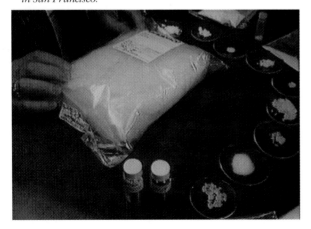

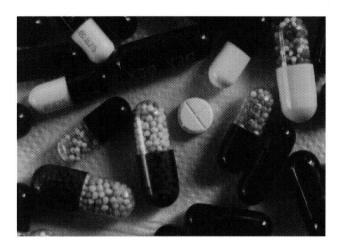

DEA display of a variety of prescription amphetamines and diet pills.

Street "Speed"

The 60's were the peak of the "speed" craze, but then the Controlled Substance Act of 1970 made it hard to buy amphetamines legally. A cap was put on the prescription use of these drugs. The street market, however, expanded to fill the need. Instead of buying legally manufactured amphetamines that had been diverted, people bought "speed" and "crank" that had been manufactured illegally.

> "I very seldom ran out in the beginning, in the 60's and 70's. It was cheap; people gave it away. It wasn't like using dope. You didn't have to get money together every day." "Speed" user

The most popular form of street speed were the "cross tops." Also called "cart wheels," these were smuggled into the U.S. from Mexico. In the early 70's they cost 5 to 10 dollars per hundred tablets. In the 90's the price is 1 to 5 dollars per tablet.

The late 1980's saw a resurgence in the availability and abuse of these illicit amphetamines particularly "crank" (methamphetamine sulfate) and "crystal" (methamphetamine hydrochloride — not to be confused with "Krystal" which is PCP). Once stymied by the tight control of chemicals needed to produce illegal amphetamines, clever street chemists now alter commonly available compounds and even use aluminum foil to produce "speed" products. However, a majority of street meth seems to be mostly look-alike drugs such as phenylpropanolamine (a decongestant), ephedrine, or simply caffeine tablets disguised to look like amphetamine products.

"Ice"

As the 1990's began, a new, highly potent, and smokable form of methamphetamine, dextromethamphetamine, called "ice," "glass," "batu," or "shabu," had taken center stage to prolong the era of upper abuse. Besides its smokability, greater strength, and longer duration of effects, "ice" had the appeal of a new fad. As with the spread of smokable crack cocaine, ice started out being marketed as a "newer, better amphetamine."

Surprisingly, perhaps because it is so intense, "ice" has not caught on as a common drug of abuse except in Hawaii. In addition, "snot," a skim from heated methamphetamine, has been tried. The reddish brown gel or oil can be smoked in a pipe or in a cigarette.

The "traditional" types of amphetamines that were or are still diverted to street use or that are manufactured illegally, are small tablets of amphetamine or methamphetamine ("crosstops," "whites") originally made in Mexico; Biphetamines ("black beauties"), a combination of several amphetamine compounds; Dexadrine ("dexys," "beans"), a dextroamphetamine tablet; Benzedrine ("bennies"), one of the classic "stay awake" amphetamine pills; and Methadrine, (or Ambar), a methamphetamine.

ROUTES OF ADMINISTRATION

Because of the extremely bitter taste of amphetamines, they are usually put in a gelatin capsule or in a piece of paper when taken orally. This route is popular because of the pain or danger of injecting or snorting the caustic drug.

Amphetamines usually cause pain in the blood vessels when used intravenously. Also, with injecting, there is the attendant risk of contaminated needles. However, I.V. use does put large quantities of the drug directly into the bloodstream and causes a more intense "high" than snorting or swallowing.

"I'd already tasted that first high and wanted to get back to it, but it was always different, each time I shot up. I started shooting when I was 13, and I was 20 before I learned you could get AIDS from it. I have it ... I'm HIV positive."
Intravenous meth user

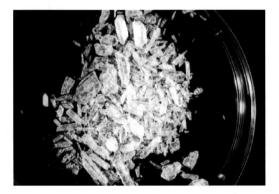
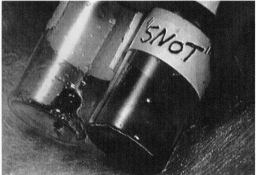

On the left are crystals of "ice," and on the right, "snot."

Snorting "meth," done the same way as cocaine, is also not as popular as oral ingestion, because of the extreme irritation and pain it causes to the nasal mucosa.

Because of these limiting effects, users have taken to smoking "crank," "crystal," or "ice," a potentially more appealing method of use than the other ways. The technique of smoking "crank" or "ice" is similar to smoking freebase cocaine (in a pipe). Smoking gets the drug to the brain faster.

Whether swallowed, smoked, or shot, "crank," "crystal," "ice," and the other amphetamines offer a cheaper substitute for cocaine. Occasionally, they are mixed with cocaine ("supercrank") to prolong the effects. Amphetamines last 4 to 6 hours compared to only 40 minutes to one-and-a-half hours for cocaine. "Ice," the newest form of methamphetamine, is alleged to last at least 8 hours, and some say up to 24 hours, after it is smoked.

Tolerance to amphetamines is pronounced. A long-term user might need 20 times the initial dose to produce the same high.

"When I first started off, I remember having a huge reaction to a small amount of it. And inside of probably a year, I could easily shoot a spoon of speed easily."
Meth user

EFFECTS

The effects of small to moderate doses include increased heart rate, respiration, and blood pressure, CNS stimulation, increased body temperature, and appetite suppression. Amphetamines can initially produce a mild euphoria and a feeling of well being, very similar to a cocaine high.

"I would inject some speed and right after doing it, you get an incredible ... rush, which some people compare with sexual feelings. And your heart pounds, and I've seen people actually pass out from having too much speed. My heart would pound, and I would sweat, and the rush would pass, and then I would just be very high energy."
Meth user

Because the effects last for hours, energy supplies are being continually squeezed from the nerve cells and eventually metabolized. Amphetamines slow the metabolism of these newly released energy supplies, unlike cocaine. This slowed metabolism accounts for the longer duration of action of amphetamines. This still means, however, that extended use or the use of large quantities will severely deplete those energy supplies. Prolonged use of amphetamines, as with prolonged use of cocaine, can therefore ultimately lead to extreme depression and lethargy.

"If I didn't have speed, if I ran out, I would become depressed; very anxiety ridden; I had suicidal thoughts; and I would sleep for long stretches of time until I had more speed. And then, I would start the whole process over again." Speed user

The neurotransmitters are also unbalanced by amphetamines, so prolonged use can induce extreme paranoia. The paranoia that occurs can result in homicidal and even suicidal thoughts in many users. This paranoid schizophrenia and/or vegetative depression (more common with high-dose intravenous use or heavy smoking) are usually not permanent. Upon cessation of use, the disturbed user will usually return to some semblance of normal, after the brain chemistry has been rebalanced. Unfortunately, this can take anywhere from a few months to a year or more.

Long-term use can also cause hallucinations, sleep deprivation, heart and blood vessel toxicity, and severe malnutrition. If the user has not built up a tolerance or takes an unusually large dose, an overdose can occur.

"I shot some speed once, and immediately had a seizure. Apparently my heart stopped beating and the person I was with was pounding on my chest; I was real sore and black and blue the next day." Methamphetamine user

Much like cocaine, amphetamines release neurotransmitters that mimic sexual gratification. Thus, they are used by those who are sexually active and prone toward multiple partners and/or prolonged sexual activity. The drug has also been heavily used in gay populations for sexual endurance. But again, because of the rapid development of tolerance, larger and larger quantities are needed to produce the same effects resulting in an actual decrease of sex drive and performance.

Because of their chemical properties and the feelings they create, amphetamines can be very seductive. Users go on binges or "runs," staying up for 3, 4, or even 10 days at a time, putting a severe strain on their bodies, particularly the cardiovascular and nervous systems. During these runs, people will try to use their excess energy anyway they can...cleaning the kitchen at midnight, taking apart a car, or painting the whole house.

"If I ran out of stuff to do, I would dump out everything in the vacuum cleaner, and vacuum it back up. I didn't like to be outside too much because I would get paranoid; I felt uneasy." Methamphetamine user

Alarmingly, it seems that the current interest in crank, crystal, and ice abuse is concentrated among adolescents and older teenagers, particularly by Asian and Caucasian American youth. One of the reasons for this popularity of the drug is that initially amphetamines induce qualities which we try to teach to young people—alertness, motivation, self confidence, socialization, excitement, ability to work long hours, and trim bodies. Unfortunately, with drug use, these desirable qualities quickly give way to the reverse effects: depression, antisocial behavior, and paranoia among others.

Effects of "Ice"

"Ice" is dextromethamphetamine base as opposed to the more common equal parts mixture of levo and dextro methamphetamine. This form of methamphetamine stimulates the brain to a greater degree than the regular methamphetamine but stimulates the heart, blood vessels, and lungs to a lesser degree. "Ice" is therefore less dangerous physically (except for overdoses), but more dangerous mentally than traditional street methamphetamines.

The decrease in circulatory effects (said to be up to 25% less than that of regular crank) is therefore conducive to users smoking more, resulting in more overdoses and in

a quicker disruption of neurotransmitters. This means more "tweaking," or severe paranoid, hallucinatory, and hypervigilant thinking along with greater suicidal depression and addictive use. Detoxification of mental and psychotic symptoms of excessive "ice" use usually takes several days longer than detoxifying from regular methamphetamine abuse.

TREATMENT FOR STIMULANT ABUSE
(Cocaine or Amphetamine)

Since withdrawal from prolonged cocaine or amphetamine use is accompanied by physical and mental depression and not life threatening or physically painful symptoms, the majority of patients who want to stop can be treated by encouraging abstinence. In fact, users should avoid all stimulants, including caffeine and tobacco.

"I think when you're using the drug, it's real easy to deny everything that's going on, and put everything on the shelf, and not cope with it. Your whole world becomes the acquiring of whatever drug you happen to be using. But when you stop, it's all there waiting for you. And, eventually, you have to deal with it."
Methamphetamine user

1991

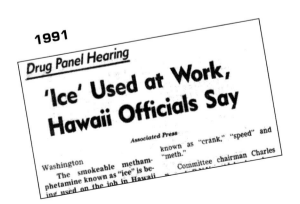

Drug Panel Hearing

'Ice' Used at Work, Hawaii Officials Say

Associated Press

Washington
The smokeable methamphetamine known as "ice" is being used on the job in Hawaii

known as "crank," "speed" and "meth."

Committee chairman Charles

STEPS OF TREATMENT

The steps of treatment are detoxification, initial abstinence, long-term abstinence, and recovery.

Detoxification and Initial Abstinence

After detoxification and treatment for any psychotic symptoms caused by prolonged use of amphetamines or cocaine, and after treatment of any life threatening symptoms such as extremely high blood pressure and heart rate, the vast majority of stimulant abusers respond positively to traditional drug counseling approaches (although a number of adaptations are made to focus on unique aspects of stimulant withdrawal such as depression and anhedonia). Compulsive stimulant users seem to do better in group counseling and in peer programs or groups like Cocaine Anonymous. (Interestingly, for some unknown reason, heroin addicts do better in one-on-one counseling.) Group counseling, individual counseling, and long-term abstinence strategies are the foundation for successful stimulant abuse treatment.

"The group keeps me honest with myself. I get to look at a lot of things and behaviors that are going on with me, and I try and keep in the now, keep thinking about staying clean today, and the group keeps me focused on my goal of each day trying to stay clean." Recovering crack cocaine user

However, a number of stimulant addicts have not been able to respond to these traditional approaches and require an initial, more intensive medical approach to bridge the detoxification/withdrawal period prior to their engagement into recovery.

Medical treatments include the use of antidepressant agents such as imipramine, desipramine, amitriptyline, doxepin, trazodone, or fluoxetine (Prozac). These affect serotonin, the neurotransmitter in the brain that deals with both depression and drug craving.

Antipsychotic medications such as Haldol, Thorazine, and others are also used to buffer the effects of unbalanced dopamine, the neurotransmitter that moderates paranoia and pleasurable sensations (feeling sated for hunger, thirst, and sex).

Sedatives such as Dalmane, chloral hydrate, Librium, phenobarbital, or even Valium are used, very carefully, on a short-term basis to treat anxiety or sleep disturbance problems.

Though still being tested, many programs have started using nutritional approaches aimed at enhancing the production of those neurotransmitters which have been depleted by heavy stimulant use thereby decreasing craving and counteracting many of the withdrawal symptoms seen in stimulant addiction. This includes the use of amino acid proteins such as Tyrosine, which is a building block (precursor) of dopamine in the brain; d,l-phenylalanine, which is used to make adrenaline and noradrenaline, and also to increase the amount of enkephalin in the brain; lecithin, which is a building block of acetylcholine; glutamine, which is a building block of GABA, the natural inhibitory neurotransmitter affected by alcohol and many sedatives; and even the judicious use of tryptophane, a serotonin precursor. Note, high-dose tryptophane has been implicated in the rare but dangerous blood disease, Eosinophilia Myalgia Syndrome.

Long-Term Abstinence

A lot of work is currently being put into the treatment of craving, the most dangerous withdrawal symptom of stimulant abuse and often thought to be responsible for the multiple relapses seen in treatment. Two major types of craving have been addressed: endogenous craving and environmentally triggered craving.

Endogenous Craving

Endogenous craving is believed to be caused by the depletion of dopamine in the nucleus acumbens of the limbic system. (The nucleus acumbens was identified in the 1950's as the potential location in the brain where the emotional addiction to all drugs of abuse occurs.) To treat this situation many medications like amantadine, bromocryptine, and L-Dopa have been used to simulate dopamine in the nucleus acumbens thereby diminishing craving for stimulants.

Environmentally Triggered Craving

Environmentally triggered craving, which is more likely to lead to relapse than endogenous craving, occurs when environmental cues like paraphernalia, white powder, money, or familiar people and places stimulate brain cells which contain memories of the drug use. The result is craving which has to be treated by intense counseling, group sessions, or desensitization techniques.

Medical sensors can record changes in skin electricity, sweating, heart rate, blood pressure, pupillary dilatation, and even an immediate, dramatic drop of two degrees or more in body temperature to document the very real physiologic changes that accompany craving.

Desensitization

One desensitization technique is to use various environmental cues to trigger this craving. Many techniques such as exercise, counseling, cold showers, etc., are then used to bring the person's responses back to normal. This technique is repeated every two to three days, and every time the individual refrains from using cocaine when experiencing these physiological changes, the craving response diminishes. After approximately 40 sessions, an addict no longer responds to most environmental cues.

Another technique is to carefully examine what happened just before the relapse occurred and to identify the environmental cues. Just recognizing the cues and examining them seems to diminish the response.

TREATMENT CONCLUSIONS

Despite a current explosion of medical approaches to the treatment of stimulant addiction, research has not been able to sustain the idea of a strictly pharmacological approach. While some compulsive users have responded well to a wide variety of treatments, more work is needed to fully develop appropriate medical intervention.

The most difficult concept for most chemical dependency clients to understand (and for many treatment personnel as well) is that recovery is often a lifetime process. Recovery can only come for most compulsive users when they alter their lifestyles to avoid or change the people, places, things, and ideas that originally led them to settle for addiction as their way of life. They have to find something they enjoy more than their initial drug use.

"Every day that I don't use drugs I have choices. Every day that I choose not to do drugs, my whole life opens up, and I am capable of things and experiences and feelings and sharing and giving and learning and growing in ways that I never was capable of before and that reinforces my desire to stay clean."
Recovering methamphetamine and cocaine user

OTHER STIMULANTS

AMPHETAMINE CONGENERS
(Ritalin, Diet Pills, etc.)

With the legal supply of amphetamines severely limited because of federal legislation, pharmaceutical companies and physicians turned to amphetamine congeners, drugs which produce many of the same effects as amphetamines but which have a different chemical structure.

The most popular of these is Ritalin, prescribed as an antidepressant. Ritalin has been used extensively as a treatment for hyperactive children. It seems a contradiction, but many stimulants, in small doses, have the ability to focus attention. However, it is clear that it should be prescribed very sparingly and only after diet changes, counseling, and therapy have failed.

The other popular group of amphetamine congeners are the diet pills such as Preludin, Ionamine, Fastin, and the like. The stimulation, the loss of appetite, and the mood elevation are similar to the effects of amphetamines with some of the same side effects: heart irregularities, toxic convulsions, restlessness, and irritability. Despite their widespread use to control appetite and shed weight, (there is significant weight loss in the first 4 to 6 months), users are often soon back to and even above their starting weights.

Advertisement for lookalike amphetamines.

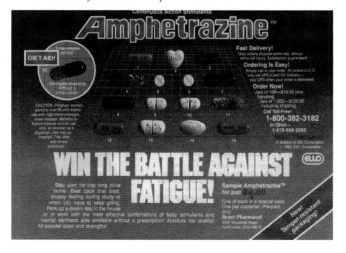

LOOKALIKES

The "lookalike" phenomenon contributed to the abuse of stimulants that began during the 1980's. By taking advantage of the interest in stimulant drugs, a few legitimate manufacturers began to make legal, over-the-counter products which looked identical to prescription stimulants.

Their various products (ephedrine—an anti-asthmatic; phenylpropanolamine—a decongestant and a mild appetite suppressant; caffeine—a stimulant) were being combined, packaged, and sold as "legal stimulants" in a deliberate attempt to misrepresent the drugs. The same chemicals were also showing up as illicit amphetamine lookalikes such as street "speed," "cartwheels," and "crank;" and as cocaine lookalikes such as "Super-caine," "Supertoot," and "Snow." The cocaine lookalikes add benzocaine or procaine to mimic the numbing effects of the actual drug.

The problem with the lookalike products is their toxicity (acting primarily on the heart and blood vessels) when taken in large quantities. Also, an amphetamine-like drug dependence develops in users who chronically abuse the drugs. The physical problems can be particularly severe since large amounts are required to get a speed, or cocaine-like high. This practice continues into the 90's.

MISCELLANEOUS PLANT STIMULANTS

Caffeine is often thought of as the principal plant stimulant other than cocaine, but worldwide, dozens of substances have been discovered that stimulate the user. In fact, in many countries, they are much more common than coffee or tea.

Khat (Qat, Shat, Miraa)

When the United States sent troops to Somalia in 1992, they were surprised to find a large percentage of the population chewing the leaves, twigs, and shoots of the khat shrub in order to get an amphetamine-like rush and stimulation. In another country, Yemen, on the Arabian peninsula, more than half the population uses khat, and the people spend over a third of their family income on the drug. It is the driving force of the economy in Somalia, Yemen, and other countries in East Africa, Southern Arabia, and the Middle East. References to Khat can be found in Arab journals in the 13th century. The leaves were used by some physicians as a treatment for depression.

The khat shrub is 10 to 20 feet tall. The fresh leaves and tender stems are chewed, then retained in the cheek as a ball and slowly chewed some more or swallowed to release the active drug. Dried leaves and twigs, which are not as potent as the fresh leaves, can be crushed for tea or made into a chewable paste. Many homes in some mideast countries actually have a room in their house dedicated to khat chewing. The main active ingredient, cathinone is most potent in fresh leaves which are less than 48 hours old.

Cathinone is a naturally occurring amphetamine-like substance that produces a similar euphoric effect along with a sense of exhilaration, energy, talkativeness, hyperactivity, wakefulness, and loss of appetite. Unfortunately, it also causes chronic insomnia, anorexia, gastric disorders, tachycardia, hypertension, and dependence. When khat is utilized to excess, users become irritable, angry, and often violent.

Chronic khat abuse results in symptoms similar to those seen with amphetamine addiction in the United States, including physical exhaustion, violence, suicidal depression upon withdrawal, and there are rare reports of paranoid hallucinations, and even of overdose deaths.

The constant factional battles in Somalia which devastated the country could be partially due to the effects of khat along with the infighting involved in trying to control the money involved in the trade. Hundreds of millions of dollars are spent on the drug, even in poor countries. In Muslim countries where alcohol is banned, khat is used in a number of social situations.

Recently, in the United States, cathinone has been synthesized in illegal laboratories, particularly in the Midwest, and sold on the street as a powerful alternate to methamphetamine. Since it is cheap to manufacture, a number of labs have sprung up. In one year in Michigan, 17 laboratories were raided. Khat, itself, has also been smuggled into the United States in large quantities.

Betel Nuts

References to betel nut use dates back more than 15 centuries. It has been widely used in the Arab world, India, Malaysia, the Philippines, and New Guinea. Marco Polo brought it to Europe in 1300.

More than 200 million people worldwide use betel nuts not only as a recreational drug but also as a medicine. The effects are similar to nicotine or strong coffee and include a mild euphoria, excitation, decrease in tiredness, and lowered levels of irritability. Some users chew from morning until night, others use it only in social situations. Some liken the practice to gum-chewing or cola-drinking in the west.

The betel nut (husk and/or meat) is chewed in combination with another plant leaf (peppermint, mustard, etc.) and some slaked lime. Unfortunately, the juice of this mixture blackens the teeth over time. In high doses, one of the ingredients, muscarine, can be toxic. However, the principal danger has to do with tissue damage to mucosal linings of the mouth. In addition, up to 7% of regular users have cancer in the mouth and esophagus. The drug can also produce psychological dependence.

Yohimbe

Yohimbine, a bitter, spicy extract from the African yohimbe tree, can be brewed into a stimulating tea or used as a medicine. It is reported to be a mild aphrodisiac. It seems to increase the activity of the neurotransmitter acetylcholine which results in more penile blood inflow. It also increases blood pressure and heart rate. Yohimbine has been reported to produce a mild euphoria and occasional hallucinations, but in larger doses it can be toxic. The bark can be bought at some herbal stores.

Ephedra

The ephedra bush, found in deserts throughout the world, contains the drug ephedrine, a mild stimulant that is used medicinally to treat asthma, other allergies, low blood pressure, and narcolepsy. Many use it to make tea. The Mormons brewed it as a substitute for coffee which was forbidden by their religion. Ephedrine, also known as marwat, has been mentioned as a stimulant tonic in China for over 4,000 years and is still sold in herbalists shops today.

CAFFEINE

Caffeine is the most popular stimulant in the world. It was first cultivated in Ethiopia and then spread to Arabia about 800 A.D. and finally to Europe by the 13th century. The drink was so stimulating that many cultures banned it as an intoxicating drug. The active ingredient, caffeine, was finally isolated in 1821 and discovered to be present in a number of plants including the cocoa bush from which we get chocolate (not the coca bush from which cocaine is derived); in tea leaves; and in cola nuts.

Caffeine, and particularly coffee, is a mild stimulant. In low doses it makes us more alert, dissipates drowsiness or fatigue, and helps us think. It can also speed up the heart rate, raise blood pressure, and irritate the stomach. As with any drug, excessive use causes other problems such as nervousness, mental confusion, irritability, muscle twitches, and insomnia.

Tolerance to the effects of caffeine does occur. We might eventually need three cups to "wake up" instead of our usual single cup with lots of cream and sugar. Also, withdrawal symptoms do occur after long-term use or high-dose use. These include headaches, fatigue, depression, sleep problems, and irritability, but fortunately, most symptoms pass within a few days.

Coffee can become habit forming, but it creates a much milder dependency than that found with amphetamines and cocaine. Generally, it is felt that daily intake levels of 500 mg (about 6 cups of coffee, 6 cola drinks, or 6 cups of tea) or greater will result in dependence and toxic problems.

Fig. 3-6

Amount of Beverage or Food	Caffeine
1 demitasse espresso	200 mg
1 cup freshly brewed American coffee	100 mg
1 No-Doz tablet	100 mg
12 ounce glass of Coca Cola (also in some orange and root beer sodas)	80 mg
4 ounce bar of chocolate	80 mg
1 cup of instant coffee	70 mg
1 cut of tea	70 mg
1 cup of decaf coffee	3 mg

Of the 100 million or so coffee drinkers in the United States, 20% to 30% consume 5 to 7 cups per day. At this dose, signs of caffeine toxicity—increased heart rate, palpitations, anxiety, high blood pressure, and insomnia—are readily apparent. Some women develop benign lumps in their breasts. Caffeine is lethal at about 10 grams (100 cups of coffee), but toxic effects start to appear after only 5 cups.

One of the questions a physician or psychiatrist will ask patients who come in with symptoms of anxiety is about their caffeine consumption since many users have an exaggerated reaction to the drug. People who are prone to panic attacks should also avoid caffeine.

Many researchers also feel that caffeine use makes it harder to lose weight. This is because caffeine stimulates the release of insulin which metabolizes sugar which then reduces the level of sugar in the blood which, in turn, triggers hunger in the user. Even diet colas can trigger this response.

Coronary heart disease, ischemic heart disease, heart attacks, intestinal ulcers, diabetes, and some liver problems linked to caffeine have been seen more often in countries with very high per capita caffeine consumption.

TOBACCO (NICOTINE)

Tobacco is a psychoactive drug. This stimulant affects many of the same areas of the brain as cocaine and amphetamines. As with cocaine, the history of the drug is also a history of the changing methods and levels of use.

HISTORY

Tobacco was used by Native Americans in religious and social rituals 1,000 years ago. After several voyages to the New World, Columbus introduced it to Europe where it was used for recreation and as a medicine. It was banned by a few European countries in the 16th and 17th centuries and in China in 1630 because it was so intoxicating. Tobacco was a major source of revenue that enabled the colonies to pursue the revolutionary war and break free of England. On the other hand, it was considered evil by many religions, and it is still banned by some religious groups such as the Mormons.

Although smoking was the original method of use, snuff and chewing tobacco became popular in the 18th century. Snuff is finely chopped or processed tobacco which is snorted or placed next to the gums so the drug can be absorbed. Chewing tobacco also became popular about that time since a user didn't have to roll a cigarette or carry a means to light it. When tobacco is chewed, the nicotine in the juice is absorbed through the gums and other mucosal tissues. The amount of smoking tobacco didn't exceed the amount of chewing tobacco until the end of World War I.

Surprisingly, since tobacco used to be so scarce and was so harsh to the lungs, it was used sparingly and was not the major health problem it is today. It was the development of milder strains of

The old peace pipe used tobacco, not marijuana, to promote friendship.

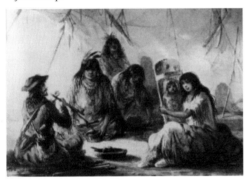

At the turn of the century, tobacco dens were as notorious as the psychedelic clubs of the 60's and the "rave" clubs of the 90's.

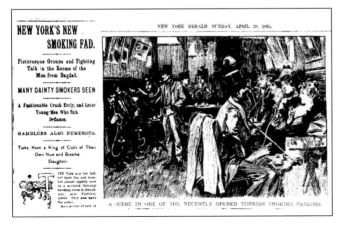

tobacco, the invention of the automatic cigarette rolling machine, massive advertising campaigns, the distribution of free samples to members of the armed forces and to college students, the recognition by governments that tobacco was a potent source of revenue, and the basic addictive properties of nicotine that greatly expanded the cigarette market (Fig. 3-7).

When a user smoked 40 cigarettes a year in the late 1800's, it was not nearly the health problem it is today when the consumption of an average smoker is 30 to 40 cigarettes a day or more than 10,000 a year. This new popularity of tobacco not only multiplied the number of smokers, it multiplied the number of dollars made from tobacco. Gross sales in the United States in 1992 approached 40 billion dollars. In 1992 in the United States, 54 million Americans, about one in five, smoked cigarettes.

EFFECTS

Nicotine, a central nervous system stimulant, disrupts neurotransmitter balance: endorphins, adrenalin, dopamine, and particularly acetylcholine. Acetylcholine affects heart rate, blood pressure, memory, learning, reflexes, aggression, sleep, sexual activity, and mental acuity; adrenalin acts as an energizer; endorphin probably acts as a mild euphoriant; and dopamine triggers the reward/pleasure center.

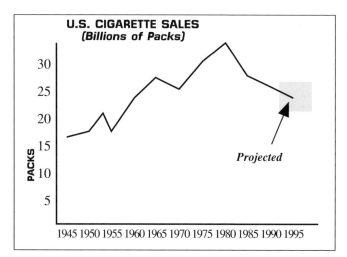

U.S. CIGARETTE SALES
(Billions of Packs)

PACKS

30

25

20

15

10

5

Projected

1945 1950 1955 1960 1965 1970 1975 1980 1985 1990 1995

Fig. 3-7 Sales of ciga-rettes have climbed from 18 billion packs a year in 1945 to a peak of 32 billion packs a year in 1980. Recently, they have dropped to 27 billion packs.

Because of nicotine's effects on neurotransmitter balance, smoking or chewing tobacco constricts blood vessels, raises the heart rate and blood pressure, decreases appetite, increases alertness, produces a very mild euphoria, partially deadens the senses of taste and smell, and irritates the lungs.

Nicotine, the most active ingredient in cigarettes, is commercially used as a pesticide. However, when tobacco is burned in a cigarette, it is not quite so deadly. Unfortunately, burning creates hundreds of other chemicals including nitrosamines that can be almost as dangerous as the nicotine.

Prolonged use of tobacco can cause lung, heart and blood vessel damage, and cancer. Diseases caused by smoking such as lung cancer, emphysema, heart attacks, strokes, and a few others are responsible for more deaths than all other psychoactive drugs combined. Each year, almost 500,000

premature American deaths are directly attributable to smoking compared to only 6 to 7 thousand deaths from heroin and cocaine. In addition another 40 to 60 thousand deaths are attributable to second-hand smoke when those who live or work with smokers have to inhale their exhaled smoke.

Worldwide, the World Health Organization estimates that smoking is responsible for 1 out of every 5 deaths, or 3 million people per year.

"I've smoked 2 packs-a-day for 36 years and I'm still alive. I'm active and I'm good at my job. In any case, I'm not going to live forever. Death is not an option so why should I give up smoking?" 54-year-old smoker

Everyone knows a 75-year-old smoker who's healthy and will use this as proof that smoking won't kill you, but one has to look at the overall statistics, and they show that on average, a 2-pack-a-day smoker will live 8 years less than someone who doesn't smoke. Almost as important as these premature death statistics is the issue of quality of life. Because of breathing complications including chronic bronchitis, greatly reduced lung capacity, and emphysema; because of poor circulation caused by the blood vessel constricting properties; and because of a dozen other imbalances cause by smoking, a smoker will have more medical complications, be less able to participate in sports, and not be able to live life to the fullest.

TOLERANCE, WITHDRAWAL, AND COMPULSION

Tolerance to the effects of nicotine, a strong poison, develops quite rapidly, even faster than with heroin or cocaine.

A few hours of smoking is sufficient for the process to begin. This rapidly induced tolerance is the key to understanding the addictive qualities of tobacco. What happens is that since tobacco is so strong and causes significant mental and physical effects including light-headedness and nausea, the body, in self-protection, immediately begins to adapt its neurochemistry to handle the toxins. Soon one comes to depend on smoking to stay "normal."

1993

Friday, April 2, 1993

Smoking's on rise after 25 years of decline: CDC

By PAUL SCHWARTZMAN

....

Fig. 3-8 *shows the various fatal illnesses caused by smoking in 1989. The figures are based on studies by the American Cancer Society and an extrapolation from the State of Oregon's extremely detailed study of smoking habits, illnesses, and deaths.*

"The first time I smoked, it was to impress a girl, When I first started smoking I got dizzy and high and had to sit down, but a year later, my 30th cigarette of the day only gave me a mild stimulation and a nagging cough. Now, all I have left is the cough ... and it costs over 2 bucks a pack." 2-pack-a-day smoker

Withdrawal from a pack or 2-pack-a-day habit after prolonged use can cause headaches, severe irritability, inability to concentrate, nervousness, and sleep disturbances, so it is not just an emotional addiction but a physical one as well. The sense of relaxation that some smokers receive from a cigarette is, in fact, the sensation of the symptoms of withdrawal being subdued. For this reason, a smoker will try to maintain a constant level of nicotine in the blood stream to maintain a feeling of "well-being." Even when smokers switch to a low tar and nicotine brand, they often increase the number of cigarettes they smoke just to maintain their target level. This need to maintain a level feeling of well-being keeps the user smoking and is the major part of the mechanism of nicotine addiction.

"I tell you, that first cigarette when I wake up is the one I enjoy most. It sets up my whole day. It gets me going." 2-pack-a-day smoker

---

SMOKING-DEATHS U.S.—1991

22.5% OF ALL DEATHS ARE LINKED TO SMOKING	**466,000**
30% OF CANCER DEATHS *(Lung cancer=132,000)*	157,000
20% OF CIRCULATORY DEATHS	176,000
45% OF RESPIRATORY DEATHS	89,000
OTHERS	44,000

Tobacco is the most addicting drug there is. Nicotine craving, in fact, may last a lifetime after withdrawal.

Warnings were first put on tobacco products in 1967 as a result of the Surgeon General's 1966 report on the dangers of smoking. Even though tobacco contains a number of cancer-causing chemicals (carcinogens), it is still sold legally. It is sold legally in spite of federal law which prohibits the sale of any product made for human consumption that is proven to cause cancer. The reason it is still legal is that a special law was passed exempting tobacco from the other law. Speculation is that the exemption was passed because of pressure from the tobacco-growing states where it is a big cash crop.

The other reason for the exemption is the fact that 54 million Americans (and who knows how many in other countries) are addicted to tobacco and constitute a large voting block.

The battle over smoking in the 90's is being fought over the issue of second-hand smoke, the smoke that is inhaled by non-users in a room with smokers. It is estimated that 1 person dies from second-hand smoke (mostly from cardiovascular disease) for every 8 who die from the direct effects.

Numerous laws have been passed in many states and at the Federal level prohibiting the use of tobacco products in a variety of spaces and buildings (e.g., sections of restaurants, airplanes, some businesses, schools, Federal buildings).

SMOKELESS TOBACCO

The two types of smokeless tobacco, moist snuff and loose leaf, are, unfortunately, still popular. A pinch of moist snuff, finely chopped tobacco as found in brands such as Copenhagen and Skoal, is stuck in the mouth next to the gums where the nicotine is absorbed into the capillaries. With loose leaf chewing tobacco as found in brands like Beech Nut and Red Man, larger sections of leaf are stuffed into the mouth and chewed to allow the nicotine-laden juice to be absorbed.

Effects

Tobacco is almost as addicting in this form as in its smoked formed even though the nicotine takes 3 to 5 minutes to affect the central nervous system when chewed or pouched in the cheek compared to the 10 seconds it takes when inhaled from a cigarette. Strangely enough, more of the nicotine reaches the bloodstream with smokeless tobacco, and the rush is somewhat more intense. The effects of chewing are almost identical to the effects when smoking, including a slight increase in energy, alertness, blood pressure, and heart rate.

The main advantage of smokeless tobacco over cigarettes is the protection it gives the lungs since no smoke is inhaled. Lung cancer rates and other respiratory problems drop dramatically. Unfortunately, there are other problems with smokeless tobacco.

"I can't think of a more disgusting habit than chewing tobacco. I broke up with my boyfriend because he was always dripping tobacco juice, spitting, and had those awful brown stains on his clothing. Ugh." 16-year-old high school student

Smokeless tobacco is irritating to the tissues of the mouth and the digestive tract. Many users experience leukoplakia, a thickening, whitening, and hardening of tissues in the mouth; their gums can become inflamed causing more dental problems, and though the risk of lung cancer is reduced, oral, pharynx, and esophageal cancer is increased. In addition, since blood vessels are still constricted, the largest health hazard of smoking, circulatory problems, is just as deadly with smokeless tobacco.

TREATMENT

The only guaranteed, successful therapy when it comes to tobacco is to never smoke, chew, or use it in any form. Abstinence is necessary because many of the neurologic and neurochemical alterations which cause addiction are permanent. This means that even 10 years after cessation of smoking, a single cigarette can trigger the nicotine craving in some users. The old phrase that described this phenomena was "habit-forming." In the 90's, the phrase is "addicting."

The two forms of smokeless tobacco are moist snuff on the left and loose leaf on the right.

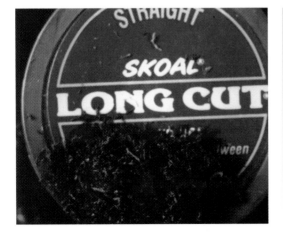
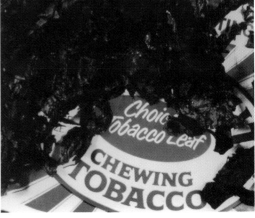

The failure rate for most therapies to stop smoking is 70 to 80 %, this in spite of the fact that 90% of all smokers want to quit. These two statistics alone are testimony to the extremely addictive properties of nicotine. In the past, the focus on treatment was the psychological components of addiction, particularly the "habit" of smoking. Unfortunately these approaches didn't fully take into account the lifetime nature of addiction and therefore recovery. They tried to apply short-term fixes, i.e., 21-day smoking cessation programs, to a long-term problem.

Recently, in recognition of the very real alterations in brain chemistry that trigger nicotine craving during withdrawal, the treatment community has focused on pharmacological treatments.

It is worth noting here that nicotine craving is much more subtle and less noticeable to the user than the other cravings that occur with drugs like cocaine, heroin or alcohol. However, the craving is extremely powerful and may be associated with what is called a self-determined nicotine state of consciousness or state dependence. State dependence means that a person will try to achieve a certain mental and physical state which may neither be pleasurable or objectionable, but it is a state with which they are familiar and one that they, and not others, have determined. Many people think that a large part of addiction is created by this desire to be in a familiar physical and mental mood even if it is damaging to the body and mind.

Nicotine Replacement

Since the main mechanism that causes craving is the drop in blood levels of nicotine which then trigger withdrawal symptoms such as irritability, anxiety, drowsiness, and light headedness, research has been aimed at nicotine replacement systems. The purpose of these systems is to slowly reduce the blood plasma nicotine levels to the point where cessation will not trigger withdrawal symptoms that will cause the smoker to relapse.

The four types of nicotine replacement systems are transdermal nicotine patches, nicotine gum, nicotine sprays, and nicotine nasal inhalers. One of the main advantages of all of these systems is that users are no longer damaging their lungs with some of the 4,000 chemicals found in cigarette smoke. This alone could save almost 200,000 lives per year in the United States. The main problem is that if relapse prevention, counseling, and self-help groups are not used in conjunction with nicotine replacement therapy, then the chances of smokers returning to their old habits is extremely high.

Nicotine patches

Nicotine patches such as Nicoderm and Habitrol are nicotine soaked adhesive patches that are applied to the skin. Patches can be worn intermittently (daytime only) or continuously. Most of them contain enough nicotine for 24 to 72 hours. The advantages of patches are the steady rate of release of nicotine, the ease of compliance, and the lack of toxic effects to tissues in the mouth or digestive track. The disadvantages are the 4 to 6 hours it takes for a patch to raise the nicotine level enough to dull nicotine craving, the cost, and the inability to alter the amount being absorbed. Also, if the user starts smoking while wearing the patch, plasma levels of nicotine can become extremely high and dangerous.

Nicotine gum

Nicotine gum such as Nicorette has the advantage of slowing the rise in nicotine levels that smoking brings. The 10 second rush of an inhaled cigarette gives way to the 15- to - 30-minute slow rise that nicotine gum provides when absorbed through the gums and other mucosal tissues. A slower rise means that craving, which is triggered by the sudden drop in nicotine levels after smoking, doesn't occur. The 15- to -30-minute rise however is considerable faster than the 4 to 6 hours it takes for a transdermal patch to work so the user has more control over the dose. The disadvantages are the user can cram a lot of gum into the mouth or not use it at all; the gum can irritate mucosal tissues; and an oral habit is maintained (users are still putting something in their mouths when the craving hits or when they are agitated rather than learning other behaviors).

Nasal spray

Nasal sprays (still undergoing clinical trials) are self administered and reach the brain in 3 to 5 minutes thereby giving more instant relief to the nicotine craving and giving more control to the user. The disadvantage is irritation to the nasal passages and the fact that the process of rapid ups and downs which reinforce addiction is still operative.

Nicotine inhalers

Nicotine inhalers (still undergoing clinical trials) give the fastest relief of nicotine craving without involving the inhalation of all the chemicals present in smoke. The problem seems to be that misuse can produce plasma levels similar to those produced by smoking, thereby perpetuating the addictive process.

TREATING THE SYMPTOMS

The purpose of symptomatic treatment is to reduce the anxiety, depression, and craving that accompany withdrawal and therefore trigger relapse. Clonidine, benzodiazepines, buspirone, Prozac, and some other antidepressants have been used to try to alleviate the symptoms of nicotine withdrawal.

Nicotine addiction researchers have found a great similarity between the symptoms of heroin withdrawal and nicotine withdrawal, particularly those associated with anxiety, so they have tried to use clonidine, a drug normally used to control both high blood pressure and the symptoms of heroin withdrawal, in order to control nicotine withdrawal. Clonidine, available in pills or in patches, acts by inhibiting the release of norepinephrine (adrenalin). This depresses the activity of the locus coeruleus, the part of the brain that controls many symptoms of heroin and nicotine withdrawal. It also controls some of the symptoms of anxiety.

Other drugs that have been tried are mecamylamine which blocks the nicotinic acetylcholine receptors; propranolol, which blocks dopamine and therefore some of the peripheral effects of nicotine; naltrexone and naloxone which are actually used for opiate craving and which block endorphins.

Most behavioral therapies which include one-on-one counseling, group therapy, educational approaches, aversion therapy, hypnotism, and acupuncture have a one-year success rate of 15 to 30%. The same problems with pharmaceutical therapies apply to behavioral therapies, and that is, unless they are long-term and unless they focus on relapse prevention training, they will not be successful. Many of the techniques used in stimulant abuse recovery are directly applicable to quitting smoking. These include:

• Desensitizing the smoker to environmental cues that trigger craving;

• Practicing alternate methods of calming oneself when under stress or going through withdrawal;

• Avoiding environments and situations such as bars where smoking is rampant;

• Finding other ways of getting the small rush or mild euphoria that nicotine provides;

• Teaching the smoker the physiology of nicotine use and addiction along with the medical consequences of smoking or chewing tobacco;

• Teaching the smoker the extraordinary benefits of quitting.

Physically some of the beneficial physiologic changes that occur on quitting are that

• Within 36 hours, blood carbon monoxide levels return to normal;

• Within 48 hours, nerve endings adjust to the absence of nicotine, and the senses of smell and taste are enhanced;

• Within a week, the risk of heart attack drops, breathing improves, and constricted vessels begin to relax;

• Within 2 weeks to 3 months, circulation improves and lung function increases up to 30%, and the complexion looks healthy again;

• Within 1 to 9 months, fatigue, coughing, sinus congestion, and shortness of breath decrease, and the lungs increase their ability to handle mucus thereby helping to clean themselves and reduce infection;

• Within 5 years, heart disease death rate returns to the rate for nonsmokers;

• Within 10 years, the lung cancer death rate drops almost to the rate for nonsmokers, precancerous cells are replaced, and the incidence of other cancers decreases.

Mentally there are other beneficial changes. Initially, there is anxiety, anger, difficulty concentrating, increased appetite, and craving due to withdrawal.

After 2 weeks most of these disappear with the exception of craving and increased appetite.

The Haight-Ashbury Clinic in San Francisco has had good results using a combination of clonidine patches, nicotine patches and/or nicotine gum in conjunction with recovery oriented counseling and group education work, all aimed at preventing relapse.

Doonesbury

BY GARRY TRUDEAU

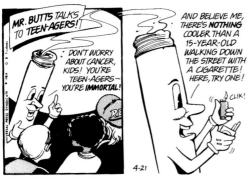
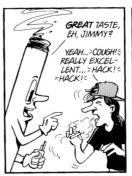
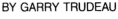
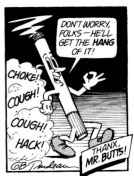

REVIEW

UPPERS

1. Uppers are central nervous system stimulants.

2. In general, uppers stimulate us by forcing the release of energy chemicals (particularly adrenalin), by increasing electrical activity in the brain, and by artificially stimulating our reward/pleasure center.

3. The basic effects of stimulants are increased energy, faster heart rate, higher blood pressure, quicker respiration, restlessness, dilated pupils, talkativeness, irritability, reduced appetite, or thirst, and variable euphoria depending on the strength of the stimulant.

4. Most problems with stimulants occur when we don't give the body time to recover from the stimulation and we deplete our energy supply.

5. Other problems with the stronger stimulants occur when we disrupt our neurotransmitter balance. We can become paranoid, have muscle tremors, become aggressive, and fall into a deep mental depression.

6. Another set of problems with the stronger stimulants comes when our stimulated reward/pleasure center tells us we don't need food, drink, or sexual stimulation. We can become malnourished, dehydrated, or unable to perform sexually.

7. A final set of problems with the stronger stimulants such as cocaine comes from overdosing: using too much at one time, or having a severe reaction to a small dose. A "caine" or "speed" reaction can cause uncontrolled heart rhythms, convulsions, ultra-high blood pressure, heart attacks, strokes, dangerously high body temperatures, psychotic episodes, coma, and eventually death, if not handled quickly by trained or knowledgeable people.

8. The principal stimulants are cocaine, amphetamines (speed), diet pills, nicotine, and caffeine.

9. Cocaine is the second most addicting stimulant (nicotine is the first). It is noted for the intensity of its stimulation, the high price, and the speed with which it is metabolized from the body.

10. Cocaine can be snorted, injected, drunk, or smoked. The smoking form is called crack, rock, freebase, or a dozen other names. Smoking is the fastest route to the brain, 7 to 10 seconds.

11. Cocaine's allure comes from the fact that it mimics natural body functions and highs. The comedown is also extremely intense, so the user keeps taking it to stay up. And finally, the brain becomes sensitized to the memory of the pleasurable effects.

12. An overdose of cocaine can be the result of as little as 1/50th of a gram or as much as 1.2 grams or more. Most overdose reactions are not fatal, but death can come from cardiac arrest, respiratory depression, and seizures.

13. Crack cocaine causes many problems because of the economics of the drug. It comes in smaller amounts; there's a large market for it; and the profits are great.

14. Amphetamines are very similar to cocaine, the main difference being that they are longer acting, take more time to metabolize, and are cheaper to buy.

15. Amphetamines were originally prescribed to fight exhaustion, depression, and obesity but were taken more often for their mood- elevating and euphoric properties.

16. Prolonged use of amphetamines can induce paranoia, heart and blood vessel problems, increased body temperature, dehydration, and malnutrition.

17. Tolerance develops rapidly with amphetamines. Amphetamine and cocaine withdrawal cause physical and emotional depression, extreme irritability, and nervousness.

18. Many diet pills and mood elevators mimic the actions of amphetamines but are not quite as strong. They can still cause many of the problems found with amphetamines. Ritalin and Preludin can be as addicting as cocaine and speed.

19. Lookalike drugs were popularized to take advantage of the desire for the now hard-to-get amphetamines and cocaine. They are composed of over-the-counter stimulants. Heavy use can cause heart and blood vessel problems as well as dependence.

20. Other plant stimulants such as Khat, betel nut, ephedra, and yohimbe have been used by hundreds of millions of people, particularly in the mideast and Africa.

21. Caffeine, particularly coffee, is the most popular stimulant in the world. Tolerance can develop with caffeine, and withdrawal symptoms such as headaches, depression, and irritability do occur, particularly if consumption is more than 5 cups a day.

22. Nicotine (tobacco) is the most addicting psychoactive drug. Fifty-four million people are addicted to cigarettes compared to 15 million addicted to alcohol. Nicotine causes more deaths than all the other psychoactive drugs combined.

23. One of the main reasons for tobacco's addictive nature, besides the slight stimulation it gives, is the need for the smoker's body to maintain a certain level of nicotine in the blood to avoid withdrawal.

24. Besides reducing the number of years of life, tobacco lowers the quality of life.

25. Smokeless tobacco is as addicting and as damaging as tobacco that is smoked.

QUESTIONS

1. What neurotransmitter is most responsible for the stimulation caused by uppers?

2. What are three major physical effects of most stimulants?

3. What are three major mental effects of stimulants?

4. Why does a user suffer appetite loss when taking amphetamines, cocaine, or diet pills?

5. What are the major problems caused by:

   a. depletion of energy chemicals?

   b. disruption of neurotransmitter balance?

   c. stimulation of reward and pleasure centers?

6. Name five kinds of stimulants.

7. What are the three most common ways to put cocaine into the body?

8. What are the major differences between amphetamine and cocaine?

9. What are the effects of an overdose of amphetamine or cocaine?

10. What are the main chemical ingredients of lookalike stimulants?

11. Name two exotic plant stimulants besides the coca and cocoa bush.

12. What are the symptoms of caffeine withdrawal?

13. Which stimulant causes the most injuries and medical problems?

14. Which stimulant causes the most deaths?

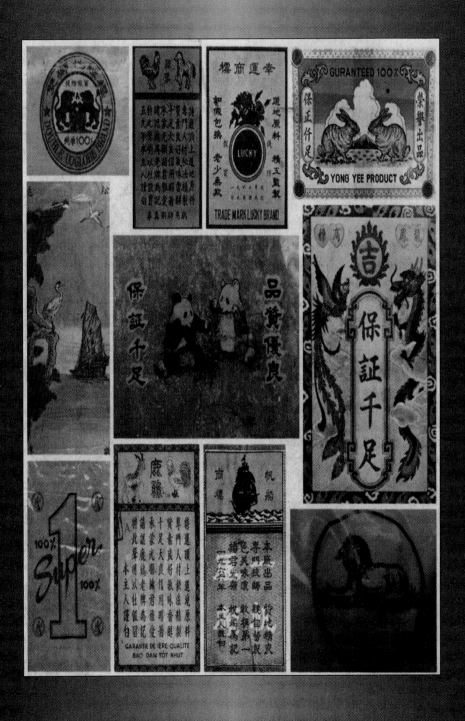

These are labels from packets of heroin produced in Asia; a perverted pride in workmanship.

DOWNERS

OPIATES & OPIOIDS AND
SEDATIVE–HYPNOTICS

CHAPTER 4

1984

Codeine Diversion Through 10 State Drugstores Charged

By ALLAN PARACHINI Times Staff Writer

Failures in inventory control systems at the Bay Area warehouse of one of the nation's largest drug chains led to the diversion of dozens of ounces and 167 million in the state's sold through Metro...

1992

New Form of Heroin Linked To Rise in Overdose Deaths

By JOEL BRINKLEY
Special to The New York Times

WASHINGTON, March 27 — An unusually potent and dangerous new form of Mexican heroin is being spread rapidly across the United States, Federal drug enforcement officials say. They assert that it has led to dozens, perhaps hundreds, of deaths by overdose, as well as to thousands of injuries in the last year.

The new heroin, which users call black tar because it resembles roofing tar in color and consistency, is increasingly dominating the nation's heroin markets. It is now sold in 27 states, up from four in 1983, according to officials...

of the Federal Drug Enforcement Administration.

It is blamed for causing the first general increase in overall heroin use in more than five years, in part because its low price has forced down other heroin prices.

The drug agency says black tar sells in some areas of the country for one-tenth the price of the heroin previously available, even though purity levels are as much as 40 times higher.

"It's a very serious problem and it's getting worse," John C. Lawn, head of...

1924

Pharmacy Board Backs 3 Drastic Bills to Correct Law Weaknesses

First Offense for Peddling of Drugs Made Felony; Hospital on Island for Addicts Urged
JANUARY 4, 1924

GENERAL CLASSIFICATION

Downers (depressants) depress the overall functioning of the central nervous system to ultimately induce sedation, muscle relaxation, drowsiness, and even coma (if used to excess). Unlike uppers, which generally function through the release and enhancement of the body's natural stimulatory neurochemicals, the diverse group of drugs classed as depressants produce their effects through a wide range of biochemical processes at different sites of the brain and spinal cord.

Some depressants mimic the actions of the body's natural sedating or inhibiting neuro-transmitters (i.e. endorphins, enkephalins, GABA), while others directly suppress the stimulatory areas of the brain. Still others work in ways scientists haven't yet fully understood. Because of these variations, the depressants are grouped into a number of subclasses based upon their medical use, chemistry, and legal classification.

The three main classes of depressants are opiates and opioids, sedative-hypnotics, and alcohol.

We will first give a thumbnail sketch of each class and later treat the first two groups in detail. Because of the complexity of the problem with alcohol abuse, alcohol will be discussed in the next chapter.

OPIATES & OPIOIDS

Opiates such as heroin, morphine, and codeine are refined from the opium poppy. Opioids such as Demerol and Darvon are synthetic, produced to mimic the effects of natural opiates. Opiates and opioids were developed for the treatment of acute pain, diarrhea, coughs, and a number of other illnesses. Most illicit use is to gain the euphoric effects, to avoid pain, and to avoid withdrawal symptoms.

SEDATIVE-HYPNOTICS

The sedative-hypnotics represent a wide range of synthetic chemical substances developed to treat nervousness and insomnia. The first, a barbiturate, was developed in 1864 by Dr. Adolph Von Bayer. Since then, thousands of different sedative-hypnotics such as Miltown, Valium, Doriden, and Quaalude have been created. All have toxic side effects and tissue dependence liability.

ALCOHOL (See Chapter 5)

Alcohol, the natural by-product of fermented plant sugars or starch, is probably the oldest psychoactive drug in the world. It has been used for a number of medical remedies, from sterilizing wounds to reducing the risk of heart attack. It has been used to reduce stress and stimulate sexuality. Alcohol is also the world's most devastating drug (second in the U.S. to nicotine) in terms of health consequences, i.e., cirrhosis of the liver, mental deterioration, ulcers, impotence; and social consequences, i.e., violence, crime, marital problems, absenteeism, and automobile accidents. In the United States alone, it is estimated that there are 15 million active alcoholics or problem drinkers.

The four minor classes of depressants are skeletal muscle relaxants, antihistamines, "over-the-counter sedatives," and lookalike sedatives.

SKELETAL MUSCLE RELAXANTS

Centrally acting skeletal muscle relaxants are actually synthetically developed central nervous system depressants aimed at areas of the brain responsible for muscular coordination and activity. They are used to treat muscle tension and pain. Though the current abuse of these products is rare, their overall downer effect on all parts of the central nervous system produces reactions similar to those caused by other abused depressants.

ANTIHISTAMINES

Antihistamines are synthetic drugs, developed during the 1930's and 1940's for treatment of allergic reactions, ulcers, shock, rashes, motion sickness, and even symptoms of Parkinson's Disease. In addition to blocking the release of histamine, these drugs cross the blood-brain barrier to induce the common and oftentimes very potent side effect of depression of the central nervous system, resulting in drowsiness. Thus, even antihistamines are occasionally sought and abused for their depressant effects.

OVER-THE-COUNTER SEDATIVES

These are depressant drugs such as Nytol, Sleep-Eze, and Sominex that are sold legally in stores, without the need for a prescription. Many brands have been marketed as sleep aids or sedatives for years. These kinds of sedatives were, in fact, first used as depressants during the 1880's. Scopolamine in low doses, antihistamines, salicylates (a natural form of aspirin), salicylamide, bromide derivatives, and even alcohol constitute the active sedating components of many of these products. As with other downer drugs, these products are occasionally abused for their depressant effects.

LOOKALIKE SEDATIVES

"Lookalike" sedatives were advertised along with lookalike stimulants in the early 80's. The great commercial success of the lookalike stimulants encouraged shady drug manufacturers to sell products disguised as prescription downers. These companies took legally available antihistamines and packaged them in tablets and capsules so they resembled prescription downers; i.e., Quaalude, Valium, Seconal. As with the other antihistamines, lookalike sedatives cause drowsiness as a side effect thereby mimicking the effects of more potent downers.

OPIATES & OPIOIDS

CLASSIFICATION

One of the oldest and best-documented class of drugs, opiates (natural derivatives of opium) and opioids (synthetic opiates) have been the source of continual, and occasionally explosive, worldwide problems. Heroin gets the most publicity, but there are many more opiates and opioids such as codeine, Demerol, and Fentanyl which have created their own set of problems and their own groups of compulsive users.

Fortunately, developments in opiate and opioid research during the 1970's, following the discovery of the body's own natural painkillers, endorphins and enkephalins, represent the most significant change to the whole field of biochemical research, pain management, and drug abuse treatment in this century by giving us a new perspective and new research tools to understand the biochemical mechanisms that govern all our thoughts and actions.

Figure 4-1 OPIATES & OPIOIDS

Drug Name	Trade Name	Street Name
OPIATES (Opium Poppy Extracts or Modified Extracts)		
Opium	Pantopon, Paregoric Laudanum	"O", op, poppy
Codeine (usually w/aspirin or Tylenol)	Empirin w/codeine, Tylenol w/codeine Codeine w/Doriden	Number 4's (1 grain) Number 3's (1/2 grain) Loads, sets, 4's & doors
Morphine	Various	Murphy, morph, M, Miss Emma
Diacetyl morphine	Heroin	Smack, junk, tar (chiva, puro, goma, puta), Mexican brown, China White, Harry, skag, Rufus, Perze, "H," dava, boy
Hydrocodone	Hycodan, Vicodin	
Hydromorphone	Dilaudid	Dillies, drugstore heroin
Oxycodone	Percodan, Tylox	Percs
OPIOIDS (Synthetic Opiates)		
Methadone	Dolophine	Juice
Propoxyphene	Darvon, Darvocet-N	Pink ladies, pumpkin seeds
Meperidine	Demerol	
Fentanyl	Sublimaze	Street derivatives are misrepresented as China White
Pentazocine	Talwin	Part of "T's and blues"
l-alpha acetyl methadol (long-acting methadone)	LAAM	Lam

HISTORY OF
METHODS OF USE

The story of opiates starts with the opium poppy, the substances made from that plant such as heroin and codeine, and the effects of those drugs on our pain and pleasure centers.

The Sumerians, Egyptians, and Chinese, more than 2,000 years before the birth of Christ, recorded the paradoxical nature of opium in their ancient medical texts, listing it as a cure for all illness, a pleasurable substance, and a poison. Over the centuries, experimentation with different methods of use, creation of new refinements of the drug, and synthesis of molecules which act like opiates have slowly increased not only the benefits of this substance but also the abuse potential.

The opium poppy (papaver somniferum) was named after Somnis, the Roman God of Sleep, and though the drug was used extensively to induce drowsiness as well as heal many illnesses, the abuse potential was low because it had a bitter taste and was only taken by mouth. Orally, the drug has to go through the entire digestive system before it enters the blood stream and makes its way to the brain 20 or 30 minutes later.

It was the introduction of the pipe from North America to Europe and Asia that set the stage for the widespread non-medical abuse of opium. Smoking puts more of the active ingredients of the drug into the blood stream faster, by way of the lungs, so the drug begins to reach the brain in as few as 7 seconds. The higher concentration of the opiate produces a stronger euphoria and sense of well-being, thereby encouraging abuse. In 1806, a German pharmacist refined morphine from opium and found it to be 10 times stronger. Morphine was a much better pain reliever, but its greater strength promoted more compulsive use than opium.

Next came the invention in 1848 of the hypodermic needle which could put high concentrations of a drug directly into the blood stream. It takes 15 to 30 seconds for an injected opiate to affect the central nervous system. If the drug is injected just under the skin or in a muscle ("skin poppin" or "muscling"), the effects are delayed 5 to 8 minutes. The refinement of morphine and the discovery·of the hypodermic needle were of benefit during the Crimean and the U.S. Civil Wars to treat wounded soldiers, but a generation of morphine addicts was created. At that time the opiate addiction was called the "soldier's disease."

....

Legally controlled field of opium poppies in India, the largest grower of opium (U.N. photo).

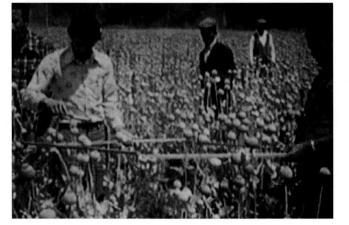

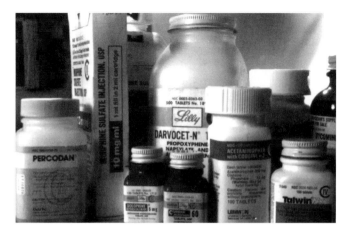

Collection of prescription opiates and opioids, still some of the most common prescription drugs.

Samples of heroin seized by the Drug Enforcement Administration on the West Coast of the United States. Note that many highly diluted samples are dyed to make them appear a purer cut of the drug, i.e., "Mexican brown" or "tar" (Courtesy of Robert Sager, DEA).

Just before the turn of the century morphine was altered chemically to produce heroin in an attempt to find a more effective pain killer which didn't have addictive properties. Unfortunately, the opposite proved to be true. Since heroin crosses the blood-brain barrier much more rapidly than morphine, the rush was more instantaneous and intense, thus creating a subculture of heroin abusers in the 20th century.

During the mid to late 1800's opiates in their many forms became so popular that hundreds of tonics and medications came on the market to treat everything from tired blood, to coughs, to diarrhea, to toothaches, before casual, non-medical use was declared illegal at the beginning of the 20th century.

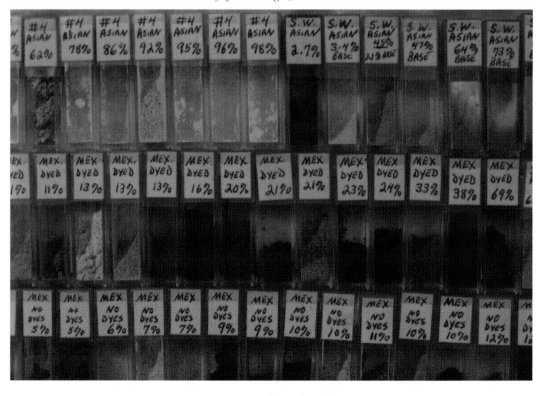

Since then, growing, processing, and distributing opiates, especially heroin, have become major sources of revenue for criminal organizations worldwide, i.e., the Chinese Triads, the Mafia, Mexican narcoficantes, the Columbian Cartel, and even African traffickers.

In addition, diversion of legitimate prescription opiates and opioids like codeine and Dilaudid, through theft, phony purchases, and forged prescriptions, has created an illegal, uncontrolled market of pills and injectibles.

There are an estimated 100,000 to 300,000 prescription opiate and opioid abusers in the U.S., compared to 300,000 to 800,000 heroin abusers. Approximately two million Americans have tried heroin.

HEROIN

Since the 1930's, heroin has captured more headlines than any of the other opiates. There are 5 to 10 million heroin abusers worldwide. A dozen countries are battling the growth, use, and exportation of heroin and other opiates on their own soil.

The area of Southeast Asia known as the Golden Triangle (Burma, Northern Thailand, and Laos) is the largest producer and exporter of heroin. It is also one of the largest users. Thailand alone has close to half a million addicts. Golden Triangle heroin, known as China White in its exportable form, can be up to 99% pure. Other Southeast Asian types of heroin are Indian, Cambodian, and Malaysian or Sri Lankan pink heroin (usually around 50% pure). India is the largest grower of opium. It is highly regulated, and the majority of the crop is used for legal medical purposes.

Since the 1940's, Mexico has been the major supplier of heroin to the United States. In the 1980's a relatively new form of Mexican heroin, known as "tar" or "black tar," has taken over most of the market. It is extremely potent, 40 to 80 % pure, but also has more plant impurities than the Asian form of the drug. A small chunk the size of a match head, which is enough for 2 to 5 doses, costs about 20 to 25 dollars. "Tar" heroin, also called "chapa pote," "puta," "goma," and "puro," is unique in that it's sold as a gummy, pasty substance rather than the usual powder form of heroin. It is also more likely to be smoked than other heroins.

"You throw up a lot more with tar. "Tar" really makes me sick to my stomach. Unfortunately, on the West Coast that's all you can find anymore." Heroin dealer/user

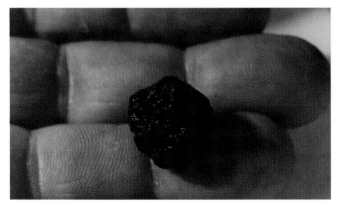

A small sample of Mexican "tar" heroin, the most common type of heroin sold in the U.S.

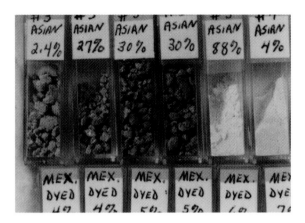

#3 Heroin from SE Asia, generally less refined and more dilute than #4 shooting heroin.

The headlines point to the worldwide increase in opium growing and expansion of the trade since much of the cocaine market has been saturated.

The region where there has been a major increase in the production and abuse of heroin is Southwest Asia. From Afghanistan, Iran, Pakistan, Turkey, and Lebanon comes a product that is known as "Persian brown" or "Perze," which can be more than 90% pure. Several of these countries that grow opium now also have exploding addict populations.

"Persian heroin is simply raw processed morphine. The process to take raw morphine and turn it into number 4 white is a very expensive and lengthy chemical process which takes experts, so dealers are just giving you less quality for ridiculous prices."
Recovering heroin smoker

In addition, several countries have major refining facilities or are major transshipment points for heroin including the Netherlands, Canada, Italy, France, and West Africa (the latter also grows its own).

There has also been a recent increase in home-grown opium in the United States. However, a few criminal organizations still control most of the trade. For example, with the return of Hong Kong to the People's Republic of China in 1997, many of the Triads (Chinese criminal organizations) that were based there have decided that their headquarters would be wiped out if they stayed, so they have increased their presence in other countries and have tried to expand their markets and the number of users. This has also led to a large increase in Asian gangs becoming involved in trafficking heroin in the United States.

They reportedly try to disguise some of their "China white" as "Mexican Brown," or "tar" so the authorities won't be as alarmed about their increased presence in the United States. They and the Mafia have also increased the importation of cheaper smokable heroin to encourage many young crack users to try it in their pipes to create a new market, much the same way that crack cocaine expanded the number of cocaine users.

At the present time, injection is the preferred means of abusing heroin in the west. Occasionally it is snorted. In most Asian and Middle Eastern countries it is smoked.

1990

Major Changes in Heroin Trade
Chinese 'triads' taking over the business, Senate panel told

By Bob Dart
Cox News Service

Washington

Centuries-old "triads" with thousands of ethnic Chinese

gives in, ironically, due in part to the success U.S. law enforcement agencies have had in prosecuting heroin traffickers from the traditional Mafia.

witnesses said. Street-level heroin came mostly from Southwest Asia and was 3 to 5 percent pure when sold in East Coast cities in the early 1980s, said Bryant. The heroin from Southwest Asia is better said

Drug Lords Diversify Into Opium Market

1990

1991

Colombia Farmers Show Signs Of Switching to Heroin Trade

By Tady Pranate
Chronicle Foreign Service

spread. A recent investigation by Colombian officials found that poppies are being grown in 30 per-

niguen and from the fertile soil and mountain climate.

The same chemical process

"Snorting it, you have to snort more and then you have to wait to take it in your system and it might take you 10-15 minutes to get loaded. When you're snorting it, you get sick, your nose runs uncontrollably, and you get stomach cramps."
Recovering heroin user

Heroin can be smoked in a water pipe or standard pipe, be mixed in a regular cigarette or marijuana joint, or be heated and the smoke inhaled. This last method is known as "Chasing the Dragon."

"If anybody has the delusion that smoking's all that much different than shooting heroin, they're in for a big surprise. It's just as easy to get addicted smoking heroin as it is shooting heroin." *Heroin smoker*

But alarmingly, a number of South American illicit cocaine suppliers have recently begun to grow opium poppies (in addition to their fields of coca shrubs) in an effort to cash in on the heroin market as well.

OTHER OPIATES & OPIOIDS

Opium

The term opiate refers to certain alkaloids or chemical compounds found in the milky fluid of the unripe seed pod of the opium poppy plant, Papaver Somniferum. There are over 25 known alkaloids in the poppy, but the two most important are morphine and codeine. Although a small amount of opium is used to make antidiarrheal preparations such as paregoric, virtually all the opium coming into this country is refined into its alkaloid constituents, principally morphine and codeine.

Codeine

One to five percent of the opium extract contains codeine. It can also be refined from morphine. Codeine is not as strong as morphine and is generally used for the relief of moderate pain (aspirin plus codeine or Tylenol plus codeine), or to control severe coughs (Robitussin AC, Cheracol). Codeine is the most widely used, legal opiate or opioid. It is also one of the most widely abused prescription drugs.

Codeine is often abused in combination with Doriden, a sleeping pill. This combination known as "loads," "sets," or "set ups," is taken orally and results in a heroin-like high. The combination has a great overdose potential because it depresses respiration and prolongs the other drug's toxic effects.

Morphine

Four to twenty one percent of pure opium is morphine. It is usually processed into white crystal hypodermic tablets and injectable solutions. It may be administered orally, under the tongue, rectally, or into a vein, into a muscle, or under the skin. Morphine still remains the standard by which effective pain relief is measured in medicine.

Dilaudid

A short acting, semi-synthetic, opioid, Dilaudid can be taken orally or injected. Once morphine is extracted from opium, a simple chemical process changes it to Dilaudid which is stronger and shorter acting than morphine. Dilaudid is used as an alternative to morphine for the treatment of severe pain. Illegally diverted Dilaudid is becoming increasingly attractive to cocaine users for use in "speedballs."

Percodan

Also used for the relief of pain, Percodan is most often taken orally. By this route, it usually takes about 30 minutes before the effects appear, and these effects last from four to six hours. Its pain-relieving effect is much stronger than codeine, but weaker than that of morphine or dilaudid.

Methadone

Methadone and some of the illicit fentanyl derivatives are long-acting opioids. Methadone is usually taken orally causing pain-killing and depressant effects that can last 4 to 6 hours. It also reduces drug craving and blocks withdrawal symptoms for 24 to 72 hours. It is the only legally authorized opioid (that is not an opiate blocker) to treat heroin addiction through a program known as methadone maintenance. Despite heavy regulation of methadone

Methadone mixed with fruit juice is ready to be drunk by heroin addicts at a methadone clinic.

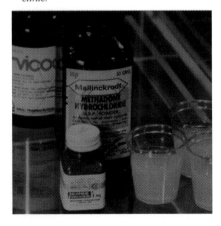

clinics and tight controls of the supply of methadone, it is still abused and results in a number of overdoses every year. Like heroin, it too is addicting and must be monitored closely to prevent diversion. (See the end of this chapter for more information on methadone maintenance.)

LAAM

LAAM is another opioid that is still being tested for heroin replacement therapy similar to methadone maintenance. Unlike methadone, its ability to prevent withdrawal symptoms lasts about 3 days.

Demerol

A short-acting opioid, Demerol is most often injected. It is a fairly strong analgesic (pain reliever) and is the abused drug of choice for some in the medical community.

Talwin (Pentazocine)

Talwin, prescribed for chronic pain, comes in tablets or as an injectable liquid. Talwin acts as a weak narcotic antagonist (a drug that counters the effects of opiates) as well as opioid agonist (drug that mimics the effects of opiates). This drug was frequently combined and injected with an anti-histamine drug ("T's and blues"). Increased vigilance and reformulation of Talwin by its manufacturer has almost stopped this problem although some abusers still take the combination orally or abuse Talwin by itself.

Darvon

Prescribed for the relief of mild to moderate pain, Darvon is often prescribed by dentists. It is taken orally with the effects lasting 4-6 hours. It too can cause an overdose or addiction.

"After 7 years of doing Darvon, I started having withdrawals after three to four hours from the last pill that I had taken, so I was addicted to my watch."
Compulsive Darvon user

Designer Heroin

These street versions of fentanyl (alpha, 3-methyl, etc.) and Demerol (MPPP), manufactured in illegal laboratories, are extremely potent and can cause drug overdoses and even nervous system damage. Sold as "China white," these drugs bear witness to a growing sophistication of street chemists who now can bypass the traditional smuggling and trafficking routes of heroin. Since these are street drugs made without controls, the "designer drugs" represent a tremendous health threat to the opiate abusing community.

"When I first got out here on the West Coast, I found out that it ['China White'] wasn't white dope at all. It was fentanyl and it wasn't even pharmaceutical fentanyl. It was bathtub fentanyl and people were dying on it."
Dealer/heroin user

Street fentanyl can be up to 3,000 to 20,000 times stronger than regular heroin. A dose the size of a grain of salt is powerful enough to kill 30 people. Recently, in Baltimore and Vancouver, there have been dozens of deaths because of this substitution.

Street Demerol, if improperly made, can contain a chemical, MPTP, which destroys brain cells and destroys most of the voluntary muscular movement by inducing the degenerative nerve condition known as Parkinson's disease. This causes a condition known as the "frozen addict," where the addict can't voluntarily move.

Naloxone & Naltrexone

These are opiate or opioid antagonists. They do not have much effect on the body except for their ability to block the effects of opiates. Naloxone is effective in treating heroin or opiate overdose while Naltrexone is used to prevent addiction. While taking Naltrexone daily, a user will not feel the effects of heroin or any other opiate or opioid. Research is also being conducted on Naltrexone's ability to reduce craving in the treatment of alcohol and cocaine addiction as well.

EFFECTS

Pain and Pleasure

Medically, physicians prescribe opiates and opioids to deaden pain, stop coughing, and control diarrhea. Non-medically, users self-prescribe opiates and opioids for the euphoria, to drown out their emotional pain, or to try to feel normal by preventing withdrawal symptoms. But to truly compre-

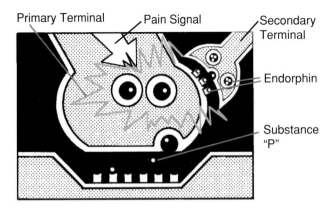

Primary Terminal   Pain Signal   Secondary Terminal

Endorphin

Substance "P"

Fig. 4-2 This diagram of a synapse shows how the secondary messenger terminal releases endorphins which then slots into the primary terminal and limits its release of substance "P."

Fig. 4-3 Heroin slots into the secondary endorphin receptor sites and the primary substance "P" receptor sites.

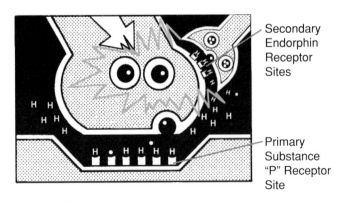

Secondary Endorphin Receptor Sites

Primary Substance "P" Receptor Site

hend opiates and opioids, it is important to understand pain and its connection to the nervous system and to understand pleasure and its connection to the limbic system.

Pain

Pain, such as the pain of burned skin, is a warning signal. It tells us if we are being damaged physically. It sends a message to our brain which in turn tells the rest of the body to protect itself, to stop the damage. The pain message is transmitted by a neurotransmitter called substance "P."

If the pain is too intense, the body tries to protect itself by softening the pain signals. It does this by flooding the brain and spinal cord with special neurotransmitters, called endorphins. These endorphins attach themselves to the membrane of the sending nerve cell telling it not to send substance "P" (Fig. 4-2).

However, many signals still get through. If the pain is still unbearable, opiates and opioids can be used. These drugs are effective because they act like endorphins. They not only prevent too much substance "P" from being released, they also block what little does get through to the receiving neuron (Fig. 4-3).

The effects of the various opiates and opioids are similar. The differences have to do with how long the drug lasts, how strong it is per gram, and how toxic it is to the body.

For example heroin, codeine, and Darvon will affect the user for 4 to 6 hours. A heroin user might shoot up 4 times a day. Fentanyl, on the other hand, will barely last an hour.

"Codeine just stops the pain and stops your nose from running. It just gets you able to function enough in order to go get you some heroin." Heroin user

Pleasure

The other major effect of opiates and opioids has to do with pleasure. Just as pain is a warning signal to keep us from damaging ourselves, so pleasure is a signal to

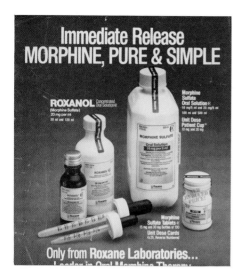

Immediate Release
MORPHINE, PURE & SIMPLE

ROXANOL Concentrated Oral Solution

Morphine Sulfate Oral Solution
Unit Dose Patient Cup

MORPHINE SULFATE Oral Solution

Morphine Sulfate Tablets
Unit Dose Cards

Only from Roxane Laboratories...

Prescription morphine is still the most effective treatment for acute and severe pain.

activate this reward center directly by slotting into the receptor sites on the receiving neurons meant for the endorphins, artificially triggering signals of pleasure.

Other Physical and Mental Effects

Opiates and opioids affect the heart, breathing, reproductive system, digestion, excretion, thinking, cough and nausea centers, eyes, voice box, muscles, immune system, in fact, every part of the body.

Some of the effects of opiates and opioids are mild but quite identifiable in the heavier user, particularly if the drug is heroin. The drug's ability to relax muscles causes eyelids to droop, the head to nod, and speech to become slurred and slowed. The walking gait is also slowed. The pupils become pinpoint and do not react to light, the skin dries out, and itching increases.

Other effects are less obvious. The cough center in the brain is suppressed, making codeine-based cough medicine the most widely used prescription drug. Opiates and opioids also affect the nausea center.

encourage us to do something that is good for the body and mind. And, just as endorphins are released naturally to block pain in the corpus striatum (a part of the brain), so they are released to activate dopamine which in turn triggers the reward/pleasure center in the limbic system, the emotional center of the brain, to tell us we're doing okay.

For example, if we succeed at a task, we feel an extra surge of pleasure because our reward center is triggered. It encourages us to keep on doing well. It is activated by the release of endorphins. If the reward/pleasure center is not being activated or if there are not enough endorphins in the system to do the job, a person will not feel good, will not feel rewarded, and will not feel pleasure. Instead, there will be a feeling of emptiness and depression.

So, some people searching for relief or a high try opiates or opioids because these drugs, particularly the stronger ones, artificially

"It hit from the feet going up to the head. I was yelling at him to take the needle out and I was on the toilet seat. I mean, I hugged that toilet bowl for hours, vomiting."
21-year-old heroin user

Other effects of opiates and opioids are even more severe. They stop diarrhea but cause chronic constipation by numbing the intestinal muscles. They also affect the hormonal system; a women's period is delayed and a man produces less testosterone; sexual desire is dulled, often to the point of indifference.

"Lots of times I don't want to be bothered by anybody, or anyone touching me, like my girlfriend. Like if she wants to hug me, kiss me, I just say, 'Don't touch me.'"
28-year-old heroin user

Neonatal effects

Because opiates and opioids cross the placental barrier between the fetus and the mother thereby sending large doses of the drug to the developing infant, pregnant users have a greater risk of miscarriage, placental separations, premature labor, breech births, stillbirths, and seizures. When a baby is born to an addicted mother, the child is also addicted, and since babies are much smaller than adults, the addiction is more severe. These symptoms can last 5 to 8 weeks, and unlike adults, babies in withdrawal can die.

Overdose

Other effects of opiates in older users can also be life threatening. Overdose occurs when so much of the drug enters the brain that the nervous system shuts down. The blood pressure drops and the heart beats too weakly to circulate blood. The lungs labor and fill with fluid. The person passes out and, unless quickly revived, will slip into a coma and die.

PROBLEMS WITH OPIATE USE

Dilution & Adulteration

One of the reasons an overdose occurs is that street drugs can vary radically in strength. Street heroin varies from zero to 99% pure. So if a user is expecting 3% heroin and gets 30%, the results could be fatal. Dilution of an expensive item like heroin with a cheap substitute like powered milk, sugar, baby laxative, aspirin, Ajax, quinine, or talcum powder is the rule and not the exception.

"The first China White I got came from Vietnam and it looked like a 20 hitter. I know that if I was shooting up then I probably would have OD'd. A 20 hitter means that you could take one gram and throw 19 grams of cut on it, and it'd still be good, it'd still get you off. With the tar that's going around now, the most you're going to get is basically a 6 hitter." Vietnam veteran

Dirty and Shared Needles

The most dangerous problem with opiates, and the one that causes the most illness and death, is dirty or shared needles. Needles are used because they put a large amount of the drug in the blood stream at one time. Needles can also inject powdered milk, procaine, Ajax, or dangerous bacteria and viruses, including the HIV virus that causes AIDS. It is estimated that 50% to 80% of all needle-using heroin addicts in the New York area test positive for the HIV virus.

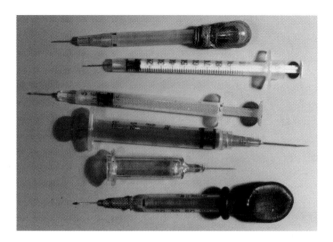

Addicts will use diabetics' syringes, eyedroppers, veterinary needles, almost anything to inject their drug.

Cost

Contrary to popular belief promoted by television and movies which show heroin addicts as derelicts, criminals, and mental cases, a majority of heroin users are gainfully employed, but, unfortunately, some still have to turn to illegal methods to pay for their habit.

"I had two other friends and one was blackmailing a pharmacist. We'd get outdated drugs they were supposed to throw away. We'd pick them up in the alley, and we'd get gallons and gallons of cough syrup and any other narcotic pills." Ex-heroin user

"Since I worked in the medical field, writing my own prescriptions was no problem except that I committed a felony every time I did it which was once a week. I never got caught, but I always lived in morbid fear that they would get me." Recovering Darvon user

Crime

The overwhelming need to support the habit financially and the antisocial behaviors such as robbery, prostitution, and dealing drugs that use of the drug engenders make involvement with the legal system inevitable.

"As I used drugs more and started putting needles in my arms and smoking heroin instead of sniffing heroin, the clientele went down, the friends I associated with became more criminal-like, and they became people who went to jail more often, and I went to jail more often." Recovering heroin user

Polydrug Use

Another danger that comes with opiate or opioid use is combining these drugs with other drugs. For example, if another depressant such as alcohol or a barbiturate is used at the same time as a shot of heroin or a tablet of codeine is taken, the effects are much greater than one would expect.

"I'd be waiting and waiting, and during the time that I was waiting, I'd be getting drunk. By the time I got around to doing my shot, I was already drunk. I'd hit up and boom, I'd be on the floor." Heroin user

Drug users also combine drugs to enhance the effect of the opiate/opioid.

"I was using a lot of heroin and the heroin wasn't working. I wasn't staying loaded long enough, so I'd make doctors for barbiturates in order to enhance the heroin."
Recovering heroin user

Finally, people use another drug to counter the effects of the opiate or opioid.

"As one person said, 'I like going up on speed; and I like taking heroin to come down; and I take cocaine to mellow out.'" Young heroin user

THE ADDICTIVE NATURE OF OPIATES & OPIOIDS

Tolerance, tissue dependence, and withdrawal, as well as pain relief and euphoria, are the main reasons for the addictive nature of opiates and opioids.

Tissue Dependence and Tolerance

Tissue dependence and tolerance occur when the body tries to neutralize the opiate by first, speeding up the metabolism, second, desensitizing the nerve cells to the drug's effects, and finally by altering the brain chemistry so it can compensate for the effects of the drug. Since tolerance occurs so rapidly with opiates and opioids, users might need 10 times their initial dose within a month of beginning use.

"I used drugs for so long, to cover all the feelings, the hurt and such, that one day, they didn't work." Young mother and recovering heroin user

Tolerance extends to all opiates and opioids. That is, if users build a tolerance to heroin, they will also have a tolerance for morphine or codeine. This cross tolerance is the basis for methadone maintenance treatment.

Withdrawal

Withdrawal occurs after two to three weeks of continuous use when an abrupt cessation will cause symptoms.

"You get deep, deep muscle and bone pains. There's no way to get comfortable, and you fluctuate between being chilly and sweating a lot. You can either be constipated or have diarrhea. You're in total body agony that nothing relieves. It's real uncomfortable. I have actually, this is not a figure of speech, I have been going through withdrawal where I said I wish I was dead." 35-year-old recovering heroin user

In general, short-acting drugs like heroin, morphine, and Dilaudid result in more severe yet short-lived (5 to 7 day) major withdrawal symptoms. Long-acting opioids like Methadone will delay the symptoms from 24 to 72 hours, but once they occur, these symptoms can last for weeks and are milder than those seen with short-acting opiates or opioids. Other opiates and opioids such as codeine, Percodan, and Darvon have withdrawal phenomena somewhere in between those two extremes.

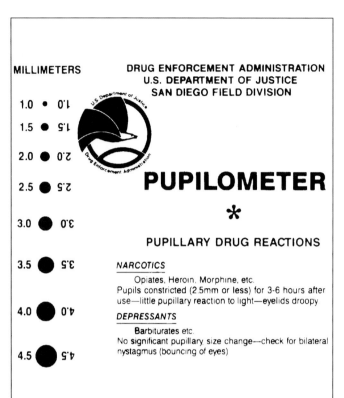

MILLIMETERS

DRUG ENFORCEMENT ADMINISTRATION
U.S. DEPARTMENT OF JUSTICE
SAN DIEGO FIELD DIVISION

PUPILOMETER

*

PUPILLARY DRUG REACTIONS

NARCOTICS

Opiates, Heroin, Morphine, etc.
Pupils constricted (2.5mm or less) for 3-6 hours after use—little pupillary reaction to light—eyelids droopy

DEPRESSANTS

Barbiturates etc.
No significant pupillary size change—check for bilateral nystagmus (bouncing of eyes)

A pupillometer is used to compare the size of pupils in a suspected drug user. Since opiates and opioids contract pupils, pupil size is a strong indicator of drug use.

It is important to remember that although opiate withdrawal feels like an incredibly bad case of the flu, it is almost never life threatening as is withdrawal from alcohol or sedative-hypnotics.

TREATMENT

Steps of Treatment

The steps of recovery, as with stimulants, are detoxification, initial abstinence, long-term abstinence, and recovery.

Detoxification

Users have to clean the drug out of their systems to give their body chemistry a chance to return to a semblance of normalcy and to give their judgment and reasoning centers a chance to clear up so they can engage in treatment. Since physical withdrawal from opiates is more severe than withdrawal from stimulants, most opiate abusers need to be involved in some kind of treatment program.

Most programs use medications, including mild opiates like Darvon, to detoxify and taper the habit. This allows addicts to have less fear of the pain of withdrawal and less pain during withdrawal. An alternative to this treatment is Clonidine. It quiets the part of the brain that gets hyperactive when one goes through withdrawal. It also suppresses withdrawal symptoms.

"The physical part of the detox is only a tiny portion. It's what happens after you get off, after you detox, that's important. Everyone around you is using, and in a lot of cases you may have financial problems. You may not even have a place to stay. There are other kinds of things that build up and cause you to want to use again." Drug counselor

Initial abstinence and long-term abstinence

After the withdrawal symptoms are controlled, the user needs help controlling the desire to use again. Environmental cues such as having cash, seeing former drug-using associates or even white powder can trigger the desire to use, even after detoxification. Long-lasting opiate antagonists, such as Naltrexone, which dull the stimulation of the reward/pleasure

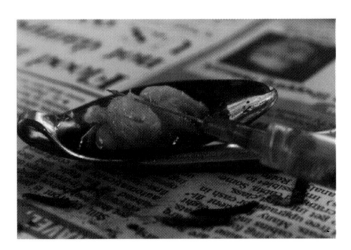

Environmental cues such as the sight of a needle and "cooking spoon," can trigger the desire to use.

center, can help the user stay clean and also seem to help decrease craving for the drug.

Initial abstinence is supported by participating in individual counseling sessions, group sessions, or self-help groups such as Narcotics Anonymous. Up to seven-day-a-week, regular attendance, at least during the first 4 to 8 weeks, is absolutely necessary to maintain initial abstinence when the craving is strongest. As successful treatment continues, fewer sessions are necessary.

Recovery

Drug counselor to a heroin addict in a counseling session:

Counselor "You can stay clean for a while. Is that what you want? You want to stay clean for a while or for the rest of your life?"

Addict: "I want to stay clean permanently."

Counselor: "Permanently drug free?

Addict: "But I can do it without attending those meetings."

Counselor: "All by yourself?"

Addict: "I mean with the medication that I take."

Counselor: "But the medications are only going to last you 21 days. They'll help you for a little while with the withdrawal of getting off heroin. But, what are you going to do when the urges come up?"

Addict: "I guess I'll deal with that when the time comes."

Counselor: "So you're just going to wait for it. You're going to wait for the urges to come on and start using then?"

Addict: "Nah, I can deal with it."

Counselor: "You're being highly uncooperative. As a matter of fact, we're going to stop the medications today because we know you're still using heroin, and we can't have you using on the program."

Addict: "I need those medications."

Counselor: "What for? It's just another drug. What you're doing is using it like another drug. I'd like for you to come back to get into that group meeting we have at 3 o'clock. Also, I want you to go to an NA (Narcotics Anonymous) meeting every day. I want you to go to these meetings and participate. Talk every opportunity you can. And also what I want you to do is bring back the signed participation card that you attended. I want you to do that. That's just part of the requirement of being in the program. See, I'm going to assume that you want to stop using drugs."

Addict: "Why can't I just get the detoxification drugs?"

Counselor: "Because we're not just a medication ⋅ program. This is a counseling and full recovery program too."

(Counselor Manuel Sanchez at the Haight-Ashbury Free Clinic confronting denial.)

Other Treatment Modalities

Methadone Maintenance

Much controversy has always swirled around the concept of opiate/opioid substitution ever since morphine addiction became a problem in the 19th century. Because of the large number of morphine addicts following the Civil War, opiate maintenance clinics multiplied. At this time, morphine was used in China to treat opium addiction.

In the early 1900's heroin was used to treat morphine addiction in Europe. This practice of using opiates to treat opiate addiction was ended in the United States (though continued in England and other countries) at the end of World War I and not revived until methadone maintenance was developed in the late 60's in New York City. This treatment modality eventually spread to hundreds of methadone maintenance clinics nation-wide in the 70's and 80's. Today, there are more than 100,000 recovering heroin addicts in methadone maintenance programs.

The theory is that methadone, a totally synthetic opioid, is not as intense as heroin, is longer lasting, and so, will keep the user from having heroin-like withdrawal symptoms for 36 to 48 hours. Heroin, on the other hand, causes withdrawal symptoms in a few hours, so the user goes through the roller coaster of highs and lows and the pain of withdrawal on a daily basis.

With methadone maintenance, the highs and lows that promote addiction are avoided. The user doesn't have to hustle for money to pay for a habit, get drugs and needles on the street, or be exposed to a high risk lifestyle. With HIV infection rates in intravenous heroin users as high as 80%, this method of harm reduction has certain benefits including forcing the addict to come to a certain location every day where counseling, medical care, and other services are available which might reduce the harm addicts do to themselves and others. Methadone also reduces an addict's craving for heroin.

The controversy arises because many chemical dependency treatment personnel don't believe drug abuse should be treated with another addicting drug on a long-term basis. Since many users seek treatment after only a short period of addiction, while their dose is still relatively low, the immediate use of methadone will further ingrain their opiate addiction. The pro-methadone advocates believe that keeping addicts from the harmful lifestyle associated with heroin addiction is more important than focusing on total recovery from opiate addiction which, in any case, is extremely difficult. Methadone maintenance has often been referred to as a political solution for a medical problem.

With either approach (methadone or immediate abstinence), retention in therapy to encourage eventual complete abstinence, helping recovering addicts find employment, assisting them to deal with their emotional and social problems, eliminating criminal behavior, and instilling in them the hope of recovery are all essential.

LAAM

Recently, the use of LAAM (levo alpha acetyl methadol) a long-acting methadone-like drug, has been used in much the same manner. LAAM will stay in the body for up to 3 days, so users further avoid withdrawal and the ups and downs of opiate addiction. Further, they do not have to go to a clinic every day. The negative side of LAAM is that it is still an addictive drug, and though fewer clinic visits mean lower treatment costs, 4 fewer visits a week to a center mean fewer opportunities to encourage recovery on a daily basis.

Buprenorphine

Another drug that is being tried for treating opiate addiction is Buprenorphine. It is an opiate agonist-antagonist. What this means is that at low doses, it is a powerful opiate, almost 50 times as powerful as heroin, but strangely enough, at high doses it blocks the opiate receptors. It enables an addict to be started on methadone, then switched to buprenorphine as a transition to a true antagonist like naltrexone. Though still undergoing clinical trials, buprenorphine should be available in the near future.

DOWNERS
SEDATIVE-HYPNOTICS

A GENERAL CLASSIFICATION

More than 150 million prescriptions are written for sedative-hypnotics each year in the U. S. These drugs are usually prescribed to diminish the possibility of neurotic reactions in unstable patients, to control anxiety, to induce sleep in chronic insomniacs, and to control hypertension and epilepsy. They are also used as mild tran-

Fig. 4-4

Name	Trade Name	Street Name
BARBITURATES		
Secobarbital	Seconal	Reds, red devils, F-40's, seccies, Mexican Reds
Pentobarbital	Nembutal	Yellows, yellow jackets, yellow bullets, nebbies
Equal parts secobarbitol & amylbarbital	Tuinal	Rainbows, tuies, double trouble
Phenobarbital	(Generic)	Phenos
Amobarbital	Amytal	Blue heavens, blue dolls, blues
Hexobarbital	Sombulex	
Thiopental	Pentothal	
BENZODIAZEPINES		
Diazepam	Valium	Vals
Chlordiazepoxide	Librium, Libritabs	Libs
Flurazepam	Dalmane	
Chlorazepate	Tranxene	
Oxazepam	Serax	
Triazolam	Halcion	
Alprazolam	Xanax	
Lorazepam	Ativan	
Clonazepam	Clonopin	
Temazepam	Restoril	
Halazepam	Paxipam	
Prazepam	Centrax	
NON-BARBITURATE SEDATIVE-HYPNOTICS		
Glutethimide	Doriden	Goofballs, goofers
Gluthemide & codeine	Doriden & codeine	Loads, sets, setups
Methaqualone	Quaalude, Sope, Parest, Optimil Somnafac	Ludes, sopes, soapers, Q
Ethchlovynol	Placidyl	Green weenies
Chloral hydrate	Noctec, Somnos	Jelly beans, Miki's, knockout drops
Methaprylon	Noludar	Noodlelars
Meprobamate	Equinil, Miltown, Meprotabs	Mother's little helper

quilizers and muscle relaxants. The effects of sedative-hypnotics are generally similar to the effects of alcohol. The basic difference between the two depressants is the concentration of the drug involved: sedative-hypnotics come in a more concentrated form than alcohol. Sedative-hypnotic withdrawal symptoms can also be more life-threatening than opiate/opioid withdrawal symptoms.

Almost all sedative-hypnotics are available as pills, capsules, or tablets though some, such as Valium, Ativan, and Pentothal are used intravenously for instant relief. The two main groups are benzodiazepines and barbiturates.

GENERAL EFFECTS & METABOLISM

Sedative-hypnotics are quite specific to those sections of the central nervous system they affect. Hypnotics such as barbiturates work on the brain stem, inducing sleep along with depression of most body functions such as breathing and muscular coordination. Sedatives such as Doriden, Quaalude, Miltown, and Valium are calming drugs. They work on a number of sites in the brain and are used as either sleeping aids or as anti-anxiety agents. Benzodiazepines, for example, act on the neurotransmitter GABA to help control anxiety and restlessness. Sedatives are capable of producing relaxation, lowered inhibitions, reduced intensity of physical sensations, body heat loss, and reduced muscular coordination in speech, movement,

and manual dexterity. Some sedatives are used as hypnotics and some hypnotics are used as sedatives, so it can be hard to separate the two functions.

Tolerance

Tolerance develops rapidly with sedative-hypnotics. However, tolerance to the mental and physical effects develops at a different rate. This means that when users increase daily intake to recapture a mental high, they might not be aware that tolerance to the physical effects, such as respiratory depression, develops at a slower rate. Thus, the daily dose taken for the mental effects comes close to the lethal dose for some sedative-hypnotics particularly the barbiturates, and any accidental overdose can cause respiratory or cardiovascular collapse and kill the user. (This is called selective tolerance and is discussed in Chapter 2.) The intake of sedative-hypnotics might reach 10 to 20 times the original dose.

Withdrawal

Withdrawal from sedative-hypnotics after tolerance has developed can be extremely dangerous. Within 6 to 8 hours after using short-acting drugs like most barbiturates, users will begin to experience withdrawal symptoms such as anxiety, agitation, loss of appetite, nausea, vomiting, increased heart rate, excessive sweating, abdominal cramps, and tremulousness. The symptoms will peak on the second or third day. With long-acting barbiturates and tranquilizers such as Valium or Librium, the peak may not be reached until the second or third week, and the onset of symptoms can be delayed for several days. Severe withdrawal symptoms include seizures, delirium, uncontrolled heart beat, and death.

Overdosing

Overdosing with sedative-hypnotics, particularly barbiturates, might include cold, clammy skin, a weak and rapid pulse, and slow to rapid, but shallow, breathing. Death will follow if the low blood pressure and slowed respiration are not treated. It is particularly dangerous to combine alcohol and any sedative-hypnotic because these combinations can cause an exaggerated depression of the respiratory center in the brain and therefore, a greater risk of death.

BARBITURATES

Though barbituric acid was first synthesized in 1868, it remained a medical curiosity for 40 years until it was chemically modified to enter the central nervous system, thus becoming psychoactive. Since then, more than 2,500 different barbiturate compounds have been created.

Effects

The slow-acting barbiturates such as phenobarbital, last 12 to 24 hours and are used mostly as daytime sedatives or to control epileptic seizures.

The shorter-acting compounds such as Seconal (reds), and Nembutal (yellows), last 4 to 6 hours and are used to induce sleep.

They can induce pleasant feelings along with the sedation (at least initially), so they are more likely to be abused.

The very short-acting barbiturates such as pentothal, used mostly for anesthesia, can cause immediate unconsciousness. The extremely high potency of these barbiturates makes them extremely dangerous if abused.

Temporary stimulation and eventual sedating effects are very similar to those of alcohol. And as with alcohol, excessive or long-term use can lead to changes in personality and emotion (mood swings, depression, irritability, and obnoxious or manipulative behavior).

Tolerance to barbiturates develops in a variety of ways. The most dramatic tolerance, drug dispositional tolerance, results from the physiologic conversion of liver cells to more efficient cells which metabolize or destroy barbiturates more quickly. This results in the need to take more barbiturates to reach or maintain the same psychoactive effects originally obtained at lower doses.

Tissue dependence to barbiturates occurs when 8 to 10 times the normal dose is taken daily for 30 days or more. Withdrawal symptoms resulting from this dependence are very dangerous and can result in convulsions within 12 hours to one week from the last dose.

BENZODIAZEPINES (XANAX, VALIUM, HALCION, ETC.)

Benzodiazepines are the most widely used sedative-hypnotic in the United States. This class of drugs was developed in the late 40's and 50's as an alternative to barbiturates. Starting with Librium, then Valium, benzodiazepines came into wide clinical use in the 60's and by the 70's accounted for more than half of all prescriptions written for sedative-hypnotics. The drugs were an innovation in the treatment of anxiety disorders, replacing barbiturates, bromides, opiates and opioids, and even alcohol which were too toxic and had too many side effects.

Effects

Several benzodiazepines are used to treat other problems in addition to their antianxiety use. Some examples: alprazolam (Xanax) is used to treat patients subject to panic attacks; triazolam (Halcion) is used to treat insom-nia; diazepam (Valium) is used to control seizures such as those that occur during severe alcohol or barbiturate withdrawal. Intravenous Valium is used as a sedative during some surgeries.

The benzodiazepines have been shown to exert their sedative effects by interacting with or acting like a naturally occurring neurotransmitter in the brain called gama amino butyric acid, or GABA for short. GABA is recognized as the most important inhibitory neurotransmitter. Drugs, like Valium, greatly increase the actions of GABA and also influence other sedating neurotransmitters such as serotonin and dopamine. By increasing the activity of GABA, benzodiazepines increase the inhibition of anxiety producing thoughts and neural messages.

Problems with Benzodiazepines

Benzodiazepines have a fairly safe therapeutic index, meaning that the amount of chemical needed to induce sedation is much lower than the amount that would cause an overdose. The problem was that while many health care professionals were hailing the supposedly "safe" new drugs and raving about patient acceptance, they overlooked its peculiarities: the length of time it lasts in the body, its ability to induce addiction at low levels of use, and the severity of withdrawal from the drug.

Benzodiazepines alone can be abused, but they are most often abused in conjunction with other

Fig. 4-5 Valium is unusual in that the liver metabolizes the drug into five other psychoactive drugs, some stronger than the original drug. These drugs can persist in the body for days or weeks.

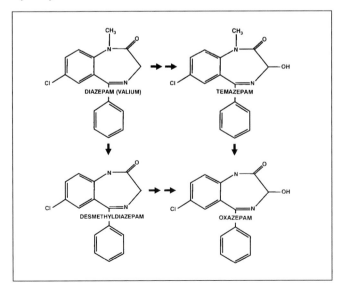

drugs. Speed and cocaine users will use a benzo to come down from excess stimulation. Heroin addicts will use a benzodiazepine when they can't get their drug of choice. An alcoholic will use them to prevent life-threatening withdrawal symptoms such as convulsions.

Tolerance

As the liver becomes more efficient in processing the drug, tolerance develops since more benzodiazepine is needed to achieve the same effects. However, age-dependent tolerance also occurs with these drugs, meaning that a younger person can tolerate much more of these drugs than someone older. The effect of a dose on a 50-year-old first-time user can be five or ten times stronger than the same dose on a 16-year-old.

Addiction

Physical addiction to the benzodiazepine can develop if the patient takes 10 to 20 times the normal dose daily, for several months or longer, or takes a normal dose for a year or more. Since many benzodiazepines are slowly deactivated by the body over a period of several days, even low-dose use can lead to addiction when these drugs are taken daily for a number of years. In addition, the pleasant mental effects and "hypnotizing" aspects of the drugs (reinforcement) can result in a mental or psychological dependence.

Withdrawal

After high-dose, continuous use for about two months, or lower-dose use for a year or more, withdrawal can be extremely severe. In fact, more people have died from Valium withdrawal than from Valium overdose. The drug is long lasting, so the symptoms will be delayed 24 to 72 hours. First, there will be a craving for the drug, then more anxiety, sleep disturbances, pacing the floor, tremulous movements, and even hallucinations. Some people even allege a temporary loss of vision, hearing, or smell while in withdrawal. The symptoms continue and peak in the first to third weeks. These can include multiple seizures and convulsions. The severe symptoms will occur in 80-90% of the users who stop taking the drug after physical addiction has occurred.

....

Valium used to be the most popular benzodiazepine. Now Xanax, used to treat panic attacks and anxiety, is the most widely used benzodiazepine.

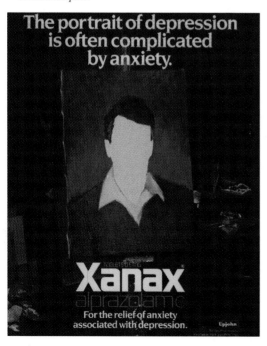

The portrait of depression is often complicated by anxiety.

Xanax
alprazolam

For the relief of anxiety associated with depression.   Upjohn

Fig 4-6 PLASMA HALF-LIFE OF BENZODIAZEPINES

Trade Name	Chemical Name	Half Life
Very long acting		
Dalmane	Flurazepam	90-200 hours
Paxipam	Halazepam	30-200 hours
Verstran, Centrax	Prazepam	30-200 hours
Intermediate acting		
Librium	Chlordiazepoxide	7-46 hours
Valium	Diazepam	14-90 hours
Clonopin	Clonazepam	18-50 hours
Short acting		
Restoril	Temazepam	5-20 hours
Xanax	Alprazolam	6-20 hours
Serax	Oxazepam	6-24 hours
Ativan	Lorazepam	9-22 hours
Very short acting		
Halcion	Triazolam	2-6 hours

Overdose

Symptoms of overdose include drowsiness, loss of consciousness, depressed breathing, coma, and death if left untreated, but it might take 50 or 100 pills to cause a serious overdose. Unfortunately, street versions of the drug, misrepresented and sold as Quaaludes, were so strong that only five or ten pills could cause really severe reactions. The relative safety of benzodiazepines does not extend to mixing them with alcohol or other depressants. People do die from just a few pills and a modest amount of alcohol.

The persistence of these drugs in the body from low or regular doses taken over a long period of time results not only in prolonged withdrawal symptoms but in symptoms that erratically come and go in cycles separated by 2 to 10 days. These previously described symptoms are sometimes bizarre, sometimes life-threatening, and all complicated by the cyclical nature of the severity. Short-acting barbiturates, on the other hand, follow a fairly predictable course where the symptoms come, and then go, and don't return. Called the "protracted withdrawal syndrome," the symptoms of benzodiazepine withdrawal may persist for several months after the drug has been terminated.

Prescribing Practices

Because of the addictive potential of benzodiazepines, regulations regarding prescribing practice have proliferated to the point that a triplicate prescription, identical to those used for opiates and opioids to control use, is now required in many states. Many physicians and psychiatrists see this as an intrusion in their practice of medicine while others in the chemical dependency treatment community see benzodiazepines as a drug with huge addiction potential or one which can cause relapse in a recovering addict.

OTHER SEDATIVE-HYPNOTICS

Quaaludes

Although widely used at one time as a sleep aid, the heavy abuse of Quaaludes led to the withdrawal of this product from the legitimate market. This led to a tremendous increase in the illicit production of Quaalude, known as bootleg "ludes," which look identical to the original prescription drug. The active ingredient in Quaaludes, methaqualone, is being manufactured by street chemists or smuggled in from Europe or Columbia. However, there is no guarantee that the street version contains actual methaqualone, and even when it does, the dosage may vary dra-

matically, making an overdose more likely. The street samples analyzed have contained everything from PCP to Benadryl (an antihistamine), to Valium. Many of the substitute drugs are more harmful than the Quaalude itself. The original prescription Quaaludes contained 300 milligrams of the active drug while street "ludes," have contained methaqualone in doses of anywhere from zero to five hundred milligrams.

The reasons for the popularity of methaqualone are its overall sedative effect and the prolonged period of mild euphoria caused by suppression of inhibitions. This disinhibitory effect is similar to that caused by alcohol.

Doriden

Doriden (glutethimide), a short-acting, non-barbiturate hypnotic, is used to treat insomnia. Though widely available and somewhat abused in the 50's, it wasn't until the 70's and 80's that Doriden became popular on the street in a polydrug combination (Doriden

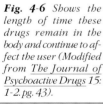

Fig. 4-6 Shows the length of time these drugs remain in the body and continue to affect the user (Modified from The Journal of Psychoactive Drugs 15: 1-2. pg. 43).

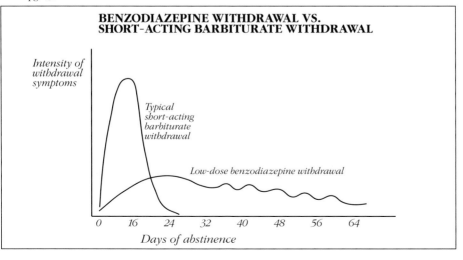

and codeine), variously known as "loads," "sets," "setups," "four by fours," "fours and doors," etc. The effect of this combination is prolonged drowsiness, relaxation, and euphoria over a period of 6 to 8 hours. The combination has led to double addiction to a sedative-hypnotic and an opiate. An additional danger with Doriden is that the drug is pulled out of the blood by the liver, concentrated in the gall bladder, released back into the intestine, and then back into the blood, causing extended, reoccurring, toxic effects which result in a greater chance of harm.

Placidyl

Called "green weenies," Placidyl is one of the older sedative hypnotics. It is still a prescription drug and is subject to limited abuse. It is about the equivalent of Doriden in potency, with similar toxic and addictive effects but is shorter acting.

Miltown

Miltown (meprobamate), first popularized in the 1950's, led to the first modern recognition of prescription abuse whereby a drug, used legally by prescription, can lead to addiction. The drug was prescribed excessively and misused in larger than prescribed amounts. It was also the forerunner of a downer cycle dominated by sedative-hypnotics. Miltown was called "mother's little helper" by street users.

DRUG INTERACTIONS

DRUG SYNERGISM

If more than one depressant drug is used, the combination can cause a much greater reaction than simply the sum of the effects. One of the reasons for this synergistic effect lies in the chemistry of the liver.

For example, if alcohol and Valium are taken together, the liver becomes so busy metabolizing the alcohol that the sedative-hypnotic passes through the body at full strength. Alcohol also dissolves the Valium more readily than stomach fluids allowing more Valium to be absorbed rapidly into the body. Valium exerts its depressant effects on different parts of the brain than alcohol. Thus, when combined, they cause more problems than if they were taken at different times.

The exaggerated respiratory depression is the biggest danger with the use of alcohol and another depressant. That combination also causes more blackouts (a period of amnesia or loss of memory while intoxicated.)

"I took my little medication with me one night, drinking in the bar. I played some pool, And that's all I remember. This was on a Sunday. When I woke up, it was Wednesday."
Recovering alcoholic

The synergistic effect causes 4,000 deaths a year. In addition, almost 50,000 people are treated in emergency rooms because of adverse reactions to multiple drug use.

CROSS TOLERANCE, CROSS DEPENDENCE

Depressant drugs also exhibit cross tolerance and cross dependence between different as well as similar chemical drug classes. Further, some depressants exhibit these characteristics with stimulant, psychedelic, and even with non-psychoactive drugs.

Cross Tolerance

Cross tolerance is the development of tolerance to other drugs by the continued exposure to a particular drug. For example, a barbiturate addict who develops a tolerance to a high-dose of Seconal is also tolerant to and can withstand high doses of Nembutal, Phenobarbital, anesthetics, opiates, alcohol, Valium, and even blood thinner medication. One explanation of cross tolerance lies in the fact that many drugs are metabolized or broken down by the same body enzymes. As one continues to take barbiturates, the liver creates more enzymes to rid the body of these toxins. The unusually high levels of these enzymes result in tolerance to all barbiturates as well as other drugs also metabolized by those same enzymes.

Cross Dependence

Cross dependence occurs as an individual becomes addicted or tissue dependent on one drug resulting in biochemical and cellular changes that support an addiction to other drugs. A heroin addict, for example, has altered body chemistry such that he or she is also likely to be addicted to an opioid (Dilaudid, Demerol, morphine, codeine, methadone or Darvon). As with this example, cross dependence most often occurs with different drugs in the same chemical family. A Valium addict is also tissue dependent on Librium, Dalmane, and Ativan. A heavy Seconal user is also tissue dependent on Nembutal, Tuinal, and phenobarbital. Cross dependence has also been documented to some extent with opiates/opioids and alcohol; cocaine and alcohol; and Valium and alcohol.

REVIEW

DOWNERS

1. Downers are central nervous system depressants.

2. The three main groups of downers are opiates/opioids, sedative-hypnotics and alcohol.

3. Other downers are skeletal muscle relaxants, antihistamines, lookalike sedatives, and over-the-counter sedatives.

4. Opiates (from the opium poppy) and opioids (synthetic versions of opiates) were developed for the treatment of acute pain.

5. Opiates include opium, heroin, codeine, morphine, Dilaudid and Percodan. Opioids include methadone, Darvon, Demerol, Talwin, and fentanyl.

6. Opiates and opioids work by mimicking the body's own natural painkillers, endorphins and enkephalins. They block the transmission of pain messages to the brain.

7. Opiates and opioids can also cause euphoria, increase nausea, depress respiration and heart rate, depress muscular coordination, and suppress the cough mechanism.

8. A physical tolerance to opiates and opioids develops rapidly, increasing the speed with which the body becomes dependent on the drug.

9. Withdrawal from opiates is like an extreme case of the flu.

People do not usually die from opiate withdrawal. They can die from an overdose. However, newborn addicted babies can die in opiate withdrawal.

10. Heroin can be injected, smoked or snorted. The concentration of street heroin is generally 3% to 4% pure, although much higher percentages have been seen recently.

11. Codeine is the most abused opiate prescription.

12. Recently, synthetic heroin (fentanyl and Demerol derivatives) have appeared on the street. The danger is that one by-product of street Demerol, MPTP, can cause Parkinson's disease, an irreversible nervous system disorder. Fentanyl derivatives are so potent that overdose occurs more frequently.

13. Sedative-hypnotics are usually prescribed to control anxiety, induce sleep, relax muscles, and act as mild tranquilizers.

14. The three main types of sedative-hypnotics are barbiturates, non-barbiturates, and benzodiazepines.

15. Barbiturates include Seconal ("reds"), Nembutal ("yellows"), Tuinal ("rainbows"), Amytal ("blue heavens"), and phenobarbital.

16. Non-barbiturate sedative-hypnotics include Doriden, Quaaludes, Miltown, Placidyl, and dozens more.

17. Benzodiazepines include Valium, Librium, Dalmane, Xanax, Halcion and a dozen more.

18. Sedative-hypnotics work on specific sections of the brain, i.e., the brainstem and midbrain, to induce sleep.

19. Tolerance to sedative-hypnotics develops rather quickly.

20. Withdrawal from a sedative-hypnotic dependence can be extremely dangerous and life threatening: convulsions, nausea, hallucinations, and major health problems are common.

21. Valium, the most widely prescribed tranquilizer, stays in the body for days, even weeks. Withdrawal from prolonged benzodiazepine use can be life threatening.

22. Quaaludes are only available from illicit sources. The drug causes an overall sedation, mild euphoria, and suppression of inhibitions.

23. Alcohol and sedative-hypnotics used together can be especially life threatening. They cause a synergistic (exaggerated) effect which can suppress respiration and heart functions to dangerous levels.

QUESTIONS

1. What are the three major categories of downers?

2. Name the four minor categories of downers.

3. What are the overall effects of downers?

4. What is the difference between opiates and opioids?

5. Name three opiates and three opioids.

6. What is the body's own, natural painkiller called?

7. What are the most common effects of opiates and opioids?

8. Name three ways heroin can be put into the body.

9. Which is more dangerous, opiate/opioid withdrawal or overdose?

10. What is China White and why is it dangerous?

11. What are the three categories of sedative-hypnotics?

12. What are reds and yellows?

13. Name three reasons why sedative-hypnotics are prescribed by physicians.

14. What are the most widely prescribed sedative-hypnotics?

15. Why is withdrawal from prolonged use of sedative-hypnotics dangerous?

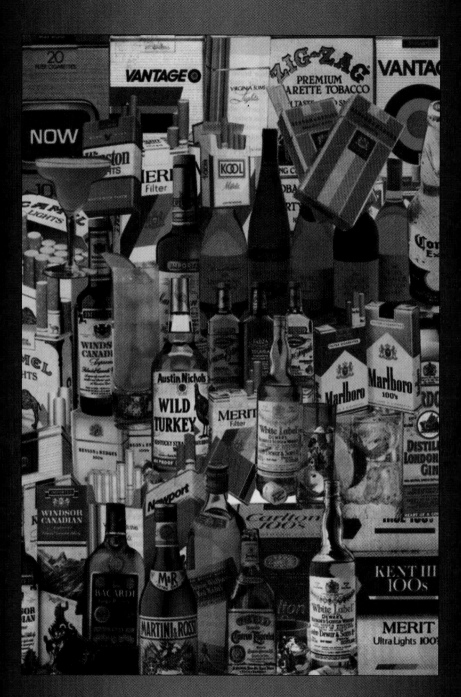

CHAPTER 5

DOWNERS

ALCOHOL

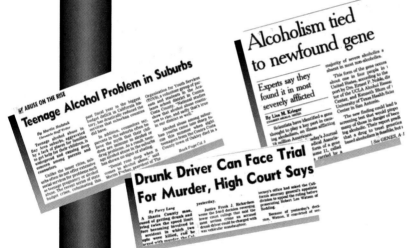

INTRODUCTION

O f all the psychoactive drugs, the most widespread abuse involves the depressant alcohol. Alcohol is legal, sold in every state in the union, and used for dozens of different occasions. It is used for social, medicinal, euphoric, disinhibitory, and tranquilizing reasons. It is used at weddings, wakes, parties, and in church. It is a major economic force in many states, and whole TV series and shows take place in a bar or have segments about drinking. For these reasons, most people place alcohol in a different category than other psychoactive drugs.

*"I don't take drugs. I have
an aspirin once a month. I
don't do drugs, and I really
don't like to be around
anyone who does. To me,
drugs are bad. I only drink."*
50-year-old "social" drinker

The contradictions about alcohol's place in society are not lost on the younger generation.

*"Alcohol is heavily social so
one of the problems that I
have with prohibition
attitudes is that society drinks
as much as we do. And
because it is legal, I feel I am
still part of society even when
loaded, whereas with illicit
drugs like marijuana, I feel I
am stepping outside of what is
acceptable."* 19-year-old
college freshman

EPIDEMIOLOGY

The statistics about the use of alcohol are startling.

Last month

• About 98 million Americans, or about 40% of the population of 250 million, had a can of beer, a glass of wine, or a cocktail;

• About 2/3 of the 5 million college students also had a drink as did half of the 2.5 million high school seniors.

Last week

• About 1.5 million college students had 5 or more drinks at one sitting.

Yesterday

• About 10 million Americans of all ages had more than 5 drinks;

• About 200 million dollars were spent at bars, restaurants, and liquor stores for those drinks;

• A champagne toast was made to 7,000 brides and grooms.

Also yesterday, unfortunately,

• About 3 million adolescents had a continuing problem with alcohol;

• From 25% to 30% of all hospital admissions were there because of direct or indirect medical complications from alcohol;

• Almost 400 million dollars was lost because of alcohol-related problems such as lost productivity and illness;

• Over 350 heavy drinkers died from medical complications of their drinking (130,000 a year);

• About 1,250 people were maimed or injured by drunk drivers;

• Around 50 drunk drivers or their passengers died;

• At least 30 people committed suicide while under the influence of alcohol;

• About half the people who were murdered were drinking as were half the murderers;

• More than half of the 300 rapes that occurred involved alcohol;

• And 20,000 of the crimes that occurred involved alcohol or other drugs.

On a more limited scale, over 35% of college students drove drunk at least once in the past year, and 6% did it 10 or more times; 35% got into a fight or severe argument at least once; and over 30% vomited more than twice.

Cultural Differences

One of the determinants of how a person drinks is the culture. For example in France and Italy, children are served watered down wine at the dinner table. Chinese families generally don't drink at home because the Asiatic biochemistry doesn't process alcohol very well. In Russia vodka is traditionally drunk between meals in large quantities. In England a trip to the pub for warm beer and darts is a tradition. Germans have Oktoberfest and celebrate the bringing in of the hops. In fact, all the major breweries in America were established by German brewers. In America, drinking is often done away from the lunch and dinner table.

Fig. 5-1 *Adult Patterns of Alcohol Use in the United States*

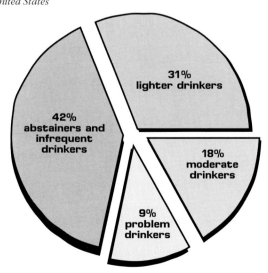

In 1992, whites continued to have the highest rate of alcohol use at 50%. Rates for Hispanics were 45% and for African Americans, 40%. Rates of heavy use showed no statistically significant differences (5.1% for whites, 5.6% for Hispanics, and 4.5% for African Americans).

Reasons for Drinking

In spite of the problems caused by alcohol and because it is legal in much of the world (except for most Moslem countries), it is readily available and used for almost every imaginable occasion or reason.

To lower inhibitions:

"I'm basically reserved, no, let's be honest and make that scared, when talking to girls, even after two-and-a-half years away from home, so I go to a mixer at the fraternity and have a couple, three, four drinks real quick, and then I'm not so afraid."
20-year-old college junior

As a medicine:

"At the rest home where my grandfather spent his last few years, they had this one closet where most of the patients had their own liquor bottle with their name on it. They were allowed 2 drinks per day for medicinal reasons. The physician on the staff figured it was cheaper than Valium."
Grandson

To facilitate business:

"The partners in the law firm where I worked had a nice bar in the office, and quite a bit of business was conducted over a drink in the conference room."
Paralegal law firm employee

As a sacrament:

"Drink all of you from this for this is my blood, the blood of the covenant which is to be shed for you for the forgiveness of sins." From the Gospel of St. Luke

As a stimulant:

"I used to work on the docks doing heavy work like lifting coffee sacks. I'd have a drink, and I'd be working faster, but then I'd look around and there still were 2 or 3 hundred sacks left. So I'd have another drink to build myself back up to get into the mood." 40-year-old longshoreman

For oblivion:

"I know people who, when they are on a heavy drinking kick, they brag, 'I can outdrink anyone and I'm proud of it. I like my booze and if it is on a weekend, why should I care. I don't care if I die at 35. I know that I am not going to live forever.' What could you possibly say to someone like that to get them to stop drinking?" 22-year-old drinker

As a sedative:

"I didn't want to confront those feelings so I'd put them aside. Next thing I know I'm feeling real hopeless, alone, and isolated, and a drink seems like a pretty good idea." 26-year-old woman

With so many uses of alcohol entwined within the fabric of society, it's no wonder that the problems associated with drinking are pervasive.

And even though it would seem that we could solve many of society's problems by outlawing alcohol or severely restricting its use, how realistic is that course? And what do you teach about alcohol in the schools or to the general public? Do you teach abstention or moderation? The question is particularly difficult in college and high school where students are not naive about drugs, are not responsive to scare tactics, and feel they are invulnerable?

"When I drink, I drink to get drunk. I drink a lot, otherwise I wouldn't drink at all because I don't like the taste of alcohol. There aren't that many casual college or high school drinkers." 18-year-old college freshman

"They have a drug and alcohol program at our school, and I guess their intentions are okay, but so much of it is clichés, and it's not too damn realistic. To ask me not to drink when I'm in college, away from home for the first time, where I'm in charge finally, where there's always a mixer or homecoming or

fooling around after class . . . it doesn't work, it just doesn't work, and it doesn't make sense, so it makes me leery of anything they say. I'm going to drink at least once, maybe several times a month. Just tell me the truth." 19-year-old college freshman

The purpose of this chapter is to present the facts about alcohol.

Fig. 5-2 Percentage of Alcohol in Certain Beverages

Wine

Red, white, rosé, champagne	12%
Sherry	20%
Vermouth	18%
Wine cooler	6%

Beer

Light lager or dark ale	6%
Malt or stout	8%
Light beer	6%

Liquors & Whiskeys

Bourbon, whiskey, scotch, vodka, gin, brandy, rum	43%
Tequila, cognac, Drambui	40%
Amaretto, Kahlua, etc.	28%
Everclear	95%

(Note: Double the alcohol content to get the proof; 40% alcohol = 80 proof.)

BIOLOGY AND PHARMACOLOGY

Alcohol is the most commonly used psychoactive drug in the world and the oldest known. It was probably discovered by accident when some fruit, perhaps a bunch of grapes or basket of plums, was left standing in a warm place allowing the fruit sugar to ferment into alcohol. Later it was found that the starch in potatoes, rice, corn, and grains could also be fermented, first to sugar, then to alcohol. The concentration of alcohol in each kind of beverage depends on the length of fermentation, the type of fruit, grain, or vegetable used, the percent of additives, and the amount of distillation.

If fruits are fermented, the product is wine. If grains are fermented, it is beer. Distilled spirits can be a distillation of fermented malt barley (whiskey), a distillation of wine (brandy), or any number of variations with an alcohol concentration 3 or 4 times that of wine, and 8 times that of beer. Local variations exist: pulque is made from the maguey cactus, and there is even a garlic wine.

METABOLISM

Alcohol is one of the few drugs that the body metabolizes at a defined, continuous rate, based upon a person's body weight, amount of alcohol drunk, the time that has passed since the last drink, and to a lesser extent the tolerance to alcohol that has come from years of drinking. Thus, we can usually

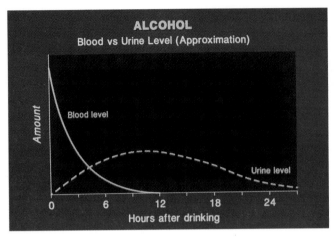

ALCOHOL
Blood vs Urine Level (Approximation)

Fig. 5-3 Graph of blood alcohol level and urine alcohol level plotted against time. In most states, .10 or .08 is the legal allowable blood alcohol limit. Some think it should be .05 for safety.

predict the amount of alcohol that will be circulating through the body and brain, and how long it will take to be metabolized by the liver and eliminated via urination, sweating, and breathing.

These are the amounts of alcohol needed to be drunk within one hour for a young, healthy, 175 lb. man to achieve legal intoxication of .10 (in many states).

Wine	Four 4-oz glasses
Beer	Five 12-oz cans
Distilled whiskey	Five 1-oz shots

However, age, medical condition, additional drugs, overall health, and a few other factors can greatly affect blood alcohol level such that even lower amounts can result in legal intoxication.

EFFECTS

"Just because I know what happens to my body when I drink doesn't mean that I don't want that to happen to my body. You also have to convince me I can feel good or have fun without drinking." College sophomore

The physical effects of alcohol as with many psychoactive drugs, are dependent on the amount and frequency of drinking, but the mental and emotional effects are more conditioned by the setting in which the drug is used and the mood of the user.

"Drinking is a way of life here. Somebody comes up and you offer them a drink; it's cordial. That's how you break the ice. I like to drink; it makes me happy." "Social" drinker

However, along with this apparent emotional stimulation comes a physical depression. The more alcohol that is drunk, the freer the user feels, but the blood pressure is lowered, motor reflexes are slowed, digestion becomes poor, body heat is lost, and sexual performance is diminished. In fact, every system in the body is affected. If truly large amounts are drunk, depression of the various systems can lead to coma or death.

PHYSICAL EFFECTS

Skeletal system: Skeletal muscular coordination decreases.

Muscular system: Normal muscular coordination is impaired.

Circulatory system: The pulse rate increases and blood vessels dilate causing increased heat loss from the body. The blood vessel dilation and lowering of blood pressure at low doses are reasons that alcohol lowers the risk of heart attacks. Notice the emphasis on low-dose. With large doses, dangerous levels of cardiac and vascular depression can occur.

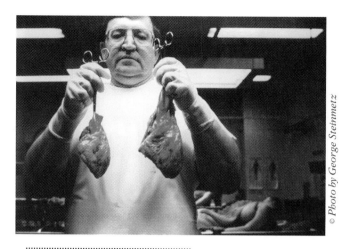

© *Photo by George Steinmetz*

The pathologist compares the heart of a light drinker with the enlarged heart of a heavy drinker. The protective effect of light drinking versus the damaging effect of heavier drinking varies with the physiology of the user.

Boris Ruebner, M.D.

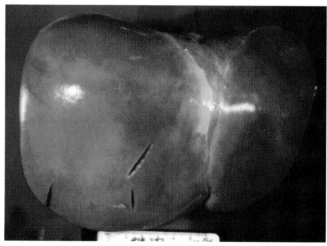

Fatty liver of a drinker. When drinking stops, the fat deposits usually disappear.

With prolonged use, high blood pressure and actual damage to heart and vascular tissues occur.

Respiratory system: Small doses initially stimulate the respiratory rate, but increased doses cause a dramatic decrease in the ability to breath normally.

Digestive system: There is an increase in digestive secretions causing irritation of the stomach. Excessive drinking can lead to ulcers. If the alcohol is drunk with a meal, particularly an oily meal, there is less irritation and less absorption of the alcohol. Excessive alcohol use also causes excess fat deposits in the liver. Chronic use can seriously aggravate hepatitis and cause hepatic cirrhosis (liver scarring).

Excretory system: Depression of small and large intestine functions can cause constipation or diarrhea. Urine production and urination increase.

Endocrine (hormone) system: Increased secretions of various hormones caused by alcohol also increase urination, raise, then lower blood sugar levels, dilate pupils, and raise blood pressure.

Reproductive system: Alcohol overuse during pregnancy increases the number of miscarriages and infant deaths. There are more problem pregnancies, and newborns are smaller and weaker. Specific toxic effects of alcohol on the developing fetus are known as the "Fetal Alcohol Syndrome," or FAS (see Chapter 8 - the section on Drugs and Pregnancy).

Boris Ruebner, M.D.

Cirrhosis of the liver takes 10 or more years of steady drinking. The toxic effects of alcohol cause scar tissue to replace healthy tissue. This condition remains permanent, even when drinking stops.

Nervous system: Alcohol is a protoplasmic poison. It can kill tissues such as liver and kidney cells on contact. In particular, it kills nerve cells. During binge drinking, 10 times as many nerve cells (100,000) die each day as die normally. This leads to many mental deficits in chronic users, anywhere from slightly reduced mental sharpness, to an inability to walk normally, a decline in intellect, and an impaired memory.

Recent studies have demonstrated a greater incidence of breast cancer in women who drink even moderate amounts of daily alcohol.

Tolerance

Dispositional tolerance and pharmacodynamic tolerance develop to try to restrict the physical and behavioral effects of alcohol. Dispositional tolerance means the body changes the way it metabolizes alcohol. Pharmacodynamic tolerance means the cells change to resist the effects of alcohol. Dispositional tolerance depends mostly on the liver. As we drink over a period of time, the liver adapts and changes. It creates more enzymes to process the protoplasmic poison, alcohol. Unfortunately, since liver cells are also being destroyed by drinking and by the natural aging process, the liver eventually becomes less able to handle the alcohol. A condition known as reverse tolerance occurs. So, a drinker who could handle two fifths of whiskey at the age of 30 will become totally incapacitated by half a pint of wine at the age of 50. Drinkers also learn how to "handle their liquor," by modifying their behavior or trying to act in such a way that they hope others won't notice they are inebriated. This is called behavioral tolerance.

Withdrawal

Mild withdrawal is often known as a hangover. It is caused by the alcohol and the additives (congeners) in the drink. Because of the additives, a beer hangover can feel worse than a vodka hangover even if the amount of actual alcohol drunk is the same. Hangover symptoms can range from a cottony mouth and a queasy stomach to headache, fatigue, upset stomach, mild physical and mental depression, lack of ability to concentrate, nausea, and a feeling that one would rather be dead. But with alcoholics, withdrawal can be even more serious.

"If I was drinking a quart a day and had a heroin habit, I would be more afraid of quitting alcohol, 'cause with drinking, you go into convulsions and you are really sick. I thought I was going to die from the pain in my stomach; the throwing up, the sweating, and the diarrhea. You don't have any energy, and you know if you just took a drink you'd feel better. And with heroin, you get some muscle cramps and you throw up and you get a little diarrhea, but you're not going to get convulsions. You're not going to die. You can die from kicking alcohol." Recovering alcohol/heroin abuser

Since the main symptoms of severe withdrawal are tremulousness, transitory hallucinations, vomiting, muscle cramps, sweating, diarrhea, and stomach pains plus any medical complications

such as malnutrition, depressed respiration, liver problems, pneumonia, or physical damage, medical care for a compulsive drinker or alcoholic needs to be a consideration of any course of treatment. In 10% of the cases there are seizures, convulsions, and delirium tremens. Untreated, the mortality rate is 8% to 24%.

MENTAL AND EMOTIONAL EFFECTS

Alcohol depresses and slows other functions of the central and the peripheral nervous systems. Initial relaxation and lowered inhibitions at low doses often become mental confusion, mood swings, loss of judgment, and emotional turbulence at higher doses.

Disinhibition

The disinhibiting effect of alcohol is one of the main reasons it is used in so many social situations. The disinhibition is caused by alcohol's action on the higher centers of the brain's cortex, particularly that part of the brain which controls reasoning and judgment. Then it acts on the lower centers of the limbic system that rule mood and emotion.

Some recent studies in the 90's have also shown that this inhibitory effect comes from alcohol's ability to disrupt brain cell membranes. This first increases the passage of neurotransmitters causing stimulation, but later it impairs the neurotransmitters' ability to bind with receptor sites resulting in depression.

....

Fig. 5-4 *Graph shows the decrease in liver capacity to process alcohol as a person ages. As the liver is taxed and poisoned by the alcohol, its capacity is diminished to the point where an older drinker can get tipsy on just one drink.*

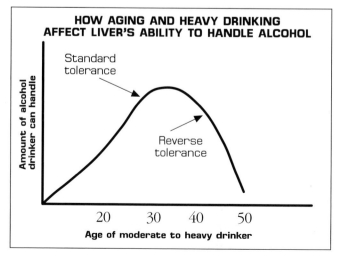

HOW AGING AND HEAVY DRINKING AFFECT LIVER'S ABILITY TO HANDLE ALCOHOL

Standard tolerance

Reverse tolerance

Amount of alcohol drinker can handle

20   30   40   50

Age of moderate to heavy drinker

"If I'm down, it picks me up. If I'm hyper, it calms me down. I could get the same thing from meditation, except meditation doesn't taste so good." "Social" drinker

The main neurotransmitters affected by alcohol are met-enkephalin, serotonin, dopamine and gama amino butyric acid (GABA). GABA is the major inhibitory neurotransmitter in the brain. By exaggerating the effects of GABA, alcohol lowers inhibitions.

The line between being relaxed, being the life of the party, and being the death of the party varies among drinkers, depending on their tolerance, their basic emotional makeup, their susceptibility to biochemical disruption, their mood, and the mood of those around them.

"You can think and say a lot of things that are crass, or disgusting, or rude when you are drunk. I don't think there is an editing process going on. It's not that you wouldn't have wanted to do some of those things when you were sober, you just wouldn't have gone and done them." 20-year-old college student

For more information on the effect of alcohol on love, sexuality, and sexual violence, including date rape, see Chapter 10.

Aggression and Violence

In the past 10 years, almost every major league baseball park and professional stadium has halted vendors from selling beer in the spectator seats. Alcohol and beer can now be purchased only at the concession stands, where a customer is limited to two drinks at a time, and no sales are allowed after the 7th inning or 3rd quarter. These changes have sharply reduced rowdiness, violence, and fights. In England and other countries where such a ban doesn't exist, fan violence, especially at soccer matches, is still a major problem.

"Well, you don't hear of any heroin addicts running their cars into people or getting in fights and cuttin' up people just from not knowing what they're doing. And when you're drunk, you do crazy things, you get violent, and you get self-destructive." Recovering alcohol abuser

Since alcohol lowers inhibitions, one of the ways it encourages violence is to encourage someone with a tendency towards violence to release pent up anger, or hatred, or desires forbidden by society, and act on them. And since alcohol disrupts judgment and reason, the common sense that would keep a person out of trouble is suppressed.

"I used to drink with a college chum, and we'd go to a bar and we'd be sitting drinking, and all of a sudden he would be picking a fight with someone at the other end of the bar...for no discernible reason. Just, bam...and we'd have to drag him off. A true Jekyll and Hyde, and a real pain in the ass." 31-year-old ex-drinker

Again, 50% of all homicides and rapes along with over 7 million crimes a year are committed under the influence of alcohol.

Self-Medication and Mental Problems

Often, alcohol is used because the person has an existing mental problem or diagnosable disorder such as major depression, schizophrenia, or bipolar illness (manic-depression), and alcohol is used to try to control the symptoms or insulate the user from the problem.

"I would pick up a beer to put me out of it. I didn't like the effect that regular psychiatric drugs such as antidepressants had on my brain, and I'd rather just put myself out with the booze than face reality." Patient with major depression and an alcohol problem

Sometimes the alcohol is used for other reasons such as overcoming boredom or controlling restlessness, and what happens is that the attempt to self-medicate by drinking or using another psychoactive drug takes on a life of its own and creates a new set of problems or aggravates an existing one.

"The problems did get worse when I was drinking. That was one reason that I never figured out that I was a manic-depressive. I figured I was depressed because I was drunk all the time." Alcoholic with manic-depression

The majority of alcoholics that come into treatment are initially diagnosed as suffering from depression. After detoxification, the figure drops to the 30% to 50% range, still a significant number. In addition, about 1/3 of alcoholics suffer an anxiety disorder.

"The alcohol, that came later on. It intensified my depression and intensified everything. I already felt bad about myself, and the alcohol just made it worse. It definitely made it worse." Recovering 16-year-old alcoholic with major depression

Again, 30% of all suicides have drunk enough alcohol to impair their judgement.

Learning and Alcohol

"Often, it's the style of drinking, not experimentation, that gets college students (as well as high school kids and young adults) in trouble. Many think the name of the game is to get drunk. They drink too fast, they drink without eating, they play drinking games or contests, or they binge drink. They drink heavily and hard on "hump day" [Wednesday] or over the weekend. But because they drink heavily only once or twice a week, they think that there is no problem. But there usually is a problem:

lower grades, disciplinary action, or behavior they regret, which usually means sexual behavior. And both males and females talk to me about having been drunk and regretting the person they were with or their conduct with that person." College drug and alcohol counselor

Forty percent of college students admit to binge drinking at least once a week. A binge is defined as having 5 or more drinks at one sitting. About half the students in one study who admitted to binge drinking admitted that their grades fell in the "C" to "F" range as opposed to the "A" to "C" range of most students. Many missed classes on a regular basis. In a national study, there was a startling, dramatic, and direct correlation between the number of drinks consumed per week and the grade point average.

Notice that women's grades start to deteriorate at slightly less than half the level it takes for men's marks to go down. Part of this is the smaller size of women and the correlation between blood alcohol level and body weight.

Some interesting statistics found in the NIDA 1992 Household Drug Survey were that the higher the level of educational attainment, the more likely was the current use (not necessarily abuse) of alcohol. Among 18- to 34-year-olds, 70% of those with college degrees were current alcohol users in 1992 compared with only 51% of those having less than a high school education. This seems a contradiction with the statistics about grade performance; however, the rate of **heavy** alcohol use in the 18 to 34 age group among those who had not completed high school was twice that of those who had completed college.

It is not the use of alcohol per se that influences grades or creates problems; it is the amount and frequency of use. Nationally, statistics show that 1 out of 10 drinkers will have lifelong problems with alcohol once he or she starts drinking. In fact, 10% of drinkers in the U.S. buy half of all alcohol sold. None of us wants to believe we are that 1 in 10.

A main purpose of this chapter is to help people decide if they are that 1 in 10 who will disrupt their lives with alcohol.

Fig. 5-5 Average Number of Drinks Per Week, Listed by Grade Average (1992)

Grade Average	Drinks Per Week		
	Males	**Females**	**Overall**
A	5.4	2.3	3.3
B	7.4	3.4	5.0
C	9.2	4.1	6.6
D or F	14.6	5.2	10.1

FROM EXPERIMENTATION TO ALCOHOLISM

"It's a kind of overlay of many different things. If you really want to drink, want to get drunk, and you want the high, that probably means that where you are when you are sober isn't as good as it could be." 22-year-old college student

The three key factors that govern addiction are heredity, environment, and psychoactive drugs.

CAUSES OF ADDICTION

Heredity

In recent years, an alcoholic marker gene has been suggested which predicts a person's susceptibility to compulsive drinking. It means that when they do use alcohol, people with this gene are more likely to become compulsive drinkers.

"My grandmother warned me, 'Our family can't drink. The only exercise your grandad got was bending his elbow. Your uncle died of cirrhosis of the liver. Your aunt died of the combination of alcohol and sleeping pills. Your dad had 5 martinis every day of his business life, and that was just at lunch.'" 31-year-old non-drinker

If one parent is alcoholic, the child is 34% more likely to be an alcoholic than children of non-alcoholics. If both parents are alcoholic, the child is 400% more likely to be alcoholic. If the child is a male with both parents and a grandfather being alcoholic, that child is 900% more likely to develop alcoholism. About 28 million Americans have at least one alcoholic parent.

People who are susceptible to developing the disease of alcoholism often get into compulsive drinking at a much quicker rate than people without that susceptibility. Many susceptible people receive an intense reaction from the alcohol with their first drinking experience. Although their first reaction to alcohol is more intense than others, predisposed alcoholics often initially have a greater tolerance to the behavioral effects of the drug. They seem to need more alcohol than others to get drunk when first starting, but their drunken state is much more intense and dysfunctional. Many have blackouts the first time they use when they don't remember what happened to them while drunk.

In the past decade, there has been increased understanding of the way alcoholism is passed on from generation to generation. Recent studies of animals, identical twins, neurological signs, body enzymes, and comprehensive reviews of an alcoholic's family history, all provide strong evidence that alcoholism is, in part, an inherited disease. Several researchers now feel that it is the human A1, A1 allele gene pair that signals the greatest vulnerability for the condition of alcoholism.

Environment

The second factor that determines people's drinking habits is environment. Environment pushes one to drink if all those around are drinking, if drinking is a respectable habit, if one is subject to heavy levels of stress, or if there are mental problems that make self-medication more likely.

"There is a serious difference between using and abusing. If people aren't happy with themselves, they'd be inclined to say, 'I want to be high right now because all this stuff sucks, and I want to get away. That's why I drink.'" 16-year-old high school student

"Peer relationships and that whole atmosphere of friendships are really important to college students, as important as autonomy. Unfortunately, some rely so heavily on alcohol to fit in that they never learn the social skills to interact with other people without drinking. They never can face disappointment or emotional pain without alcohol as a buffer. We're talking about arrested development, impaired development. After college, many continue to rely on alcohol to make the hurt go away. As the pain gets bigger, the drinking problem will get bigger. They've never developed the skills to cope with the people and problems that are part of everyone's life." College drug and alcohol counselor

Psychoactive Drugs

The final factor that determines drinking habits is the drug itself. Long-term use of alcohol changes the body so it comes to need the alcohol to stay "normal." This tolerance and physical dependence are what used to be called "habit-forming."

"There is not a night (and it doesn't matter if it's a school night) where there aren't at least 5 houses with a raging party going on." 17-year-old high-school student

The Alcoholic Mice and the Sober Mice

There are classic experiments that help explain the close connection between heredity, environment, and alcohol.

Years ago, two strains of mice were bred to help researchers understand alcoholism. One of the strains of mice was alcoholic (Fig. 6-a), that is, the mice preferred alcohol to water. Given the choice of a cup of water to a cup of alcohol, they always drank the alcohol. The other strain of mice was sober (Fig. 6-b). Given the same choice, the mice always chose the water. They couldn't even stand a few drops of alcohol in their water.

In the experiment, the researchers first took a group of the sober, alcohol-hating mice and injected them with high levels of alcohol (Fig. 6-c), the equivalent of what an adult human being would drink if he or she were a heavy drinker. Within a few weeks, these once sober mice came to prefer alcohol. In fact, if not stopped, they would drink themselves to death (Fig. 6-d).

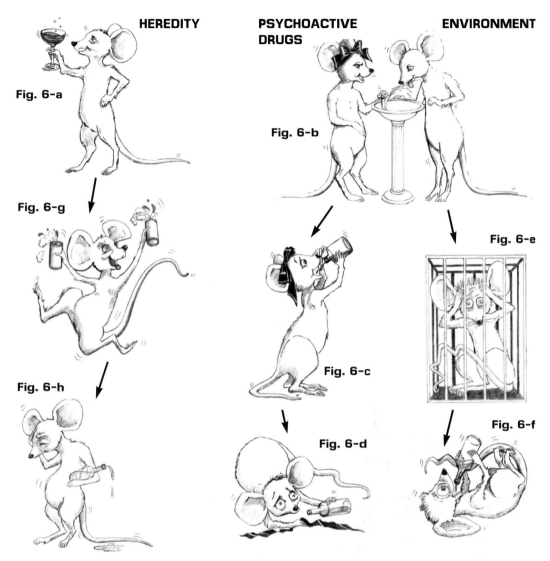

HEREDITY

Fig. 6-a

Fig. 6-g

Fig. 6-h

PSYCHOACTIVE DRUGS

Fig. 6-b

Fig. 6-c

Fig. 6-d

ENVIRONMENT

Fig. 6-e

Fig. 6-f

The researchers then took another group of the sober, alcohol-hating mice and subjected them to stress by putting them in very small, constrictive cages for intermittent periods of time (Fig. 6-e). Within a few weeks, this group of sober mice also came to prefer alcohol to water (Fig. 6-f). In essence, sober mice had been turned into alcoholic mice through stress (environment) and through excessive use of alcohol.

The mice whose heredity made them prefer alcohol, kept on drinking if alcohol was available to them. (Fig. 6-g). They would have kept drinking until they died. (Fig. 6-h). Even when they were subjected to aversive electrical shocks aimed at preventing them from drinking the alcohol, they continued to drink.

What was most interesting was that when the alcohol and stress were stopped, the originally sober mice did not return to their normal drinking habits. They had been transformed into alcoholic mice. And when the brains of the three groups of mice were examined (the hereditary alcoholic mice, the stress-induced alcoholic mice, and the drug-induced alcoholic mice), all had approximately the same alcoholic brain chemistry. This research suggests that the neurochemical disruption caused by heredity, environment, and/or psychoactive drugs can lead to the same type of serious addiction.

Addiction is not just a disease of the alcoholic.

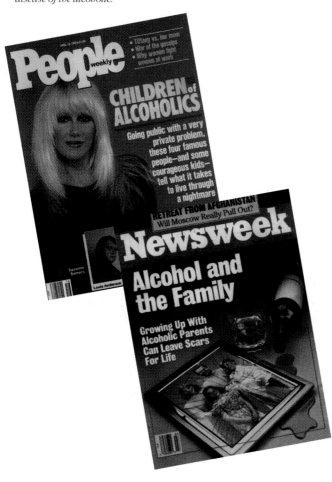

Addiction

In 1992, a medical panel from the American Society of Addiction Medicine and the National Council on Alcoholism and Drug Dependence defined alcoholism as follows:

"Alcoholism is a primary, chronic disease with genetic, psychosocial, and environmental factors influencing its development and manifestation. The disease is often progressive and fatal. It is characterized by impaired control over drinking, preoccupation with the drug alcohol, use of alcohol despite adverse consequences, and distortions in thinking, most notably denial. Each of these symptoms may be continuous or periodic."

"I don't consider myself an alcoholic. I drink a lot. I have five drinks a day ... and that's an average. It's hardly ever less than three. But, it's never interfered with my work. It's never interfered with my health." Avowed "social" drinker in denial

Polydrug Abuse

Most illicit drug users also drink for a variety of reasons:

• To increase the action of a drug (alcohol with Valium for exaggerated depressant effects);

• To subdue the effect of a stimulant;

• To substitute for another drug they can't get. (If heroin supplies are short, the addict will drink to subdue the symptoms);

• To continue the high (marijuana and alcohol are very common at parties);

• To self-treat withdrawal symptoms from addiction to another drug (alcohol after a methamphetamine binge).

Polydrug abuse has become so common that treatment centers have had to learn how to treat simultaneous addictions. Although the emotional roots of addiction are similar no matter what drug is used, the physiological and psychological changes that each drug causes, particularly during withdrawal, often have to be treated differently. For example, if a client of the Haight-Ashbury Clinic has a serious alcohol and benzodiazepine problem, the Clinic has to be extremely careful detoxifying the client. That is because Librium, a benzodiazepine, is one or the drugs used to control the symptoms of delirium tremens caused by alcohol withdrawal.

The other danger of polydrug abuse as mentioned in the previous chapter is drug synergism or the magnification of the effects of two drugs taken together. A benzodiazepine and alcohol exaggerate each other's depressant effects, usually leading to extreme respiratory depression. Four to eight thousand deaths a year, plus fifty thousand emergency room visits, can be attributed to drug synergism.

TREATMENT

Denial

Denial on the part of the alcoholic or compulsive drinker is the biggest hindrance to beginning treatment. Until drinkers admit to themselves that they have a problem, the information presented to them isn't absorbed. The drinker doesn't believe the facts apply to him or her. One reason denial is so common with the use of alcohol is that the change in people's drinking habits that cause them to become compulsive drinkers often takes years to develop (10 years on the average).

Not only do problem drinkers deny they have a problem, those around them won't confront the situation either. In a survey of alcoholics who presented themselves for treatment, only 22% had been warned by their doctors about the consequences of their drinking.

Denial also occurs because alcoholics have no memory of the negative effects they experienced while in an alcoholic "blackout." Thus, they don't believe that alcohol has harmed them. Further, alcohol impairs judgment and reason in all users making them less likely to associate any problem with their drinking.

As with stimulants and opiates, treatment consists of detoxification, initial abstinence, long-term abstinence, and recovery.

Detoxification

For a heavy drinker, physical withdrawal is very uncomfortable but usually not dangerous. Symptoms can usually be handled by aspirin, rest, liquids and any one of hundreds of hangover "cures" that have been handed down from generation to generation. However, it must be mentioned that the most often used home remedy to treat hangover, "the hair of the dog," is the unhealthiest. This is the suggestion to drink more alcohol. Although this remedy works, it just promotes the continued negative health problems of drinking. The immediate withdrawal symptoms usually go away within a day or two.

For the alcoholic, the potentially life-threatening symptoms can be handled with a variety of sedating drugs: barbiturates such as phenobarbital, benzodiazepines such as Librium, paraldehyde, chloral hydrate, and the phenothiazines. Since several of these drugs are addictive, they should be used sparingly and on a very short-term basis. Normally tapering is done on a 5 to 7 day basis but can be extended to 11 to 14 days.

Along with emergency medical care, withdrawal and detoxification can be handled through emotional support and basic physical care such as rest and nutrition (thiamine, folic acid, multi-vitamins, amino acids, electrolytes, and fructose). Many of the problems will start to repair themselves with detoxification, but for the long-term drinker, some of the damage is irreversible: liver disease, enlarged heart, cancer, and nerve damage, among others.

Initial Abstinence

A common treatment for initial abstinence is the use of Antabuse. Antabuse is a drug that will make people ill if they drink alcohol. This is used for about 6 months or longer to help get them through initial abstinence when they're most likely to relapse. A more important part of this process is encouraging them to go to Alcoholics Anonymous meetings or other support group meetings, in addition to individual therapy, to support them emotionally. One procedure is to have the user go to 90 Alcoholics Anonymous meetings in 90 days (called a 90/90 contract).

Psychological denial is an integral part of the disease of alcoholism, so much so that the key step to treatment is breaking through the denial, even more than simply detoxifying the user.

Long-Term Abstinence

In treatment, one often encounters someone known as a "dry drunk." This person is not actually drinking alcohol, but still has the craving and mind set of the alcoholic. So, the purpose of this stage of treatment, besides keeping the drinker dry (avoiding relapse), is to begin healing the emotional scars, confusion, and immaturity that kept the person drinking for so many years.

In many cases, abstinence from alcohol brings to the fore many of the problems that were covered by the alcohol or other drug, so depression, anxiety, or life problems are constant, grinding motivators for relapse. Treatment for coexisting mental and emotional problems are part of long-term abstinence treatment.

Recovery

Since the development of compulsive drinking habits and addiction takes many years to acquire, it makes sense that recovery has to be an equally long-term process, usually lasting a lifetime. Many treatment centers advertise 30-day drying-out programs implying that detoxification is the key to recovery rather than being a small, initial step in a long process. The body's chemistry has been permanently changed by years of drinking, so the recovering alcoholic is always susceptible to relapse.

PREVENTION

In talking about prevention, a decision has to be made about what needs to be prevented.

• Do we want to prevent all drinking (Just say "No.")?

• Do we permit experimentation and casual drinking and try to prevent abuse (responsible drinking)?

• Or do we just want to prevent the more disastrous effects of alcoholism?

The different methods of prevention that have been tried are

• Limiting the supply (prohibi-

tion, taxation, state-run stores, age limitations);

• Increasing legal penalties (drunk driving, spousal-abuse laws);

• Educating young people about the physical and mental effects of alcohol;

• Scare education about the disastrous effects of alcohol with the message, "This could happen to you."

The method of prevention has to be responsive to the culture, religion, and level of drug awareness of the people being addressed. If a community's religion prohibits alcohol in any form, lessons on responsible drinking would be a very small part of the curriculum. If the audience is college students in an average university setting, then teaching about the effects of alcohol (particularly binge drinking) along with the idea of responsible drinking, would make more sense.

Legal penalties also make sense if they are directed at the harmful effects of drinking rather than at drinking itself. For example, stiffer drunk-driving laws, especially when injury is involved, or evenly applied spousal-abuse laws (since most wife-beaters are drunk when they abuse their wives) have proven effective.

The problem is that there also have to be effective intervention techniques, sufficient treatment programs, and a recognition that alcoholism is a progressive disease that, if left untreated, will destroy the individual.

"If you can convince someone that you can understand the emotion and pain connected with how they are feeling, it is then more possible to convince that person to stop drinking. But, if you just talk at them, your chances are slim to none." 19-year-old college peer counselor

Finally, prevention and education begin in the home, so if the parents drink to excess, if the message they give their children is inconsistent, if there is violence in the home, and if there is no education in the home, then what schools or society does to prevent problems with alcohol loses much of its effectiveness.

*"I know parents who say, 'Don't drink at all,' and others that say, 'Don't drink **it** all,' because they don't want their kids to drink up all their liquor. If you have a good friendship with your parents and you respect what they think, you'll listen to what they say. But, half the kids I know, their parents will buy them liquor."* 19-year-old college sophomore

Did Prohibition Work?

Most people claim that Prohibition (1919-1933) didn't work. They point to the increase in crime, the speakeasy, and the flouting of the law as proof that Americans wanted to continue drinking. Others say that Prohibition did work in that it gave many Americans a chance to dry out and break the cycle of alcoholism.

Some statistics might be illuminating:

• Death rates from cirrhosis of the liver fell from 29.5 per 100,000 men in 1911 to just 10.7 in 1929;

• Families had about $1 billion more to spend on consumer goods;

• Per capita consumption measured in gallons of pure alcohol went from 2.6 gallons in 1910 to .97 gallons just after prohibition, to 1.56 gallons six years later. In 1987, the figure had crept back up to 2.54 gallons (the actual amount of beverages containing alcohol that are drunk is approximately 30 gallons per person).

So, the drying out of America did keep the level of alcohol consumption below preprohibition levels for almost 40 years.

Several conclusions are possible. First, alcohol in and of itself will promote compulsive use, and the sheer benefit of detoxification alone will help compulsive users control their drinking. Next, the children who grew up during prohibition didn't have the constant example of everyone drinking around them all the time, so that possibly delayed their resumption of the practice and habit. Finally, it makes one realize that the case for or against prohibition isn't as clear-cut as either side would like us to believe.

PROHIBITION

Benefits	Bad Effects
Reduced consumption	Growth of organized crime
Less compulsive use	Increased price of the drug
Less money wasted	Increased contempt of laws
Less family violence	Adulterated product

ALCOHOL ASSESSMENT TEST

These are some of the past behaviors of people already in treatment for alcoholism. If you recognize several of these behaviors in a friend, classmate, or relative, suspect that they have a problem with alcohol.

1. They know which convenience stores are open and how late they can sell alcohol.
2. They say "It's none of your business" when you or their girlfriend or boyfriend tells them they're drinking too much.
3. They are late to first period class because of a hangover.
4. They say they can't be an alcoholic since they've only been drunk on the weekends this semester.
5. They say they can drive better drunk than most people sober.
6. They are proud they can hold a bottle of scotch like their dad, without passing out.
7. They drink to give them confidence in social occasions.
8. They think they are wittier or more charming once they have had a few drinks.
9. They like to play drinking games.
10. They keep an emergency six-pack of beer in the back of their closet.
11. They call anyone who doesn't drink a wimp.
12. They know they can stop drinking anytime they want to, they've just never had any occasion to try.
13. At a party they finish off a drink that has been left unattended.
14. They drink before they go to a party and will have a drink after they get home.
15. They've been arrested for drunk driving.
16. They constantly urge others around them to have another drink.
17. They loudly announce how they are sticking to the quota they have set for themselves.
18. They find many excuses to celebrate with a drink including not drinking for a day.
19. They have a quick drink in the kitchen while the guests are in the living room.
20. They always offer to replenish the supply of booze.
21. They are always near the bottles at a party.
22. All their friends drink.

The most important thing to remember about the above behaviors and attitudes is that the people are either not aware of what they are doing or vigorously deny that it is a problem. Most drinkers have this magic shield of denial around their attitudes and behaviors that becomes more impervious to reason the more it is attacked.

(In Chapter 11, the process of intervention is discussed.)

DOWNERS—ALCOHOL

1. About 98 million Americans have at least one drink a month.

2. Alcohol is used to lower inhibitions, as a medicine, to cover up problems, as a relaxant, or for a dozen different reasons.

3. Alcohol is the oldest psychoactive drug known. It is legal and found in beer, wine, and hard liquors.

4. Initially, alcohol suppresses inhibitions, so it seems to act like a stimulant. As the depressant effect takes over, however, it slows reflexes, depresses respiration and heart rate, and disrupts reasoning and judgement.

5. As a person grows older, the liver and body are less able to handle the same amount of alcohol, so the person gets drunk sooner.

6. Withdrawal from overuse (hangover) is usually not life threatening. Withdrawal from prolonged heavy use of alcohol can cause hallucinations, tremors, vomiting, life-threatening convulsions, and irregular heart rates.

7. Fatty liver, cirrhosis of the liver, circulatory problems, nervous system damage, cancer, and digestive problems are some of the long-term medical effects of excessive drinking.

8. The main neurotransmitters affected by alcohol are GABA, serotonin, and met-enkephalin.

9. Alcohol can cause violence by lowering inhibitions in people with a tendency to violence.

10. Many people with mental problems use alcohol to self-medicate to control the symptoms of their illness.

11. There is a direct relationship between the amount of alcohol drunk and grades: the more alcohol drunk, the lower the grades.

12. The three factors that determine the way a person drinks are heredity, environment, and psychoactive drugs.

13. People with a tendency to alcoholism probably have an alcohol marker gene. If one or both parents are alcoholic, the chances are much greater that the child will become an alcoholic.

14. Tests with mice show that intense consumption of alcohol or extreme stress can cause teatotaling mice to prefer alcohol to water.

15. Alcohol addiction is a chronic, progressive disease characterized by lack of control over drinking, preoccupation with alcohol, use despite adverse consequences, and denial. It can be fatal if not controlled.

16. Medical treatment is often necessary for extreme cases of withdrawal.

17. Alcoholism takes years to develop and recovery can take a lifetime.

18. Education and prevention programs need to be culturally specific since each society's attitude towards alcohol is different.

19. Alcohol and sedative-hypnotics used together can be especially life threatening. They cause a synergistic (magnified) effect which can suppress respiration and heart functions to dangerous levels.

20. Four to eight thousand people in the United States die each year from the synergistic effect of alcohol and another depressant. An additional 50,000 people are treated in emergency rooms because of polydrug abuse.

QUESTIONS

1. What percentage of college students drink at least once a month?

2. Name three ways people use alcohol.

3. Why do many people think alcohol is a stimulant?

4. What is reverse tolerance in regards to alcohol?

5. Name three serious medical side effects of excessive drinking.

6. Name two neurotransmitters affected by alcohol.

7. How does alcohol use encourage violence?

8. How do people with mental problems or a true mental illness use alcohol?

9. Explain the alcohol marker gene.

10. Name two criteria for a diagnosis of alcoholism?

11. Why is recovery a lifetime process?

12. What is the relationship between the culture of the user and the style of drug education?

13. What is a synergistic effect, and why is it dangerous?

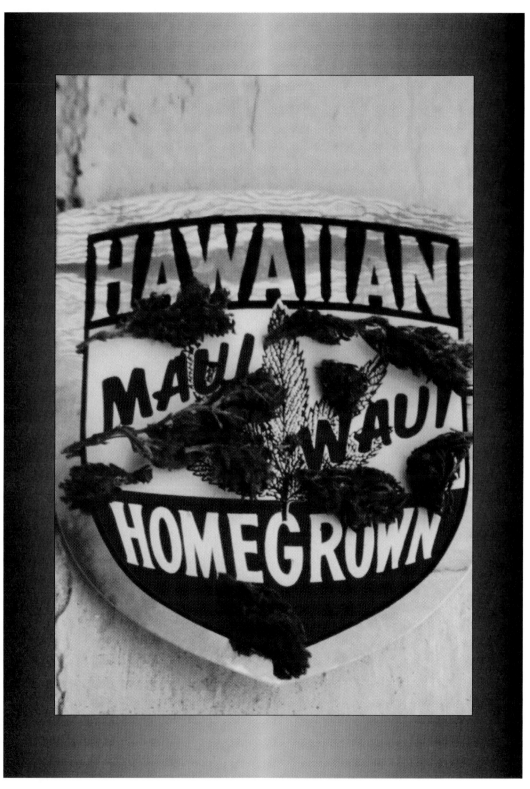

Although illegal throughout most of the world, the desire to advertise is still strong among some growers, particularly in Hawaii.

CHAPTER 6

ALL AROUNDERS

1988

Navajo Woman Sues State Over Use of Peyote

Associated Press

Sacramento
   A Navajo woman from Fresno is suing the state for rejecting her application to become a prison guard because she had eaten the hallucinogenic plant

1934

Brooklyn's Narcotic Farm

URSDAY, OCTOBER 18, 1934   23

Marajuana Field

AMAZING DISCOVERY NEAR BRIDGE

POLICE RAID

CRAFTY DETECTIVE WORK; 2 ARRESTS

1992

Ecstasy Has Its Price

New 'Rave' drug is causing deaths in England

BY PETER MILLERSHIP

London
   "YOU'RE childishly happy. No money problems, no women problems. You're just lost in high-energy dance culture," says 18-year-old Marcus. Two hours ago he swallowed Ecstasy, to go better known as the synthetic drug craze to Raving — the latest music and drug sweep Britain. And at 2 a.m. Saturday in a central London basement nightclub, a 'Rave' is in full

swing, and Marcus and his friends are Ecstasy.
   Youngsters decked out in fluorescent wear dance convulsively, staring as they their hands hypnotically to heavy-rhythm "housed" or mixed by disc jockeys

   Tens of thousands of British teenagers each week to all-night Raves, sometimes at venues, to take drugs with names like Dis cuits, Triple X and Denis The Menace

   Popularized in the late 1980s, Ecstasy known as the "Love Drug", became it can

CLASSIFICATION

Uppers stimulate the body and downers depress it. All arounders (psychedelics) can act as stimulants or depressants, but mostly they distort the perception of the world, and create a world in which logic takes a back seat to intensified sensations. From alphabet soup psychedelics (LSD, PCP, MDMA) to naturally occurring plants used in religious ceremonies (peyote, mushrooms, belladonna), all arounders represent a diverse group of substances.

Historically, amanita mushrooms were eaten in India and pre-Columbian Mexico, belladonna was drunk in ancient Greece and Medieval Europe, marijuana was inhaled and eaten in ancient China and Egypt, and poisonous ergot, found in wheat mold (a natural form of LSD) was accidentally eaten in renaissance Europe.

In the 20th century, even though psychedelics can be found in every country, the majority of these drugs are grown and used in the Americas and Africa (marijuana is the major exception). Hundreds of primitive tribes, such as the Aztecs and Toltecs in the past, and the Kiowa and Huicholes in the present, have used or are using peyote, psilocybin, yage, morning glory seeds, and dozens of other substances for religious, social, magical, and medical reasons.

Recently, there has been an upsurge of interest in psychedelics such as LSD, MDMA ("ecstasy," "rave"), and even psychedelic mushrooms ("shrooms") containing psilocybin. The percentage of high school seniors who have tried LSD is the same as those who have ever tried cocaine (about 9% in 1992). Interest in marijuana, the most widely used psychedelic, continues at the same level of use over the past several decades (1/3 of the total population and 41% of the high school class of 1992 have tried it).

The four main classes of psychedelics are the indole psychedelics such as LSD and psilocybin which mimic certain brain hormones; the phenylalkylamines such as mescaline and "ecstasy," that closely resemble molecules of adrenaline and amphetamines; the anticholinergics, such as belladonna, that block acetylcholine; those in a class by themselves, such as PCP; and the cannabinols, found in marijuana (hemp) plants, that affect acetylcholine.

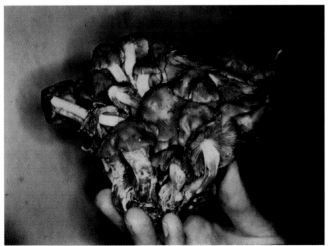

Allan Richardson

....

One of the 75 species of mushroom containing psilocybin. The "shroom" can be used fresh or dried.

Fig 6-1 ALL AROUNDERS - PSYCHEDELICS

Common name	Active ingredients	Street names
Indole Psychedelics		
LSD (LSD 25 & 49)	Lysergic acid diethyl-amide	Acid, sugar, window pane, blotter, illusion
Mushrooms	Psilocybin	Shrooms, magic mushrooms
Tabernanthe Iboga	Ibogaine	African LSD
Morning glory seeds or Hawaiian wood-rose	Lysergic acid amide	Heavenly Blue, Pearly Gates, wedding bells
DMT synthetic or from yopo beans, epena, or Sonoran desert toad	Dimethyltryptamine	Businessman's special, cohoba snuff
Yage, Ayahuasca, Caapi	Harmaline (also mixed with DMT)	Visionary vine, vine of the soul
Phenylalkylamine Psychedelics		
Peyote cactus	Mescaline	Mesc, peyote, buttons
STP, (DOM) (synthetic)	4 methyl 2,5 dimethoxy-amphetamine	Serenity, tranquility peace pill
STP-LSD Combo	Dimethoxy-amphetamine with LSD	Wedge series, orange and pink wedges, Harvey Wallbanger
MDA, MDMA (MDM), MMDA, MDE, etc.	Variations of methylene-dioxy amphetamine	Rave, love drug, XTC, ecstasy, Adam, Eve
2CB	4 bromo 2,5 dimethoxy phenethylamine	
U4Euh	4 methyl aminorex	Euphoria
Anticholinergics		
Belladonna, mandrake, henbane, datura (jimson weed, thornapple), wolfbane	Atropine, scopolamine, hyoscyamine	Deadly nightshade
Artane	Trihexypheneidyl	
Cogentin	Benztropine	
Asmador Cigarettes	Belladonna alkyloids	
Other Psychedelics		
PCP	Phencyclidine	Angel dust, hog, peace pill, krystal, krystal joint, ozone, Sherm
Keta-jet, Keta-lar	Ketamine	
Nutmeg and mace	Myristicin	
Amanita mushrooms (fly agaric)	Ibotenic acid, muscimol	Soma
Kava root	Alpha pyrones	Kava-kava
Cannabinols (marijuana, etc.)		
Marijuana	THC-tetrahydro-cannabinol	Grass, pot, weed, Acapulco gold, joint, reefer, dubie, etc.
Sinsemilla	High potency, seedless flowering tops of female marijuana plant	Sens, skunk weed, ganja
Hashish, hash oil	THC (refined from marijuana)	Bhang

GENERAL EFFECTS

Unlike stimulants and depressants, which have many well-researched legal counterparts (i.e., sedative-hypnotics, alcohol, cocaine, amphetamines), psychedelics are manufactured or grown illegally, so much of the information about the effects are anecdotal or the result of surveys rather than extended scientific testing. In addition, many drugs which are represented as one psychedelic may actually be another cheaper psychedelic, a stimulant, a depressant, or even a placebo. Some common examples of misrepresentation are PCP sold as mescaline or THC (the active ingredient in marijuana); or regular mushrooms sprinkled with LSD and sold as psychedelic mushrooms; or snuff sold as hashish.

Generally, psychedelics interfere with neurotransmitters such as dopamine, acetylcholine, adrenaline, and especially, serotonin. Serotonin, which affects mood, is particularly influenced by the indole psychedelics such as LSD.

Fig 6-2 Chemical models of MDA, PCP, DMT, and LSD, sometimes called the "alphabet soup" psychedelics.

More than with stimulants or depressants, the effects of psychedelics are uncommonly dependent on the size of the dose. A drug like LSD is thousands of times more powerful, by weight, than a similar amount of peyote.

Experience with the drug along with the basic emotional makeup of the user, the mood and mental state at the time of use, and the surroundings in which the drug is taken are also crucial. For instance, a first- or second-time psychedelic user may become nauseous, extremely anxious, depressed, and totally disoriented while an experienced user may have euphoric feelings or some mild delusions. A user with a tendency towards schizophrenia or major depression could get a really bad reaction from LSD because it might exaggerate any unstable tendencies. Someone who is basically aggressive might become violent when using PCP, whereas a young and immature user of marijuana could become more childlike.

Physical Effects

LSD and most other hallucinogens stimulate the sympathetic nervous system. This results in a rise in pulse rate and blood pressure. They can produce sweating and palpitations or trigger nausea. The stimulation of the brainstem, specifically the reticular formation, can overload the sensory pathways, making the user very conscious of all sensation. Disruption of visual and auditory

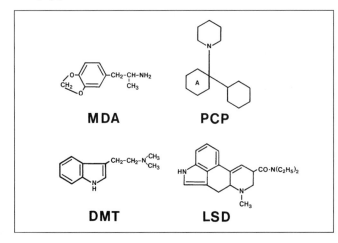

MDA   PCP

DMT   LSD

centers can cause effects ranging from flashes of light to melting walls. An auditory stimulation such as the sound of music might jump to a visual pathway, causing the music to be "seen" as shifting light patterns, or visual impulses might shift to audio ones, resulting in strange sounds. This crossover or mixing of the senses is known as synesthesia.

Emotional Effects

Psychedelics have a strong effect on mood by affecting the emotional center (the limbic system). They also suppress the memory centers and other higher cerebral functions such as judgment and reason. Since a user's reaction varies so much with psychedelics, the effects of each drug will be discussed individually.

It's important to note the difference among an illusion, a delusion, and a hallucination. An **illusion** is a mistaken perception of a real stimulus. For example a rope can be misinterpreted as a snake or smooth skin as silk. A **delusion** is a mistaken idea that is not swayed by reason. An example is someone who thinks he can fly or thinks he has become deformed or ugly. A **hallucination** is a sensory experience that doesn't relate to reality, such as seeing a creature or object that doesn't exist. With LSD and most psychedelics, illusions and delusions are the primary experiences. With mescaline and PCP, hallucinations are the primary experience.

INDOLE PSYCHEDELICS

LSD (LYSERGIC ACID DIETHYLAMIDE)

History

"Acid," "blotter," "barrels," "sunshine," "illusion," and "window panes" are just some of the street names for LSD, a synthesized form of an ergot fungus toxin which infects rye and wheat. Tested and developed in the late 1940's at Sandoz Pharmaceuticals by Dr. Albert Hoffman, LSD was investigated as a therapy for mental illnesses and as a weapon for chemical warfare. It was popularized by Dr. Timothy Leary, originally a professor at Harvard who did LSD research, and by others in the 60's as a way to "explore consciousness and feelings." Dr. Leary's slogan, "Tune in, turn on, and drop out," was used in endless newspaper articles and TV news shows leading to the suspicion that the media was as much responsible for the rise and fall of LSD as was its identification as the drug of the hippie generation in the 60's. Scientific research virtually ceased in the early 70's, and it wasn't until recently that any research on LSD or psychedelics in general has been allowed.

LSD continued to lose favor in the 80's, but in the 90's there has been a renewed interest in its use. Besides the usual reasons for using a drug like LSD (experimentation, peer pressure, availability, and curiosity), there are three oth-

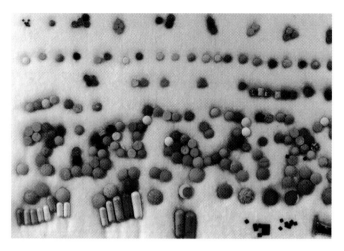

The effective dose of LSD is so small that it can be delivered in many guises. Tablets can be swallowed; saturated bits of gelatin, impregnated; blotter paper or sugar cubes can be chewed and absorbed or swallowed.

ers. One is the proliferation of "rave" clubs and parties where MDMA, LSD, and amphetamines are utilized. The other reason is that standard drug testing usually does not test for LSD, and even when tested for, the effective dose is so small that it is almost impossible to detect. Instead of taking amphetamines for stimulation, many G.I.'s and others who want to use drugs but are afraid of testing, use low-dose LSD for the stimulatory rather than the psychedelic effects. Finally, low-dose "blotter acid," 30 to 50 micrograms of LSD, results in less toxic reactions than before. Because it is less toxic and is a stimulant, users sometimes take it on a daily basis.

The majority of LSD is manufactured in Northern California, mostly in the San Francisco Bay area. The labs are hard to find since the quantities of raw material needed to make the drug are very small. Indeed, the entire U.S.

supply for one year could be carried by one person. Crystalline LSD is dissolved in alcohol, and drops of the solution are put on blotter paper or in a sugar cube, and chewed or swallowed. It has also been put into microdots or tiny squares of gelatin and eaten or dropped onto a moist body tissue and absorbed.

Currently, LSD is being used by younger Americans. Studies now document its use by even grammar school students while they are in the classroom. Indeed, these studies also demonstrate that LSD is the drug most often abused by junior high and high school students while they are sitting in class. This is because low-dose use results in less detectable physical symptoms than alcohol or marijuana and because the drug is relatively inexpensive, costing 3 to 7 dollars a hit.

In the 60's "acid heads" were usually in their early twenties, and many were searching for a quasi-religious experience. In the 90's, the target user group is younger teenagers, and they mostly just want to get high. To reach this group, illegal manufacturers even use Donald Duck, a teddy bear, and other cartoon characters printed on the blotter paper. In 1990, about 10% of high school seniors said they had tried LSD at least once. About 2% said they use it on a monthly basis.

Pharmacology

LSD is remarkable for its potency. Doses as low as 25 micrograms (mics), 25 one millionths of a gram, can cause mental changes (spaciness, decreased perception of time, mild euphoria) and mild stimulatory effects. Effects appear 15 minutes to one hour after ingestion and last 6 to 8 hours. The usual psychedelic dose of LSD is 150 to 300 micrograms. Low-dose use of 30 to 50 micrograms acts more like a stimulant than a psychedelic. Tolerance to the psychedelic effects of LSD develops very rapidly. Within a few days of daily use, a person can tolerate a 300 microgram dose without experiencing any major psychedelic effects. Cross tolerance can also develop to the effects of mescaline and psilocybin.

Recently, a new version of the drug called LSD-49 (instead of the old designation, LSD-25) has appeared on the streets. Called "illusion," it seems to give more intense visual effects than an equal amount of the original LSD-25.

Physical Effects

LSD can cause a rise in heart rate and blood pressure, a higher body temperature, dizziness, dilated pupils, and some sweating, much like amphetamines.

> *"We had some acid which we called the 'Victor Mature LSD' because it made you grind your teeth like he did in the movies. That was because it had so much speed in it."* Ex-acid user

Mental Effects

Mentally, LSD overloads the brainstem, the sensory switchboard for the mind, causing sensory distortions (seeing sounds, feeling smells, or hearing colors), dreaminess, depersonalization, altered mood, and impaired concentration and motivation. Users see many light trails, like after images in cheap televisions where there is always an after image of whatever is happening on camera (this after effect is known as the "trailing phenomena").

> *"In a real strong acid, the old ones, you'll see the walls melting like candles, and water running down the wall. That kind of distortion, not a complete hallucination or anything real solid like a bottle where you wonder whether it's there or not. The thing that got me really crazy was hearing a dog or airplane or passenger car miles away, and you didn't know whether that was real or a delusion. There was what we called the psychedelic hummmm ...."* Recovering drug user

It becomes difficult to express oneself verbally on LSD. Single word answers and seemingly nonassociated comments (non-sequiturs) are common. A user might experience intense sensations and emotions but finds it difficult to tell others what he or she is feeling.

One of the greatest dangers of LSD is the loss of judgement and impairment of the process of self-preservation. This coupled with slowed reaction time and visual distortions can make the driving of a car or a simple camping trip a chancy proposition.

"I stuck my hand in this flame and then I went, 'Uh-oh, my hand is in the flame,' and I pulled it out and I thought it didn't burn, but later that night, my hand started blistering and I'm going, 'Oh no, I got burned.'" Ex-LSD user

Bad Trips
(acute anxiety reactions)

The amount of acid, the surroundings, the user's mental state, and physical condition all determine the reaction to a drug. Because of its effect on the emotional center in the brain, a user is open to the extremes of euphoria and panic. Inexperienced or even experienced users who take too high a dose, can feel acute anxiety, fear over loss of control, paranoia, and delusions of persecution or feelings of grandeur leading to dangerous behaviors like bungee jumping without a cord.

A sheet of blotter acid (LSD); each perforated square contains a drop of LSD, anywhere from 30 to 50 micrograms of the drug. In the 60's and 70's they contained 100 to 300 micrograms.

"You would all of a sudden look at a clock and say, 'All right, I'll come down now.' And then, the writing would still be on the wall and you'd still be hearing the sounds and you'd go, 'No, I'm not going to come down. I'm never, never going to come down. I'm never going to be sane again. They're going to lock me up.'" Ex-acid user

Mental Illness and LSD

Much of the early research as well as enthusiasm for LSD as an adjunct to psychotherapy has decreased over the years. Proponents of psychotherapeutic use claim that the drug-stimulated insights afford some users a shortcut to the extended process of psychotherapy where uncovering traumas and conflicts from the unconscious helps to heal the patient. Opponents of this kind of therapy say that the potential and actual side effects of LSD more than outweigh any benefit.

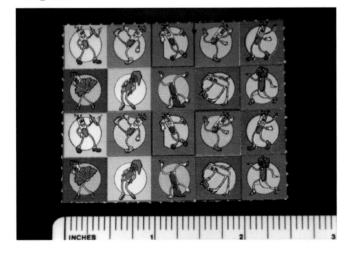

Fig. 6-3 Treatment for Bad Trips

The Haight-Ashbury Clinic uses the following ARRRT guidelines in dealing with a person experiencing a bad trip:

A equals acceptance—first, gain the user's trust and confidence.

R equals reduction of stimuli—get the user to a quiet, non-threatening environment;

R equals reassurance—educate the user that he or she is experiencing a bad trip and assure the person that he or she is in a safe place among safe people and that he or she will be all right;

R equals rest—assist the user to relax (use stress reduction techniques and allow him or her to rest);

T equals talk down—discuss peaceful, non-threatening subjects with the user, avoiding any topic which seems to create more anxiety or a strong reaction.

Two words of caution in using the ARRRT talk-down technique.

1. If the user seems to be experiencing severe medical, physical, or even emotional reactions which are not responding, medical intervention is needed. Get the person to a hospital or bring in emergency medical personnel experienced in treating the bad-trip reaction.

2. Although most psychedelic bad trip reactions are responsive to ARRRT, PCP may cause unexpected and sudden violent or belligerent behavior. Caution must be exercised in approaching a bum tripper suspected of being under the influence of PCP.

The best treatment for someone on a "bad trip" is to talk him or her down in a calm manner, without raising one's voice or appearing threatening. Avoid quick movements and let the person move around so there is no feeling of being trapped.

Counselor: "You took some acid a few hours ago."

LSD user: "You did?"

Counselor: "No, you did. You're at the talk-down room at the concert. We're from the clinic. Everything's safe, it's going to be okay."

LSD user: "Okay, yeah . . . It's too strange."

Counselor: "How do you like the music so far?"

The popular picture of someone using LSD just one time and becoming permanently psychotic or schizophrenic is incorrect. In is, in fact, an unusual occurrence. What usually happens is that there is a preexisting mental instability, and LSD use nudges those tendencies into more severe mental disturbances or cause users to experience their mental illness at an earlier age. The use may also provoke a relapse in someone who has previously suffered a psychotic episode or disorder. Also, some otherwise normal users can be thrown into a temporary but prolonged psychotic reaction or severe depression that requires extended treatment.

In addition, prolonged trips (extended LSD effects) devoid of other psychiatric symptoms have also occurred. Though very rare, these reactions can be emotionally crippling and may last for years.

A small number of users experience mental flashbacks of sensations or a bad trip they had under the influence of LSD. The flashbacks, which can be triggered by stress, the use of another psychoactive drug, or even exercise, recreate the original experience (much like the post-traumatic-stress phenomenon). This sensation can also cause anxiety and even panic since it is unexpected and the user seems to have little control over its recurrence. Most flashbacks are provoked by some sensory stimulus: sights, sounds, odor, touch, etc.

MAGIC MUSHROOMS (PSILOCYBIN and PSILOCIN)

Psilocybin and psilocin are the active ingredients in a number of psychedelic mushrooms found in Mexico, the U.S., South America, Southeast Asia, and Europe. These mushrooms were especially important to Native American cultures in Mexico and some other areas in Pre-Columbian America and were used in ceremonies dating as far back as 1000 B.C. They are still used today, although persecution by the Spaniards who conquered many Latin Countries in the 16th and 17th centuries drove the ceremonial use of them underground for hundreds of years. It wasn't until the 1950's that much was known about the ceremonies, conducted by shamans or curandera (medicine men or more often women). The ceremonies include eating or drinking the psychedelic substances to get intoxicated along with hours of chanting in order to have visions, treat illness, solve problems, or get in contact with the spirit world.

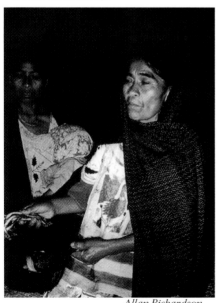

A curandera *blessing mushrooms before use in a sacred ceremony.*

Allan Richardson

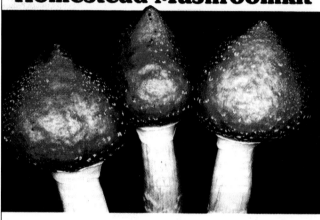

Grow Wild Mushrooms Forever With The Homestead Mushroomkit

Seven years ago, the **Homestead Book Company** introduced the first **Psilocybe Cubensis Mushroomkit**.

☐ Deluxe Psilocybe Cubensis

One of the many ads encouraging the home cultivation of mushrooms to avoid the potentially lethal problem of harvesting poisonous mushrooms by mistake.

Pharmacology

The active ingredients of the mushrooms, called Teonanacatl ("divine flesh") by the Aztecs, are found in perhaps 75 different species of mushrooms from three genera: Psilocybe, Panaeolus, and Conocybe. Fifteen species have been identified in the U.S. Pacific Northwest. Psychic effects are obtained from doses of 10 to 60 mg and generally last for 5 to 6 hours. Both wild and cultivated mushrooms vary greatly in strength, so one strong plant might have as much psilocybin as 10 weak ones. When ingested, the psilocybin is converted to psilocin, also present in the mushrooms. However psilocybin is almost twice as potent as psilocin and is more able to cross the blood-brain barrier. Its chemical structure is similar to that of LSD.

Effects

Most mushrooms containing psilocybin cause nausea and other physical symptoms before the mental effects take over. The mental effects include visceral sensations, changes in sight, hearing, taste, and touch, and altered states of consciousness. There seem to be less disassociation and panic than with LSD. Prolonged psychotic reactions are rare. However, the mental effects are not consistent and depend on the setting in which the drug is taken. In the United States, casual users of mushrooms report a sensation similar to LSD.

"We ate some of the dried mushrooms and didn't feel anything for a while then all of a sudden, we were into the sensations. We got the giggles, and visually it was like watching a strobe light show. Our vision was slowed like something would happen and then we would see it. After the first time, the trips were never as good." Ex-tripper

There is a small market in mail order kits containing spores for growing mushrooms in a closet or basement. Some users also tramp the countryside looking for a certain species. Unfortunately, the major danger in "shroom" harvesting is mistaking poisonous mushrooms for those containing psilocybin. Some of those (i.e., Amanita Phalloides) can cause death or permanent liver damage within hours of ingestion. Further, grocery-bought mushrooms laced with LSD or PCP are a common misrepresentation problem to those seeking the magic mushroom experience.

IBOGAINE

Produced by the African taber-nanthe iboga shrub, ibogaine is a long-acting psychedelic and stim-ulant. In low doses it acts as a stimulant, and in higher doses it can produce psychedelic effects and a self-determined catatonic reaction which can be maintained for up to 2 days. It is rarely found in the United States although it has been synthesized in laborato-ries. Its use is generally limited to native cultures in western and Central Africa such as the Bwiti of Gabon. They use it to help them stay alert and motionless while hunting. They also claim they have ancestral visions.

Recently there has been re-search into the use of ibogaine to treat heroin addiction. Anecdotal reports, as well as a few limited studies, claim that just a few treat-ments eliminated withdrawal symptoms and craving for opiates. The theory is that ibogaine pre-vents the increase in dopamine caused by use of heroin and co-caine. The claim is that many of the changes are permanent. Since dopamine stimulation of the re-ward/pleasure center is one of the reasons for compulsive use of drugs, the use of ibogaine in treat-ment deserves further research.

MORNING GLORY SEEDS (ololiuqui)

These seeds from the turbina (morning glory plant) or Hawaiian wood rose, contain an LSD-like substance, lysergic acid amide, in low concentration. Used by Indians in Mexico before the Spanish arrived, several hundred seeds have to be taken to get high so the nauseating properties of the drug are magnified. In sufficient quantities, the seeds cause LSD-like effects, but it is not particu-larly popular among those who use psychedelics.

Morning glory seeds are sold commercially, but to prevent mis-use, many of these seeds are dipped in a toxic substance. The seeds have names such as Heavenly Blue and Pearly Gates.

DMT

Dimethyltryptamine is a natu-rally occurring, easily synthe-sized psychedelic substance. Since digestive juices destroy the active ingredients, the drug is usually powdered and snorted or occasionally smoked. The syn-thetic form is usually put into a joint or cigarette and smoked. Occasionally it is injected.

DMT causes intense visual hal-lucinations, intoxication, and of-ten a loss of awareness of surroundings lasting about 30 minutes or less. The short dura-tion of action gave rise to the nick-name "businessman's special" for the synthetic version.

South American tribes have used it for at least 400 years. They pre-pare it from several different plants as a snuff called yopo, co-hoba, nunu, vilca, cebil or epena. They blow it into each other's noses through a hollow reed and then dance, hallucinate, and sing.

Recently, newspaper reports have sensationalized a new source of a variant of DMT, 5-MeO-DMT, the venom of the Sonoran Desert toad. Contrary to anecdotes about people licking the toad to get high, the substance is milked onto cigarettes, dried, and smoked.

YAGE

Yage, a psychedelic drink made from an Amazonian vine (ayahuasca, or "vine of the soul"), causes intense vomiting, diarrhea, and then a dreamlike condition which usually lasts up to 10 hours. The active ingredient is thought to be harmaline, an indole alkaloid found in several other psychedelic plants such as the herb, Syrian rue, from China.

Native cultures often mix yage with many DMT-containing plants in order to intensify the effects of their psychedelic drink. It has been recently discovered that harmaline protects the DMT from being deactivated by gastric enzymes thus allowing DMT to be effective when taken orally.

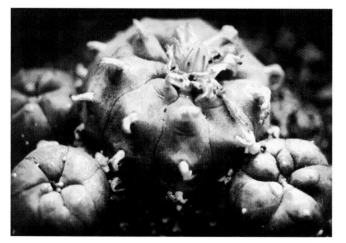

A mature peyote cactus (Lophophora williamsii) is ripe for harvesting. Each button (the top of the cactus) contains about 45 milligrams of mescaline. It can take from 2 to 10 buttons to get high.

PHENYLALKYLAMINE PSYCHEDELICS

This class of psychedelics is chemically related to adrenaline and amphetamines although many of the effects are quite different. Whereas the effects of amphetamines will peak within half an hour, much sooner if smoked, effects of henylalkylamines take several hours to reach their peak. Effects of phenylalkylamines also take longer to reach their peak than effects of indole psychedelics such as LSD.

MESCALINE (PEYOTE)

Mescaline is the active component of peyote and San Pedro cacti. They are still eaten in religious practices by the Northern Mexican tribes such as the Huichol, Tarahumara, Cora and the Southwestern Plains Indian tribes such as the Comanches, Kiowas, and Utes. In addition, the Native American Church of North America, with a claimed membership of 250,000, also uses the peyote cactus as a sacrament.

The use of peyote stretches as far back as 300 B.C. Over the centuries, the Aztecs, Toltecs, and Chichimecas and several meso-American cultures were using it for religious purposes. When the Spaniards invaded the New World and encountered the use of peyote, they regarded it as evil and the hallucinations as an invitation to the devil. They tried to abolish its use but never succeeded. In the 1800's its use spread north to the United States where about 50

North American tribes were using it in the early 1900's.

Effects

The tops of the peyote cactus are cut at ground level or uprooted. They are eaten fresh or dried into peyote or mescal "buttons." The bitter, nauseating substance is either eaten (7 to 8 buttons is an average dose) or boiled and drunk as a tea. They can also be ground and eaten as a powder. The effects of mescaline (which was isolated in the laboratory about 1890) last approximately 12 hours and are very similar to LSD with an emphasis on colorful "visions." Synthetic mescaline is thin; its needlelike crystals are sold in capsules. Users term it the "mellow LSD," but real hallucinations are more common with mescaline than with LSD. Each use of peyote is usually accompanied by a severe episode of nausea and vomiting although some users can develop a tolerance to these effects. As with most psychedelics, tolerance to the mental effects can also develop rapidly.

A peyote ceremony might consist of ingesting the peyote buttons, then singing, drumming, chanting hymns, and trying to understand the psychedelic changes in order to have spiritual experiences. Many participants also have hallucinatory visions of a deity or spiritual leader whom they are able to converse with for guidance and understanding.

Since the reaction to many psychedelics depends on the mind set and setting as much as on the actual properties of the drug, use of a mind-altering substance in a structured ceremonial setting will induce more spiritual feelings than if it's used at a rock concert. Some people would liken the difference to taking wine during the sacrament in church or during Passover as opposed to drinking a pint at a tail-gate party.

Many legal challenges have been made concerning the legality of using a psychedelic substance for a religious ceremony. In 1990, the U.S. Supreme Court ruled that the use of a psychoactive drug such as peyote during religious ceremonies is not protected by the Constitution and that states can ban its use. For this reason, many ceremonies are held in secret.

DESIGNER PSYCHEDELICS (MDA, MDMA, MMDA, MDM, MDE, ETC.)

This set of synthetic drugs uses laboratory variations of the amphetamine molecule. First discovered over 70 years ago, the drugs can cause feelings of well being and euphoria along with some stimulatory effects, side effects, and toxicity similar to amphetamines. The differences among the drugs have to do with duration of action, extent of delusional effects, and degree of euphoria. MDA was the first of these compounds to be widely abused, but in the 90's MDMA has taken over that distinction.

MDMA ("ecstasy," "rave," "XTC," "X," "Adam," "Eve," etc.)

This compound, chemical name 3,4 methylenedioxymethamphetamine, is shorter acting than MDA (4 to 6 hours versus 10 to 12 hours) and can be swallowed or injected, much like amphetamines though it is usually sold in capsule or tablet form. A capsule costs anywhere from 10 to 25 dollars and has been manufactured illegally since it was banned in 1985 by the U.S. federal government.

Physical Effects

MDMA has many stimulant effects similar to amphetamines such as increased heart rate, faster respiration, excess energy, and hyperactivity. Others claim that it has the opposite effect and calms these bodily functions. Some of this contradiction has to do with the amount ingested. The more that is used, the greater the physical effects. Since tolerance develops rapidly to its mental effects, increased doses can result in greater physical harm.

Mental Effects

Twenty minutes to one hour after ingestion, MDMA causes stimulatory and mild distortions of perception, but most often, according to some users, it calms them and increases their empathy with others. It doesn't give the visual illusions most often associated with psychedelics. It can trigger nausea, loss of appetite, and the clenching of jaw muscles. Physical dependency is generally not a problem, but as with amphetamines and cocaine, psychological dependence can cause compulsive use. If it is used daily, tolerance develops rather quickly, as with the amphetamines.

Toxicity

Major problems seen with MDMA abuse consist of a high body temperature resulting from the effects of the drug plus dehydration and physical exertion which have caused death in some users. High-dose use also results in high blood pressure, and seizure activity much like that seen in amphetamine overdose. Following an "ecstasy" experience, users have also been known to become extremely depressed and suicidal. Despite the claim that the drug does not produce major psychedelic reactions, high-dose use has resulted in an acute anxiety reaction ("bum trip," prolonged reaction, and even flashbacks).

This card, with information on drug abuse treatment, is similar to the "rave party" invitation cards.

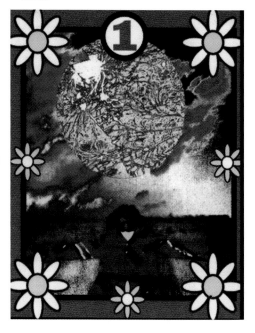

In recent experiments, it was found that MDMA damages serotonin neurons in the brain. Since it releases less adrenalin than most amphetamines, a user doesn't receive as much sympathetic nervous stimulation of heart rate and blood pressure.

"Rave Clubs"

One of the dangerous effects of MDMA, becoming overheated and dehydrated, has much to do with the way the drug is being used. Starting in 1990 in Europe, particularly in the Netherlands and England, and quickly spreading to the United States, there has been an upsurge in "rave clubs," dance and party clubs where drug taking is common. Anywhere from a few hundred to thousands of young people attend these "gatherings." Some of the clubs are legal and some are nomadic; flyers will be handed out during the week for a party at an empty warehouse that weekend. Rave clubs have become so popular that they have become a big business enterprise.

These clubs harken back to the psychedelic ballrooms of the 60's where not only light shows, the music of the times, and current hip fashions were on display, but where marijuana, LSD, amphetamine, and almost any other abused drug were common. In the "rave clubs" of the 90's, the drugs of choice are MDMA, LSD, amphetamines, marijuana, volitile nitrites, and of course alcohol. Combinations of these drugs are also being used, i.e., "ecstasy" and LSD called "X's and L's;" "flip flops," or "candy snaps;" speed-balls of "ecstasy" and heroin; "ecstasy" and methamphetamine, "ecstasy" and the so called "smart drugs" such as ephedrine or vasopressin or amino acid. Further, there has been an increasing use of other psychedelic drugs at these "raves" such as "euphoria", 2CB, CBR, and "illusion."

Since many drugs are so dependent on set and setting, the question about the upsurge in interest in MDMA and other drugs that are used in a social setting is "Do they do what proponents of the drug claim or is it just the friendly atmosphere that exists in a dance club that triggers most of the effects?" This seems to be true when stimulants are involved since users have extra energy that has to be expended. Similarly, some researchers say that MDMA helps people receive psychological insights. Opponents claim that a glass of wine or a good Alcoholic's Anonymous 12-step meeting will also provide insights.

STP (DOM) (4 methyl 2,5 dimethoxy amphetamine)

STP, also called the "serenity, tranquility, and peace pill," is similar to MDA. It causes a 12-hour intoxication characterized by intense stimulation and several mild psychedelic reactions. There are, however, reports that it is a "thicker," "duller" trip than those experienced while on mescaline or LSD. The combination of STP and LSD, called "pinks" and "purple (or orange)wedges," was popular in the late 60's but is rarely seen in the 90's. This is perhaps a good thing since the combination resulted in a high incidence of psychotic episodes in the 1960's.

ANTICHOLINERGIC PSYCHEDELICS

BELLADONNA, HENBANE, MANDRAKE, DATURA (JIMSONWEED,THORNAPPLE)

The history of these plants goes back thousands of years. From ancient Greek times to the Middle Ages, and to the Renaissance, the effects of the psychoactive substances in these plants, mostly scopolamine, hyoscyamine, and atropine, have been used in magic ceremonies, sorcery, witchcraft (black mass), and religious rituals. Belladonna, henbane, and mandrake were the plants most used. They've also been used to mimic insanity, as a poison, and even as a beauty aid by ancient Greek, Roman, and Egyptian women because they dilate pupils. In fact, "belladonna" in Latin means beautiful woman. Datura is more widely grown and references to it are found in Chinese, Indian, Greek, and Aztec history.

One of the effects of these plants is to block acetylcholine receptors in the central nervous system. Acetylcholine helps regulate reflexes, aggression, sleep, blood pressure, heart rate, sexual behavior, mental acuity, and attention. This disruptive effect can cause a form of delirium, make it hard to focus, speed up the heart, create an intense thirst, raise the body temperature to dangerous levels, and dilate the pupils. Anticholinergics also create some hallucinations, a separation from reality, and a deep sleep for up to 48 hours. They are still used today by some native tribes in Mexico and Africa. Synthetic anticholinergic prescription drugs like Cogentin and Artane, which are used to treat Parkinson's disease symptoms, are diverted and abused for their psychedelic effects. Further, even Belladonna cigarettes (Asmador), used to treat asthma, are abused by youths in search of a cheap high.

AMANITA MUSHROOMS (Fly agaric)

Most members of this family of mushrooms, except the fly agaric and the panther mushroom, are deadly. The effects of the non-poisonous ones have been described as causing dreamy intoxication, hallucinations, and delirious excitement though there are also some dangerous, physical toxic effects as well. The effects start a half hour after ingestion and can last for four to eight hours.

The amanita mushroom is mentioned in sacred writings in India in 1500 B.C. where it is referred to as the god Soma. Statues of the mushroom from 100 A.D. from Mexico indicate its early use in the Americas. Amanita has also been used by native tribes in Siberia, but its use is limited in the modern age because of the unpredictability of its effects and because many deadly mushrooms can be mistaken for it.

NUTMEG, MACE

At the low end of the "desirable" psychedelic drug spectrum, nutmeg and mace, both from the nutmeg tree, cause varied effects as mild as a floating sensation to a full blown delirium. So much has to be consumed that the user is left with a bad hangover and a severely upset stomach.

The active chemicals in nutmeg and mace are variants of MDA (methylenedioxyamphetamine). About 20 grams of brown nutmeg is still ingested by prisoners who have limited access to other psychedelic drugs. Since this dose exposes a user to the nauseating and toxic effects of other chemicals in nutmeg, its abuse is extremely rare outside prisons.

OTHER PSYCHEDELICS

PCP

Phencyclidine or PCP, also called "angel dust," "peep," "KJ," "Shermans," or "ozone," is usually misrepresented as THC or mescaline. Two other names used for PCP are "ice" and "krystal," which are also the street names for methamphetamine. Many users end up with PCP instead of the methamphetamine they were looking for, and the unexpected effects can be hazardous.

PCP was originally created as a general anesthetic for humans. However, the frequency and severity of PCP toxic effects soon limited its use to veterinary medicine. Now, the only supplies are illegal. PCP can be smoked in a joint, snorted, swallowed, or injected. Its psychic effects have been described as mind-body disassociation or sensory deprivation. It appears to distort sensory messages sent to the central nervous system. It stifles inhibitions, deadens pain, and results in an experience which has been described by users as a separation of the mind from the body.

PCP ("angel dust") comes in liquid, crystal, pill, or a powder. It is often smoked in a Sherman cigarette or sprinkled on a joint. It can also be snorted, swallowed, or injected. It is often misrepresented as THC, the active ingredient in marijuana.

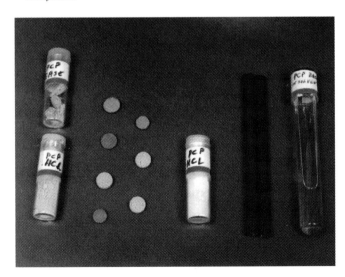

"If you smoke it, depending on how strong the joint is, you just kind of get a floating sensation about one minute after you take your first few tokes. And you get a really numbed sensation. I mean, there are actual rooms I go in that don't exist. Some people would call it a psychotic state." Recovering PCP user

Since PCP is so strong, particularly for first time users, the range between a dose that produces a pleasant sensory deprivation effect and one that induces catatonia, coma, or convulsions is very small. Low dosages (2 to 5 mg) first produce mild depression, then stimulation. Moderate doses (10 to 15 mg) can produce a desirable sensory-deprived state. They can also produce extremely high blood pressure and very combative behavior. Other adverse reactions to moderate doses include an inability to talk, a rigid, robotic attitude, tremors, confusion, agitation, and paranoid thinking. Dosages just a little higher, above 20 mg, can cause catatonia, coma, and convulsions. Large PCP doses have also produced seizures, respiratory depression, cardiovascular instability, and even kidney failure. PCP also induces amnesia in someone under its influence.

"I've had seizures before on it and banged my head really hard, continually on hard objects and got lots of bumps and everything and felt them the next few days but never felt pain while I was doing it." Recovering PCP user

The effects of a small dose of PCP will last one to two hours, but the effects of a large dose can last much longer (up to 48 hours), longer than those produced by a similar dose of LSD. Further, current evidence shows that PCP is retained by the body for several months in fatty cells. The PCP stored in fat can be released during exercise or fasting, resulting in a true chemical PCP flashback. The flashback also results because of the drug's recirculation from the brain, to the blood, to the stomach, to the intestines, then back to the blood and brain. This is called enterogastric recirculation.

PCP is not widely used by the general street population because of the frequency of bad trips associated with it. PCP is often sold as THC or mescaline to unsuspecting drug users. When the psychic effects kick in, the surprised user can have a bad trip. However, PCP can cause an emotional addiction resulting in high levels of abuse in certain populations.

In cities with large Hispanic populations, the arrests for PCP use are extremely high. Also, some studies of patients handled by Los Angeles County psychiatric emergency units found PCP in a large percentage of patient urine samples despite the fact that it was rarely reported as having been used by patients on admittance to the crisis center.

KETAMINE (Ketalar, Ketaject, Super-K)

This close relative of PCP, Ketamine, is still available by prescription. It is used as a surgical anesthetic to control severe pain such as pain from burns and is not as closely watched as other restricted drugs. It's usually injected but can be evaporated to solid crystals, powdered and smoked, snorted, or swallowed. Although it has appeared as a street drug, it is currently most often abused by veterinarians.

CANNABINOLS

MARIJUANA

The marijuana plant, also called a Cannabis or hemp plant, produces a useful fiber used to make rope, paper, an edible seed, an oil, and a number of medicines. It also produces several psychoactive substances, and various parts of the plant, including the buds (resinous flowers), leaves, and stems, can be smoked or eaten to alter the physical and mental states of the user.

Marijuana is also written about endlessly, researched in dozens of laboratories, smoked in hundreds of countries, and forbidden by thousands of laws. Add to this the fact that the street marijuana of the 90's is more potent than the marijuana of the 60's, and one can see why confusion reigns in medical, political, legal, and user circles as to the danger of the drug.

Since marijuana was declared illegal, there has been a running battle between growers or users and law enforcement officials.

Epidemiology

In the general population, 67 million Americans have tried marijuana, and 10 million use it at least once a month. Slightly more men than women smoke the drug. Monthly use by U.S. high school seniors (18-years-old) surveyed in 1990 was 14%, whereas daily use was about 2% to 3%. In 1978, the peak of marijuana use, 37% of high school seniors used it on a monthly basis.

Worldwide, according to the United Nations, marijuana in its many forms is used by more than 200 million people.

History of Use

Three uses of marijuana have determined its historical development: as a medicine, as a fiber source, and as an intoxicant. Records of its use in various medications can be found as early as 2700 B.C. in China. It was a euphoriant in 1500 B.C. in India. It was a valuable export item in the American colonies in the 18th century and during World War II. We could detail the history of marijuana and the applicable laws, but this section will focus on an objective look at the actual effects of the drug.

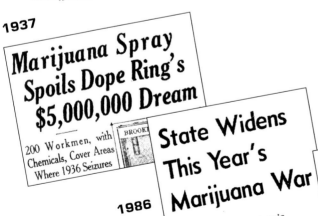

1937

Marijuana Spray Spoils Dope Ring's $5,000,000 Dream

200 Workmen, with Chemicals, Cover Areas Where 1936 Seizures

1986

State Widens This Year's Marijuana War

By Birney Jarvis

The state's Campaign Against Marijuana Planting will expand its eradication program to two more Northern Cal-

U.S. Cuts Off Medical Use Of Marijuana

1990

AIDS, cancer patients got pot from FDA for pain

By Carolyn Skorneck
Associated Press

Pharmacology

At last count, researchers had discovered 400 to 500 other chemicals in a single cannabis plant. At least 30 of these chemicals have been studied for their psychoactive effects. Further, delta 9, tetrahydrocannabinol (THC), thought to be the most psychoactive chemical in marijuana, is found to be converted into over 60 other psychoactive metabolites by the liver.

Anti-marijuana propaganda, popular in the late 30's and 40's, depicted the drug as the devil (Moloch) incarnate and its peddlers as servants of the devil. Learned men and judges are shown with their backs turned to the problem, ignoring or denying its existence.

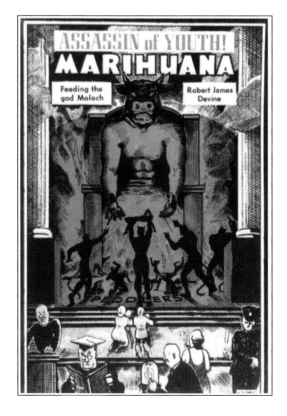

Botany

There are three species of marijuana (Cannabis); the most common, and most psychoactive, is Cannabis sativa. Another species is Cannabis indica, a plant that used to have a lower concentration of THC. New modifications have resulted in a stronger variety of this plant called "skunk weed." Cannabis ruderalis, a short species of the cannabis plant, has virtually no psychoactive ingredients.

The Cannabis sativa plant has many variants which can be grown almost anywhere in the world. The biggest change in growing methods has been the sinsemilla growing technique. Contrary to popular belief, sinsemilla is not a separate plant.

The sinsemilla technique, which involves separating female plants from male plants before pollination, is used to increase the THC concentration of any kind of cultivated Cannabis. Female plants produce more THC when unpollinated and seedless ("sinsemilla" is Spanish for "without seeds"). Male plants produce only a tiny amount of THC.

The major difference between the street marijuana of the 80's and 90's is its greater potency compared with the street marijuana of the 60's and 70's. The concentration of THC, the active ingredient, has shot up from a 1% to 3% in the 60's and 70's to 8% to 14% in the 90's. So, all the studies done in the 60's and 70's with a less potent form of the drug or with refined THC (using a weaker strength as a standard) are inaccurate and understate the psychoactive effects.

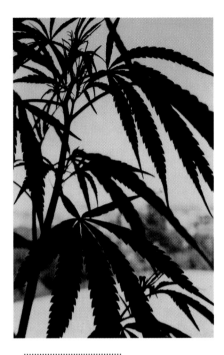

Female flowering top of Cannabis sativa with relatively long, slender leaf projections.

Marijuana leaves, flowers, and even stems can be crushed and rolled into cigarettes. They can also be used in food or in drinks. The leaves can also be chewed. In India, marijuana is divided into three different strengths, each one of which comes from a different part of the plant. Bhang is the stem and leaves with the lowest potency. Ganja is made from the stronger leaves and flowering tops, and charas, or hashish, is the concentrated resin (rich in THC) from the plant.

The sticky resin, which contains most of the THC, can be collected and pressed into cakes. This concentrated form called hashish is usually smoked in special pipes called bongs or hookahs or can be added to a "joint" to enhance the potency of leaves weaker in THC. Since hashish is more concentrated, it is easier to smuggle.

Hash oil can be extracted from the plant (using solvents) and added to foods. Most often it is smeared onto rolling paper or dripped onto crushed marijuana leaves to enhance the psychoactive effects of marijuana joints. Hash oil (red oil) can contain 20% to 30% THC.

THC has also been extracted and purified for use in medicines. Synthetic THC, Marinol, was approved for use in the U.S. in 1985, but its use is severely limited. In fact, the medicinal use of marijuana was referred to almost 5000 years ago in ancient Chinese medical texts. At the turn of the century, drug companies such as Parke Davis, Squibb, Lilly, and Burroughs Wellcome manufactured extracts of the marijuana plant for use in various medicines.

The Effects

Within 20 minutes of smoking, marijuana can induce (depending on the strength) a sedating effect in which the user is a bit confused and mentally separated from the environment. It produces a feeling of deja vu where everything seems familiar but really isn't. There is also a detachment, aloof feeling, drowsiness, and difficulty concentrating. Stronger varieties of marijuana can produce a giddiness, stimulation with increased alertness, major distortions and perceptions of time, color, and sound. Very strong doses can even produce a sensation of movement under one's feet and visual delusions.

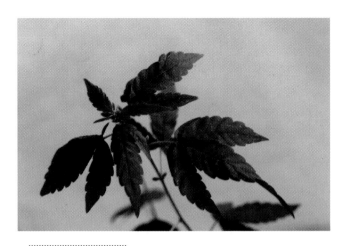

Immature Cannabis indica with shorter, stouter leafs.

"The highs are different depending on what kind it is and what kind of mood you're in. I've smoked it at times and not got high at all." Marijuana smoker

Like most psychedelics, the mental effects of marijuana are very dependent on the mood of the smoker and the surroundings. Marijuana acts almost as a mild hypnotic, exaggerating mood and personality, and making smokers more empathetic to other's feelings but also making them more suggestible.

"Sometimes you can't just let out feelings when you're straight. But if you're with your girlfriend or someone close, you can let out your feelings and talk about the way you feel." 17-year-old marijuana smoker

Marijuana can act as a stimulant or depressant depending on the variety and amount of chemical that is absorbed in the brain, but most often, it acts as a relaxant, making users sleepy, drowsy, and more inner-focused so they are less socially interactive.

"It makes time go by fast, or sometimes slows it down, depending on if you're bored." Female marijuana smoker

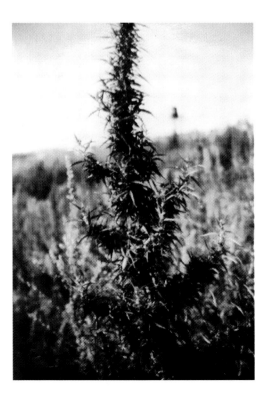

Cannabis ruderalis from Southern Siberia. Small and large fields of this species are common.

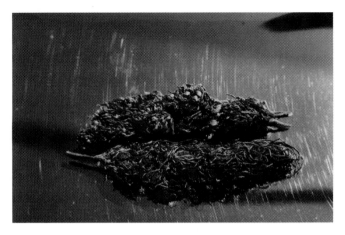

Two marijuana buds grown by the sinsemilla technique; the technique involves weeding out the male plants before pollination begins. This works because pollinated female plants quit producing the resin that contains THC.

A poster distributed by CAMP (Campaign Against Marijuana Planting). Law enforcement officials have aggressively attacked the illegal cultivation of marijuana since the early 1970's. Many growers now cultivate their crop indoors, in greenhouses and large warehouses to avoid detection.

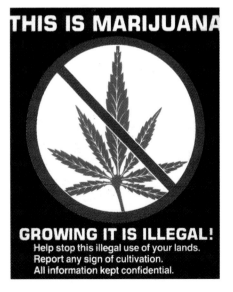

The loss of a sense of time is responsible for several of the perceived effects of marijuana. Dull, repetitive jobs seem to go by faster. In Jamaica, some cane field workers smoke ganja (marijuana) to make their hard and repetitive jobs pass by more quickly. On the other hand, high school students who smoke marijuana while studying get easily bored and often abandon their books leading to poor performance.

Marijuana also impairs tracking ability (the ability to follow a moving object, such as a baseball) and causes the trailing phenomenon where you see an after-image of a moving object. This, plus the sedation, impairment of judgment, and short-term memory loss caused by marijuana, makes it difficult to perform tasks which require multiple and interactive steps such as flying an airplane or programming a VCR.

"I don't do it when I play sports, especially serious sports, or when I'm going out with the kids at P.E. It slows you down." Teenage marijuana smoker

A major concern of health professionals is the damaging effect that marijuana smoking has on the lungs and breathing passages. A single joint contains the same amount of tar and other noxious substances as approximately 14 to 16 filtered cigarettes. These toxins irritate the throat and lungs. Frequent "pot" smoking has been associated with an increased risk of lung cancer, bronchitis, and emphysema. Some evidence also sugas a treatment for glaucoma), and decreased nausea (capsules and joints are also used for cancer patients undergoing chemotherapy).

Marijuana causes a temporary disruption of the secretion of the male hormone testosterone. That might be critical to a user with hormonal imbalance or somebody in the throes of puberty and sexual maturation. It also slightly decreases organ size in males.

Extreme reactions can lead to acute anxiety or temporary psychotic reactions when individuals believe that they have lost control of their mental state. There's often paranoia or a belief that they have severely damaged themselves or that their underlying insecurities are insurmountable.

One great concern about marijuana is the discovery that it persists in the body for up to six months after a single joint is smoked though the major effects are over within 4 to 6 hours after smoking. These residual amounts in the body may disrupt some physiological functions for a much longer period though research is skimpy on this point.

Urine tests of chronic users will test positive for THC for several months after they have quit using the drug. A casual or one-time use of marijuana may result in positive tests for several weeks. However, some users try to stretch the truth too much when they have a positive result by claiming they had one joint 6 months ago. Urine drug testing is nowhere near that sensitive. (Fig. 6-4)

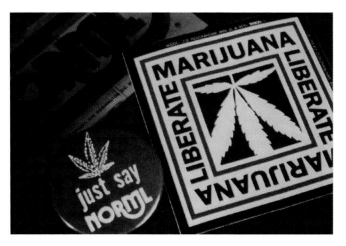

Bumper sticker, patch, and button from NORML, the National Organization for the Reform of Marijuana Laws whick began in 1971 with funding from the Playboy Foundation. It currently has chapters in 22 states. Their main goal is to legalize marijuana for medical and recreational purposes.

gests that heavy use can depress the immune system, making users susceptible to a cold, the flu, and other viral infections.

Other physical effects include an increased heart rate, decreased blood pressure, decreased pressure behind the eyes (Marinol capsules or marijuana joints are used

Fig. 6-4 *Chart shows the blood level and urine level versus time after use. Drug testing usually only measures marijuana in the urine.*

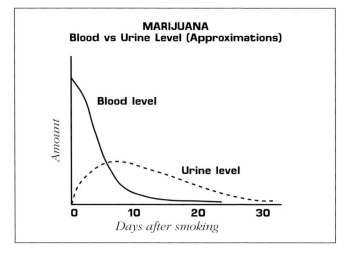

Marijuana and Learning

"If you go home and have homework to do that night and you say, 'O.K. I'm going to get stoned before I do my homework,' you're never going to get your homework done." High school student

Marijuana has been shown to slow learning and disrupt concentration. It has a specific effect on short-term memory. Short-term memory, in contrast to long-term memory, is a processing of information to be retained for only a short period of time such as a grocery list, a proper assortment of tools for a certain job, or facts crammed into the head for an upcoming exam. Marijuana greatly impairs a person's ability to retain this information. However, it has very little effect on long-term memory which is the processing of information for a long period of time such as a theory in physics that has been studied for several weeks. This explains why some honor students have been able to maintain their good grades while using marijuana on a regular basis while others end up flunking out.

"If I didn't smoke none of it when I went to school, I would have done a lot better, but if someone has some stuff you haven't had for a while and says 'What about a dubie?' you just light up some and go to class real stupid." Teenage marijuana smoker

Although more research is needed into what some researchers call an "amotivational syndrome," many chronic users show a certain apathy and lack of motivation. They have a tendency to avoid problems, which in turn delays their emotional maturation and growth.

"If you smoke a joint, then it's like there's 24 waking hours in a day. You feel every hour. If someone says, 'Look, you've got to hurry up and get this letter,' or 'You've got to hurry up and move something around,' you really don't care. It's like being on pause." Recovering marijuana user

The way this mechanism operates is similar to other drugs. What happens is that a drug is used as a shortcut to a pleasing physical sensation or to counteract boredom or emotional pain. If users then come to depend on this method for gaining pleasure or avoiding pain, rather than learning how to receive pleasure and satisfaction naturally, or face up to and deal with painful situations directly, they will habituate their minds and bodies to this course of inaction. Not only do they stand still in maturation and growth, they actually regress because the "threshold of pain" becomes less and less, and even mildly uncomfortable situations are avoided through drugs. Eventually, other coping behaviors to handle even these minor situations are "unlearned." Using drugs to deal with one's challenges to their growth results in delayed maturation.

"Before, when I had a problem, I would either have a beer, smoke a 'dubie' or run from it. I didn't face my problems, and the more that I ran, the bigger they became. And then other problems would come along and add to them. The situation escalated until I became a permanent couch potato." Recovering marijuana user

The other factor is that marijuana, thought of as "the mirror that magnifies," often exaggerates natural tendencies in the user. So, if a smoker has a slight tendency to avoid homework or cut a class, the drug will escalate that behavior.

A number of long-term users report the sensation of coming out of a fog when they finally give up daily use of grass.

"It feels good if you quit for a while. You just don't use it for a long time. It does feel better if you don't smoke it every day." Habitual marijuana user

Tolerance

Tolerance to marijuana occurs in a rapid and dramatic fashion. Although high-dose chronic users can recognize the effects of low levels of THC in their systems, they are able to tolerate much higher levels without some of the more severe emotional and psychic effects experienced by a first-time user.

"If you smoke it and smoke it, you can't get no higher after a while; it's just a waste of money." Marijuana smoker

Withdrawal

Chronic use of marijuana has now been demonstrated to cause a mild physical withdrawal syndrome. Symptoms include headaches, anxiety, depression, restlessness, sleep disturbances, change in brain waves, craving for the drug, and irritability. These problems may persist for several weeks after quitting the drug.

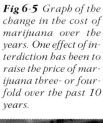

Fig 6-5 Graph of the change in the cost of marijuana over the years. One effect of interdiction has been to raise the price of marijuana three- or four-fold over the past 10 years.

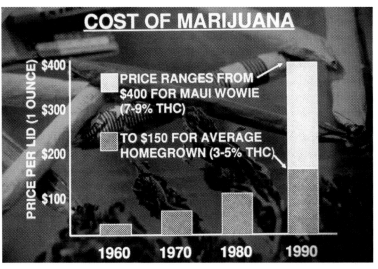

"Sometimes it burns you out to the point that you can't get up for work the next morning. It's what I call, 'the marijuana hangover.'" Factory worker

Addiction

The 1990's has made us take a different view of the addiction potential of this substance. Today, many people smoke the drug in a chronic, compulsive way and have difficulty discontinuing their use. Like cocaine, heroin, alcohol, nicotine, and other addictive drugs, marijuana does have the ability to induce compulsive use in spite the negative consequences it may be causing in the user's life. Finally, all available research on marijuana was based on a THC calculation of 20 mg per marijuana cigarette (considered in the 1960's to be a high-dose exposure). Current street "joints" are routinely analyzed to contain 40 mg or more of THC. Thus, researchers really aren't sure what they're dealing with in the marijuana of the 90's.

Is Marijuana a Gateway Drug?

In anti-drug propaganda movies like "Reefer Madness" and "Marijuana, Assassin of Youth," the claim was that marijuana physically and mentally changed the users so they became helpless addicts. The exaggeration of this idea led to an undermining of drug education because many people smoked marijuana and didn't becoming raving lunatics or depraved dope fiends. The experimenters who had tried marijuana said, 'I tried marijuana

and that didn't happen, so I guess they're lying about all the drugs."

This exaggeration and resultant ridicule, particularly by the younger generation, of propagandistic or scare films and books, probably caused more drug abuse than it prevented. It also obscured an important idea, that is, the real role marijuana use plays in future drug use and abuse.

"I used to say that everyone in my high school used marijuana, but then I realized I was only hanging around with kids who used marijuana so of course I thought everyone used. Then I talked to my brother who's straight, and he said no one he knew used marijuana. Then I realized he only hung around kids who were drug free, like himself." Highschool marijuana user

Marijuana is a gateway drug in the sense that if people smoke it, they will probably associate with others who smoke marijuana or use other drugs, so the opportunities to experiment are greater. Incidently, the history of most addicts clearly demonstrates that the first drug they ever used or abused was either tobacco or alcohol — the real gateway drugs.

ALL AROUNDERS

1. The most commonly used psychedelics are marijuana, LSD, PCP, peyote, psilocybin (magic mushrooms), and MDMA (or other variations of the amphetamine molecule).

2. A major physical effect of psychedelics, other than marijuana, PCP, or anticholinergics, is stimulation.

3. The most frequent mental effects of psychedelics are intensified sensations (particularly visual ones — illusions and delusions), mixed up sensations (synesthesia), suppressed memory centers, and impaired judgment and reasoning.

4. The effects of all arounders are particularly dependent on the size of the dose, the emotional makeup of the user, the mood at the time of use, and the user's surroundings.

5. LSD is extremely potent. Doses as low as 25 micrograms (25 millionths of a gram) can cause some psychedelic effects.

6. Like many other psychedelics, LSD overloads the brainstem, the sensory switchboard for the mind, and creates illusions and delusions.

7. Psilocybin is the active ingredient in "magic mushrooms."

8. After initial nausea or vomiting, visual illusions and a certain altered state of consciousness are the most common effects of mushrooms.

9. Mushrooms and peyote buttons have been used in religious ceremonies by many Indian tribes.

10. Mescaline is the active ingredient of the peyote cactus.

11. Eating peyote buttons or drinking them in a prepared tea causes color-filled visions and vivid hallucinations after an initial nausea and physical stimulation.

12. Belladonna and other nightshade plants contain scopolamine and atropine. In low doses, these substances cause a mild stupor, but as the dose increases, delirium, hallucinations, and a separation from reality are common.

13. PCP (angel dust) is an anesthetic, now illegal, which, besides deadening sensation, disassociates users from their surroundings and senses.

14. Effects of PCP include amnesia, extremely high blood pressure, and combativeness. Higher doses can produce tremors, seizures, catatonia, coma, and even kidney failure.

15. Marijuana, which is usually smoked, can also be eaten.

16. Current street marijuana is 3 to 7 times more potent than the marijuana of the 60's and early 70's.

17. The sinsemilla technique of growing Cannabis sativa or Cannabis indica is a major reason for the increase in potency of marijuana.

18. Smoking marijuana can cause a dreamlike effect, a certain sedation, and a mild self-hypnosis making users more likely to exaggerate their mood and react to the surroundings.

19. Some of the negative effects of marijuana are lowered testosterone levels, a decrease in the ability to do complicated tasks, a temporary disruption of short-term memory, decreased tracking ability (an impairment of eye-hand coordination), and a loss of the sense of time.

20. Large amounts of marijuana can cause anxiety reactions, paranoia, and some illusions.

21. Chronic marijuana users show a certain apathy, a tendency to neglect life's problems.

22. When stopping chronic marijuana use, one can suffer withdrawal symptoms, which include headache, anxiety, depression, restlessness, sleep disturbances, and continued craving for the drug.

QUESTIONS

1. Name five psychedelics.

2. What factors are most important in determining the effect of a psychedelic on the user?

3. What is the most common physical effect of most psychedelics?

4. What sense is most affected by psychedelics?

5. What part of the brain is overloaded by LSD?

6. What is the difference between the LSD of the 60's and the LSD of the 90's? What is the major difference in the effects?

7. What is a "bad trip?"

8. What is the best way to treat someone on a bad LSD trip?

9. What is the difference between a flash back and a prolonged trip?

10 . Where in nature is psilocybin found?

11. What is the most uncomfortable physical effect of psilocybin (magic mushrooms) and peyote?

12. From which plant is mescaline extracted?

13. What are the major effects of scopolamine and atropine?

14. What are the major effects of a low-dose of PCP? What about a moderate to high-dose?

15. What is the biggest difference between a marijuana cigarette from 1970 and one from 1993?

16. What are hashish and hash oil?

17. What are the known negative effects of marijuana?

18. Does tolerance to marijuana develop?

19. What are the withdrawal effects when chronic use of marijuana is stopped?

20. What is the "trailing" phenomena?

21. What is synesthesia?

22. Describe the differences between an illusion, a delusion, and a hallucination.

23. List four dangers which result from the use of "ecstasy," (MDMA).

24. Name five drugs which are often abused at "rave" parties.

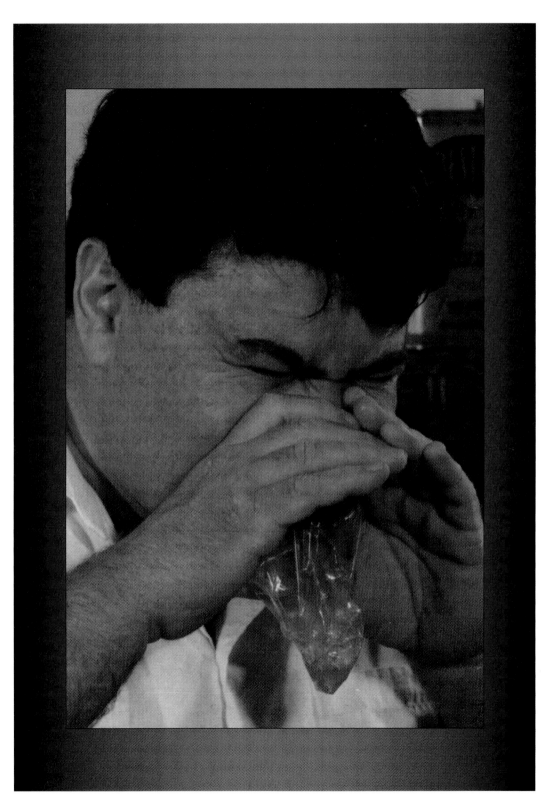

A "huffer" inhales the fumes from an organic solvent in a plastic bag.

CHAPTER 7

INHALANTS
AND OTHER
DRUGS*

By Michael Holstein, Ph.D.

1986

Odorizer Nitrites' AIDS Link Studied

By JOHN BRENNAN

This column has previously warned about the misuse of room odorizers (as a supposed sexual stimulant). The active ingredient in these products is a volatile nitrite, the most popular being isobutyl nitrite. These nitrites are similar to, but not the same as, nitrites used in the treatment of heart problems. They are marketed under various names (which I am purposely not listing). Side effects of these products include: dizziness, headache, irregular heartbeat, fainting, low blood pressure and increased eye pressure. These nitrites have also been associated with severe blood problems.

1894

GAS ALWAYS ON TAP.

An Office Where Nitrous Oxide Gas
Is Regularly Administered
to Patients.

CALLED COMPOUND OXYGEN.

Analysis Made for the Herald Shows
Two-Thirds Nitrous
Oxide.

INTRODUCTION

Inhalants include a number of substances that are either gases, liquids that give off fumes, or aerosol sprays. Inhalants are different than substances which are heated or burned and then smoked. Inhalants are used for their stupefying and intoxicating effects although excess use can produce slight psychedelic effects. Sometimes they are classified as deliriants. The practice of abusing an inhalant is called "huffing," and the users are called "huffers."

The three main types of inhalants are organic solvents, volatile nitrites, and nitrous oxide. These gases and liquids, especially the organic compounds, are present in a wide variety of substances found around the home, in the garage, and in the workplace. Organic solvents are used in glues, gasoline, plastic cement, varnish remover, paints, paint thinner, lighter fluid, and nail polish remover. The nitrites used to be sold over-the-counter as so called "room fresheners," and nitrous oxide is still used as an anesthetic or aerosol propellant. Some aerosols, which can be sprayed to produce a foggy mist, are inhaled for their gaseous propellants rather than their primary contents.

Inhalants are absorbed through the lungs into the blood stream, which carries chemicals rapidly to the brain. Their intoxicating effects are often quick-acting (7-10 seconds), intense, and short lived, lasting no more than 30 minutes to an hour. Some only last a couple of minutes.

HISTORY

The practice of inhaling gaseous substances to get high goes back to ancient times. The Greek oracle at Delphi was said to breathe in vapors from the earth before uttering her prophecies. In the Judaic world, burnt spices, gums, herbs, and incense were inhaled during religious ceremonies, a practice shared by other Mediterranean, African, and Native American peoples.

Our modern version of inhalant abuse began in the late 1700's with the discovery of nitrous oxide ("laughing gas"), chloroform, and ether. Later, at the turn of the 20th century, when petroleum began to be refined and manufactured into new products such as solvents, thinners, and glues, many more substances began to be inhaled for their intoxicating or euphoric effects. Shortly after World War II, the abuse of glue and metallic paints rose dramatically, particularly in the U.S. Midwest and in Japan. Huffing has persisted as a drug abuse problem into the 1990's where inhalants are responsible for up to 1,200 deaths each year in the United States.

EPIDEMIOLOGY

Since inhalants, especially organic solvents, are readily available and inexpensive, they provide a cheap, quick high, especially for those who are young and/or poor. However, middle-class, urban, and health care professionals also abuse inhalants.

"In college we'd have `Whippet' parties where someone would go and get 6 or 7 of those small nitrous oxide cylinders and we'd pass them around. By the time it came around again, you'd be down from the giddy, stupid feeling."
25-year-old ex-student

In a recent survey asking respondents whether they had ever used an inhalant, the most frequently abused substances were typewriter correction fluid, glue, gasoline, and spray paints. When a mixture of substances is involved, the solvents toluene and trichloroethylene are the most frequently involved ingredients.

"We got a 911 call about a kid in a coma. It seems that three of them were inhaling a waterproofing spray, and this one kid did too much. Basically he starved his head for oxygen because the spray temporarily replaced the oxygen. It took him 3 months to fully recover." Emergency medical technician

Use by Sex and Age

Generally, more young people than adults abuse inhalants in the 1990's, and among 12- to 17-year-olds, more young women than young men. In older populations, more men abuse than women, and the numbers of overall abusers decline by 2/3 or more after the age of 25.

Overall, about 1 million Americans are currently using inhalants, and about 10 million have tried them. Use in the United States is heaviest in the West, followed by the South, Northeast, and North Central.

Ethnically, earliest use is highest among Hispanics and lowest among whites.

Besides price and availability, the other reasons people use an inhalant are

- The packaging is convenient and doesn't look illegal;

- The substances themselves are generally legal;

- The high comes on quickly and leaves the body almost as quickly;

- It's a temporary substitute for more expensive drugs like marijuana, LSD, or even alcohol.

FORMS OF INHALATION

Although there have been reports of people spraying aerosols onto bread and eating the bread, or inserting small bottles of inhalants such as typewriter correction fluid into their nostrils, the more common forms are

- Sniffing: breathing in the inhalant directly from the container; sniffing puts the vapor into the lungs in contrast with snorting which puts solids (cocaine, for example) in contact with the mucosal lining of the nose;

- Huffing: soaking a rag with dissolved inhalant, putting the rag in one's mouth, and inhaling; also, inhaling from a solvent-soaked rag;

- Bagging: placing the inhalant in a plastic bag, covering the nose and/or mouth with the bag, and inhaling;

Fig. 7-1 Percent of Americans who have used inhalants.

NIDA Household Survey on Drug Use 1992

Age	Ever Used	Used Last Year	Used Last Month
12-17	1,171,000	701,000	338,000
18-25	2,737,000	652,000	237,000
26-34	3,505,000	409,000	149,000
35 & up	2,372,000	276,000	162,000

• Spraying: spraying the inhalant directly into the nasal or oral cavity.

Directly ingesting and spraying inhalants are particularly toxic methods. They expose a user's fragile membranes to the caustic effects of these substances, put a harmful amount of pressure into the lungs, and even cause a physical freezing effect as the substances vaporize quickly, taking heat from everything around them.

"In the classes I take care of, we have a problem with kids soaking their collars with this waterproofing spray and then getting loaded in class by sniffing them. It is a cheap high for 4th graders who can't afford other drugs." Kansas elementary school nurse

ORGANIC SOLVENTS

These solvents are called "organic" because they are carbon and hydrocarbon-based compounds. Refined from petroleum, they are used as fuels, aerosols, and solvents, and they include such common materials as gasoline and kerosene; paints, paint thinners, and lacquers; nail polish remover; spot removers; glues and plastic cements; lighter fluid; and a variety of aerosols.

These organic solvents are quick-acting because they are absorbed into the blood almost immediately after being inhaled, and then they move to the liver, brain, and other tissues. Some solvents are exhaled by the lungs, in which case a tell-tale odor from the inhalant remains on the breath. Other solvents are excreted by the kidneys.

Inhaling these substances produces a temporary stimulation and reduced inhibitions before the central nervous system (CNS) depressive effects begin: dizziness, slurred speech, unsteady gait, and drowsiness are seen early on. Impulsiveness, excitement, and irritability may also occur.

"I asked this kid who came into the office if he sniffed gas, and he got indignant and said, 'I don't sniff it, I huff it.' This kid reeked of gas fumes, answered in words of one syllable, and had dropped out of school at the age of 14. He was really unkempt and dirty. If something radical doesn't happen in terms of his accepting treatment, I don't think he'll make it to the age of 18." High school drug counselor

If, because of high dosage or individual susceptibility, the CNS becomes more deeply affected, illusions, hallucinations, and delusions may develop. The user may experience a dreamy stupor culminating in a short period of sleep. The effects resemble alcohol or sedative intoxication (inhalant abuse has been called "a quick drunk"), though psychedelic effects may also occur, depending on the inhalant.

The intoxicated state may last from minutes to an hour or more, depending on the kind and quantity of substance inhaled. Headaches and nausea may follow as part of an inhalant hangover. After prolonged inhalation, delirium with confusion, psychomotor clumsiness, emotional instability, impaired thinking, and coma have been reported. Both low-level and acute or high-level exposure to organic solvents usually involve reversible brain and neurologic effects.

Chronic abuse is characterized by lack of coordination, loss of weight, weakness, inability to concentrate, and disorientation. Since chronic abuse can involve extremely high concentrations of fumes, sometimes thousands of times higher than industrial exposure, mental and neurologic effects may be irreversible, though not usually progressive after abuse ceases. For example, chronic abuse of toluene can result in dementia, spasticity, and other CNS dysfunctions, whereas occupational exposure to toluene has not produced similar effects.

Complications may result from the effect of the solvent or other toxic ingredients such as lead in gasoline. Injuries to the brain, liver, kidney, bone marrow, and particularly the lungs can occur and may be from either heavy exposure or from individual hypersensitivity. Death occurs from respiratory arrest, cardiac arrhythmias, or asphyxia due to occlusion of the airway. Some of these substances have been shown to produce cancerous growths, especially those of the blood, when used chronically.

Toluene

Probably the most abused solvent, toluene is a component of many substances — glues, drying agents, solvents, thinners, paints, inks, and cleaning agents. Chronic abuse can affect balance, hearing, eyesight, and, most often, neurological functions and cognitive abilities. In one study of chronic abusers of toluene in spray paint, 65% had neurologic damage. Heavy use results in deafness, trembling, and dementia.

Trichloroethylene

This is the most common solvent used in typewriter correction fluids, paints, and spot removers. Like the other organic solvents toluene and acetone, this substance causes overall depression effects and moderate hallucinations. The toxic effects are similar to those of toluene.

Gasoline

Gasoline sniffing, common among solvent abusers especially on Native American reservations, introduces various components of gasoline into the system, including solvents, metals, and

....
Some of the more common organic solvents are spray paint, typewriter correction fluid, glue, and spot remover.

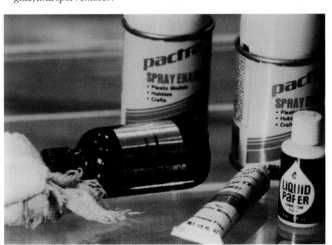

chemicals. Symptoms include insomnia, tremors, anorexia, and sometimes paralysis. When leaded gas is inhaled, symptoms can also include hallucinations, convulsions, and chronic, irreversible effects of lead poisoning.

Warning Signs of Possible Inhalant Abuse of Organic Solvents

Especially in the early stages, inhalant abuse is difficult to spot. Here are some signs of possible abuse:

— chemical odor on body and clothes, or in room;
— red, glassy or watery eyes, and dilated pupils;
— slurred speech;
— staggering gait and lack of coordination;
— inflamed nose, nosebleeds, and rashes around nose and mouth;
— loss of appetite;
— intoxication;
— seizure.
— coma.

Source: Drug Enforcement Administration

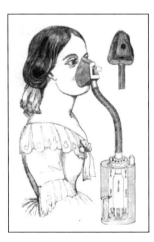

....

This mask was used by genteel inhalers at oxygen or nitrous oxide parties in the 1800's.

ANESTHETICS

In 1772, Joseph Priestly discovered nitrous oxide. "Inhalant parties," featuring the euphoric effects of the gas, were held. Humphrey Davy, a noted physician of his day, noticed at one of these parties that the gas had pain-killing ability and recommended it be used as an anesthetic during surgery. The euphoric effects of this and other gases such as chloroform, ether, and oxygen were sought starting in the 1800's. Abuse of nitrous oxide was even reported among Harvard medical students in the 19th century.

Abuse continues today by young experimenters as well as among middle class and affluent groups, including dentists, doctors, anesthesiologists, hospital workers and health-care professionals who abuse nitrous oxide, halothane, and other anesthetics like ether, ethylene, ethyl chloride, and cyclopropane.

Nitrous Oxide

Currently available in large blue painted gas tanks for dental offices where it is used as an anesthetic and in bakeries where it is used as a propellant in whipping cream aerosol cans and small metal cylinders, nitrous oxide is abused for its mood-altering effects. Within 8 to 10 seconds of inhalation, the gas produces a giddiness and stimulation often accompanied by silly laughter. The maximum effect lasts only two or three minutes. There is a buzzing or ringing in the ears along with a sense that one is about to collapse or pass out. These feelings quickly cease when the gas leaves the body.

Gas cartridges (capsules) of nitrous oxide, sold for whipping cream but often diverted to the inhalant abuser were sold with the trade name "Whippets." Their sale is severely restricted now.

"This one kid's dad was a dentist so he'd rigged some deal where he got this "blue nun," this 4-foot tank of nitrous oxide from the office. He filled a bunch of balloons with the gas and we'd pass them around and breath it in." 20-year-old

Fig. 7-2 INHALANTS

PRODUCT	CHEMICALS
Organic Solvents and Sprays	
Airplane glue	Toulene, ethyl acetate
Rubber cement	Toulene, hexane, methyl chloride, acetone, methyl ethyl ketone, methyl butyl ketone
PVC cement	Trichloroethylene
Paint sprays	Toulene, butane, propane, fluorocarbons, hydrocarbons
Hair sprays, deodorants	Butane, propane, fluorocarbons
Lighter fluid	Butane, isopropane
Fuel gas	Butane
Dry cleaning fluid, spot removers, correction fluid, degreasers	Tetrachloroethylene, trichloroethane trichloroethylene
Polish remover	Acetone
Paint remover/thinners	Toulene, methylene chloride, methanol
Local anesthetic	Ethyl chloride
Analgesic/asthma sprays	Fluorocarbons
Gasoline	Gasoline (leaded or unleaded)
Volatile Nitrites	
Room odorizers, "Locker Room," "Rush," "Quicksilver," "Bolt," "poppers"	(Iso)amyl nitrite, (iso)butyl nitrite, isopropyl nitrite
Nitrous Oxide	
Whipped cream propellant, Whippets, laughing gas, "Blue Nun," "nitrous"	Nitrous oxide
Other Anesthetics	
Chloroform	Chloroform
Ether	Ether

Dangers from the abuse of nitrous oxide if inhaled directly from a pressurized tank, include exploded or frozen lung tissue and frostbite of the tips of the nose and vocal cords. This risk is minimized when the gas is inhaled from a balloon inflated with the gas. Long-term exposure can cause central and peripheral nerve cell and brain damage due to lack of sufficient oxygen in the blood since nitrous oxide replaces the oxygen. Symptoms of long-term exposure include numbness, loss of balance and dexterity, and weakness and numbness in the arms and legs. Also, there is the danger of passing out and getting hurt from the fall. Further, nitrous oxide use can lead to physical dependence.

Halothane

Halothane is a prescription surgical anesthetic gas, sold under the trade name Fluothane. Its effects are therefore extremely rapid and powerful enough to induce a coma for surgery. Because of its limited availability, it has been most often abused by anesthesiologists and hospital personnel.

Isobutyl and butyl nitrite, sold under various trade names from the 1970's, were some of the first successful designer drugs. For example, a prescription drug, amyl nitrite, was chemically rearranged to create a legal derivative and sold as a room odorizer to circumvent drug laws.

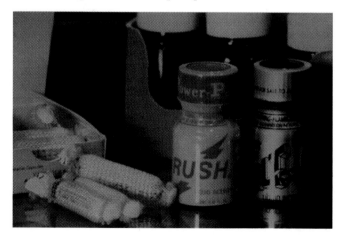

VOLATILE NITRATES

Amyl nitrite has been used medically for over a century to relieve heart-related chest pains. Amyl nitrite as well as butyl and isobutyl nitrite dilate blood vessels, so the heart receives more blood. Other effects include a rush of blood to the brain and the relaxation of smooth muscles in the body. Effects start in 7 to 10 seconds and last for about 30 to 60 seconds. Blood pressure reaches its lowest point in 30 seconds and returns to normal at 90 seconds.

"My friend used to use poppers at 'raves' because he thought it helped his dancing, made him more lively, but instead he got dizzy, fell over, and broke his nose. He was the 'rave' of the evening." 17-year-old "raver"

On inhalation, there is a feeling of a fullness in the head and a "rush" similar to that felt with nitrous oxide. There is also a mild euphoria. (First-time users have reported feeling panic attacks.) This may be followed by severe headaches, dizziness, and giddiness. A tolerance develops rapidly to the gas, though excessive, prolonged use may cause nitrite asphyxiation, and possibly death. An increase in heart rate and palpitations make nitrite inhalation risky. First aid for the headaches includes abstinence. Overdose requires that respiration and blood flow be maintained, occasionally CPR, and, if a person passes out, elevating the feet higher than the head.

Nitrites are thought to enhance sexual activity and are sought after especially by urban male homosexuals, for both their euphoric and physiological effects which include relaxation of smooth muscles such as the sphincter muscle. Repeated use may impair the immune system and thus increase susceptibility to HIV infection. There is some evidence that nitrites inhibit the functioning of the white blood cells and that the activity of these killer cells is suppressed. In addition, nitrites may change some body chemicals into carcinogens.

OTHER DRUGS

It's amazing what substances and methods people will use to get high: inhaling typewriter correction fluid, drinking hair tonic, eating nutmeg, ingesting C4 (a plastic explosive), smoking herbal medicines, and swallowing antihistamines. Steroids, cough suppressants, over-the-counter diet pills, and even ginseng root are also abused. It's not only the inherent qualities of the drug but also society's attitude toward the substance that determines which drugs are available for abuse. For example: heroin was prescribed as a cure for alcoholism and even morphine addiction. Cocaine was available in soda pops (e.g. Coca-Cola) to "perk us up" until it was restricted in 1914. Marijuana growing and its medicinal use were legal until 1938.

And then there's the imagination of street chemists who can either synthesize drugs that were once legally available such as Quaaludes, PCP, and Fentanyl or can create il-

legal drugs such as MDMA, MDE, and cathinone (synthetic khat). The danger, of course, is that street drugs have not been tested and are not made under any kind of control so irregular doses, unexpected effects, or contaminants in the manufacturing process can have a disastrous effect on the unsuspecting user.

For example, in the 80's, a group of heroin users who had supposedly been sold a synthetic Demerol derivative, MPPP, were later found to have an 80% incidence of Parkinson's disease symptoms (rigid muscles, loss of voluntary body control) caused by contamination of the drug with MPTP, a byproduct of sloppy synthesis in the laboratory. In addition, the strength can be dozens of times stronger than the expected dose leading to overdoses such as those that occurred in 1993 in Baltimore, where street Fentanyl killed thirty people. As more and more untested synthetic drugs produced by illicit chemists hit the street, we can expect to witness more tragedies like the MPTP nightmare or the Baltimore overdoses.

MISCELLANEOUS DRUGS

Camel Dung

Some Arab countries produce hashish by force feeding ripe marijuana plants to camels. Their four chambered stomachs compact the marijuana into hashish camel dung.

C4 Explosive

Modern veterans have been known to ingest C4 or cyclonite plastic explosives for their psychedelic effects. Tremors and seizure activity can result but usually not an explosion as it takes a blasting cap to set off the chemical.

Embalming Fluid (formaldehyde)

Mortuaries have been broken into and robbed of their embalming fluid. It can either be directly abused (inhaled for its depressant and psychedelic effects) or it can be used in the manufacture of other illicit drugs. Some users soak marijuana joints or cigarettes in the fluid and smoke it. Called "clickers," "clickems," or "Sherms," the mixture gives a PCP-like effect. Formaldehyde, the main ingredient of embalming fluid is a known carcinogen.

Gasoline

In spite of the toxicity of leaded or unleaded gasoline, a few kids and adults have been known to mix it with orange juice and drink it; they call it "Montana Gin." The life expectancy of these abusers is particularly short.

Ginseng Root

Ginseng has been used for thousands of years as an herbal tonic or health aid. Today, the plant extract is also used to help develop muscles rapidly. The root does contain small amounts of anabolic steroids but can cause blood problems in massive doses.

Kava Kava

The roots of the South American Piper Methysticum plant are chewed or crushed to a soapy liquid and drunk. The milky exudate of the root contain at least 6 chemicals (alpha pyrones) that produce a drunken state similar to that of alcohol to the observer. Users claim that the effects are more pleasurable, relaxing, and psychic than alcohol without the hangover. Since saliva seems to be an important ingredient in the preparation of this drug, its use has not found popularity.

Raid, Hair Spray, and Lysol

Abusers puncture the aerosol cans, draining out the liquid, which they swallow mainly for their alcohol content. These items are rarely abused in the general population, but find more use in rural, isolated areas where access to alcohol is limited.

M-99

M-99 is a powerful, injectable opiate which is 400 to 1,000 times stronger than morphine, sold under the trade names of M-99 or Immobilion. This drug is used in veterinary practices to immobilize large animals. Its abuse seems limited to the veterinary professionals since it is highly toxic. In fact, when it is abused, the user will also have a needle into a vein, ready to administer the antidote, Narcan.

Dextromethorphan (Robitussin D.M., Romilar, and other cough syrups)

This chemical has been known to be a psychedelic compound for twenty-five years. A full 6 ounces of the liquid is ingested to get a proper dose of dextromethorphan. This also provides the user with 6 ounces of up to 20% alcohol so the effects are that of a drunken deliriant.

SMART DRUGS

Higher I.Q. points in a pill? Better long-term memory in a "health drink"? Smart drugs ("SD's") are the drugs, nutrients, drinks, vitamins, extracts, and herbal potions that manufacturers, distributors, and proponents think will boost intelligence, improve memory, sharpen attention, and increase concentration, detoxify the body, especially after alcohol or other drug abuse, and energize the user. Proponents range from AIDS activists to health faddists, New Agers, anti-aging questors, and members of the technoculture who feel they are on the edge of a new field of mental development. Consumers of smart drugs are estimated to number 100,000, with 10,000 the estimate given for smart-drink users.

For some consumers, smart drinks are non-alcoholic, usually a mixture of vitamins or powdered nutrients and amino acids in fruit drink purchased in a "smart bar" for $4 to $6 or at a health foods store. More recently, smart drinks and drugs have contained combinations of medications usually prescribed for Parkinsonism, Alzheimer's disease, or dementia. It is felt that these drugs more effectively rebalance the brain after abusing drugs, for instance MDMA during a "rave," and will also slow or reverse the aging process. The consumers are typically young (17-25) urban students or professionals looking for an intellectual edge or more stamina to work or party harder.

Vitamin supplements and nutrient products, once purchased through ads in New Age magazines, are now sold through health-food stores. Critics of these supplements and products attribute their success to either a placebo effect (only the expectation, not the product produces the effect) or the caffeine or sugar that is part of the ingredients.

Americans have begun to import powerful pharmaceuticals called "nootropic" drugs ("nootropic" means "acting on the mind") from Europe where many can be purchased that are not yet approved by the Food and Drug Administration (FDA) for sale in the U.S. Critics of these and other prescription drugs, including researchers, doctors, and the FDA, point out that, at the very least, claims for the efficacy of the drugs have not been substantiated. Advocates argue that since these and other smart drugs improve mental ability for people suffering from debilitating mental disorders, they can enhance mental capacity in normal people too.

Fig. 7-3

Active Ingredient	Trade Name
Prescribed for debilitating mental disorders (FDA approved)	
ergoloid mesylates	Hydergine
selegiline hydrochloride	Eldepryl
phenytoin	Dilantin
vasopressin	Diapid
Prescription drugs (not FDA approved)	
piracetam	Nootropil
aniracetam	Draganon
fipexide	Attentil
vinpocetine	Cavinton
Lucidril	

SMART DRINKS, made with amino acids such as
phenylalanine
choline
taurine
l-cysteine
l-carnitine
Arginine
Tryptophan

OTHER SMART NUTRIENTS
ephedra
ginkgobiloba
ginseng
kelp
sarsaparilla

POLYDRUG ABUSE

"Alcohol was the great buffer for coke. Pills were also good, but booze ... because coke is such a social thing and so is alcohol, the two just mix so beautifully together. For me, my drinking just came alive at that time, and it was usually never one without the other."
Cocaine/alcohol abuser

Polydrug use and abuse can be intentional or accidental. The user might want to exaggerate or temper the effect of a drug, or the doctor, treating a patient for a variety of illnesses with different medications, might forget about such factors as drug synergism, cross dependence and cross tolerance. People can overdose or become addicted to doses of a drug that are usually too small in and of themselves to cause problems. For example, people who drink alcohol find that they are having trouble with sleep and take a sedative. They would have an increased liability of addiction or overdose to both drugs. And though each drug works on different parts of the brain, the physical addiction comes from the combination of the drugs' effects. In fact, most studies of drug abusers in this country show that addicts abuse a multitude of different drugs that are available to them. They may have a preference for cocaine but will take alcohol, Valium, heroin, marijuana, or any sedative to help them deal with the hyperactivity caused by cocaine.

REVIEW

INHALANTS AND OTHER DRUGS

1. The three main types of inhalants are organic solvents, volatile nitrites, and nitrous oxide.

2. Volatile solvents consist of fluids such as gasoline, kerosene, airplane glue, nail polish remover, lighter fluid, carbon tetrachloride, and even embalming fluid.

3. The effects of volatile solvents, mostly depressant, include dizziness, stupor, and slurred speech. Impulsiveness and irritability give way to hallucinations and delusions. Eventually, delirium, clumsiness, and impaired thinking occur.

4. Prolonged use of volatile solvents, especially leaded gasoline, can lead to brain, liver, kidney, bone marrow and especially lung damage. Death can occur from respiratory arrest or cardiac irregularities.

5. Volatile nitrites, "poppers" such as butyl or isobutyl nitrite, are sold as Bolt, Rush, and Locker Room. The major effects are muscle relaxation and blood vessel dilation causing a blood rush to the head. Dizziness and giddiness also occur. Too much can lead to vomiting, shock, unconsciousness, and blood problems.

6. Nitrous oxide, usually used as an anesthetic in the dentist's office, produces a temporary giddiness that lasts for just a couple of minutes. Inhaling directly from the tank can cause frozen lung tissue and blown out lungs.

7. Other substances used to get high have included embalming fluid, gasoline in orange juice, hair spray, and even camel dung.

8. Smart drugs are a mixture of vitamins, powdered nutrients, and amino acids. Some prescription drugs used to treat diseases of aging such as Parkinson's Disease or Alzheimer's Disease are also used.

QUESTIONS

1. What are the three main types of inhalants?

2. Name three different types of volatile solvents.

3. Name three different volatile nitrites.

4. What are the major effects of volatile solvents?

5. What are the major effects of volatile nitrites?

6. Name three unusual drugs that people use to get high.

7. What are the usual ingredients of smart drugs?

8. What is a "speedball"?

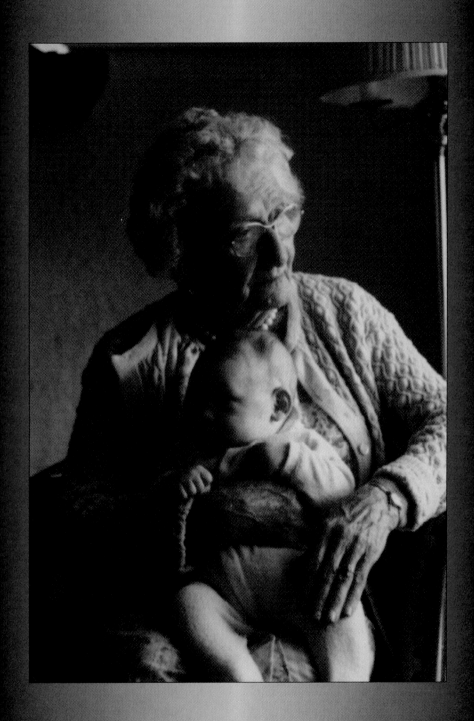

CHAPTER
8

CRADLE
TO GRAVE

1984
Study of Smoking's
Effect on Fetuses

nant women — a treatment group
that was counseled to stop or cut
down on smoking and a control
group that was only observed.

altimore

A 2½-year study of preg-
nant women has provided
strong new evidence
cigarette smoking is harm-
to the fetus, researchers
yesterday.

The study, conducted on 935
nant women in the Baltimore
showed women who stopped
smoking while pregnant
uced infants significantly
birth to longer than newborns
er and who continued smoking
bers who continued smoking
eir usual level, researchers said.

"I think this is very strong ev-
that the fetal growth is reed by maternal smoking,
Sexton, an associate professor
University of Maryland
ool of Medicine and co-author
study, financed by the National
tutes of Health.

Women were selected who
smoked at least 10 cigarets a day
before their pregnancy. They represented a broad range of race, education, income and age.

Sometime during their pregnancies, 20 percent of the contro
group and 43 percent of the treat
ment group quit smoking. Nineteen
percent of the treatment group an
13 percent of the control group ru
down on smoking.

The results showed that the in
fants born to mothers in the treat
ment group had a mean birt
weight of 3278 grams — 92 gram
heavier than the control group b
mothers in the group babies were
treatment group babies were 0.
centimeters greater in length.

1993
Population Shift
In HIV Infections

**39% of people with the virus
are minorities, survey shows**

*By Sabin Russell
Chronicle Staff Writer*

In another indication of the
changing demographics of the
AIDS epidemic, a new San Francisco survey estimates that 39
percent of those infected by HIV
are members of minority groups.

Since the start of the AIDS epidemic a decade ago, the overwhelming majority of cases in San
Francisco have occurred among
gay white men.

The latest survey shows that
gay white men continue to represent the most cases of full-blown
AIDS, but that racial minorities

number of cases that had actual
progressed to AIDS — a proce
that can take 10 years.

In 1993, the city Department
Public Health reported that mino
ities represented 25 percent of a
tual AIDS cases — a snapshot
the AIDS epidemic now. The ne
report — showing a 39 perce
HIV infection rate — shows whe
the epidemic is heading.

The new report is consiste
with the findings of earlier studi
revealing high rates of unsafe se
among young gay blacks and la

1980
How medicines can
turn the elderly
into drug abusers

By Susan Paynter

INTRODUCTION

The biggest change in drug abuse over the past 30 years is the gradual lowering of the age of first drug use. In 1992, a national survey by the University of Michigan found that although high school seniors were in general reducing their illicit drug use, 8th grade use was slowly rising. One indication is that 11.2 % of eighth graders reported trying marijuana in 1992, up from 10 % the year before. In addition, 10.8% tried stimulants such as amphetamines up from 10.3% a year ago, and 9.5% tried inhalants. The use of alcohol though is still the number one problem.

Psychoactive drugs are used at every age:

- The fetus absorbs her mother's cocaine (through the umbilical cord);

- The 8-year-old tries some scotch at the household bar;

- The 14-year-old smokes marijuana after class;

- The college student uses "speed" to stay awake for an exam;

- The mother with 3 kids hides in her room and smokes a rock of crack;

- The office worker takes a Valium to be able to put up with her job;

- The 50 year-old salesman smokes and drinks because he's bored;

- And the 74-year-old borrows his neighbors pain-killers to relieve his own arthritic pain and anxiety over his health.

Fig. 8-1 National Institute of Drug Abuse Household Survey 1992

Age Group	Ever Used	Used Past Year	Used Past Month
12-17 21 million			
Illicit Drug	16.5%	11.7%	6.1%
Cigarettes	33.7%	18.2%	9.6%
Alcohol	39.3%	32.6%	15.7%
18-25 28 million			
Illicit Drug	51.7%	26.4%	13.0%
Cigarettes	68.7%	41.1%	31.9%
Alcohol	86.3%	77.7%	59.2%
26-34 38 million			
Illicit Drug	60.8%	18.3%	10.1%
Cigarettes	74.8%	38.8%	33.7%
Alcohol	91.7%	79.0%	61.2%
35 & up 118 million			
Illicit Drug	28.0%	5.1%	2.2%
Cigarettes	76.8%	28.8%	25.3%
Alcohol	87.0%	62.6%	46.5%
Total 205 million			
Illicit Drug	36.2%	11.1%	5.5%
Cigarettes	71.0%	31.2%	26.2%
Alcohol	83.0%	64.7%	47.8%

The other point to note about the survey is the prevalence of alcohol and tobacco use. In comparison, the use of the illicit drugs might seem minimal, but like the proverbial bull in a China shop, the 12 million Americans who used illicit drugs in the past month have an exaggerated effect on all levels of society especially in regards to economic loss, crime, and violence.

It is important to understand that drug use and abuse occur at all ages, so any treatment, education, or prevention program should be continued throughout a person's lifetime: teaching pregnant mothers not to use; showing 8-year-olds how alcohol affects their studying; educating a college athlete on the health effects of amphetamines or steroids; teaching young people about the synergistic interactions of drugs; letting the Valium user know about withdrawal convulsions; getting a drinking salesman to use an employee assistance program; enlightening senior citizens as to the dangers of borrowing or mixing medications; and teaching all ages about natural highs, the most gratifying way to rectify the emotional turmoil or boredom that causes most people to abuse drugs.

In this chapter we will examine the consequences of drug use during pregnancy, in school, on the job (includes a section on drug testing), and by the elderly. We will also examine the most dangerous consequence of drug use, AIDS.

PREGNANCY

by Anthony J. Puentes, M.D.

OVERVIEW

Drug and alcohol use during pregnancy is a growing national problem. The number of infants with drug and alcohol-related birth defects has increased dramatically over the past several years. For example, in the San Francisco Bay Area, there has been a five to tenfold increase in the number of babies born addicted to drugs such as heroin, cocaine, and PCP. One 1992 survey at San Francisco hospitals showed that 65 babies per month are born toxic for "crack" at birth, and most of the mothers have had no prenatal care, so when they come in, in some cases, they're coming in ready to deliver.

Drug abuse during pregnancy occurs in women of all ethnic and socio-economic backgrounds. A recent national study indicates that 11% of all pregnant women in this country are using drugs like alcohol, cocaine, crack, marijuana, sedatives, heroin, amphetamines, and PCP. Fetal Alcohol Syndrome (FAS) is the third most common birth defect and the leading cause of mental retardation in the United States.

Medical research has established that most psychoactive substances, when ingested during pregnancy, may be harmful to the developing fetus. The exposure of a fetus to harmful drugs is an issue of critical concern, and the problems associated with substance abuse during pregnancy are now beginning to be understood.

Maternal Complications

Drugs and alcohol abuse during pregnancy puts women at high risk for a long list of medical and obstetrical complications during pregnancy. Anemia, sexually transmitted diseases, hepatitis, and poor nutrition are among the most common. The use of intravenous drugs, such as heroin or amphetamines, puts women at risk for other complications such as endocarditis (a heart infection), or even fetal death. The use of contaminated needles further increases the risk of a woman's becoming infected with the AIDS virus and passing the disease to her fetus. Eighty percent of children with AIDS in the United States were born to mothers who were or are I.V. drug abusers or sexual partners of I.V. drug abusers. The life expectancy of an infant born with AIDS is less than two years.

Multiple drug use is now commonplace and can further complicate a pregnancy. A typical pregnant drug addict is in poor health and presents herself for treatment late in pregnancy. She often has had no prenatal care or medical intervention and often lives a chaotic lifestyle.

Fetal and Neonatal Complications

Since psychoactive drugs are able to cross one of the most impervious barriers of the body, the blood-brain barrier, they can easily cross the placental barrier, the membrane separating the baby's and the mother's blood (Fig. 8-2). So, when a pregnant woman uses drugs, her fetus will also be exposed to the same chemicals. In addition, many drugs can pass into a nursing mother's breast milk and expose a developing infant to dangerous chemicals.

Because of the infant's or fetus's metabolic immaturity, each surge of effects from the psychoactive drug that the mother receives may be prolonged in the fetus. Thus, psychoactive drugs can be expected to cause greater problems for the fetus than for the mother.

Medical research on the effect of drugs on the fetus is extremely difficult to perform and has only been seriously undertaken in the last 10 to 15 years. Knowledge is being accumulated through inference from animal research and observations of women who have admitted to drug use or have been in treatment for drug abuse during pregnancy.

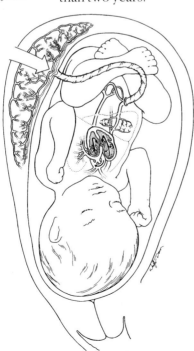

Fig. 8-2 *The developing baby and its circulation are protected by the placental barrier which screens out agents that would affect the fetus. All psychoactive drugs breach this protective barrier and affect the baby usually more than the mother, particularly when the drug is stored in the amniotic fluid.*

The health of the fetus can be affected by a variety of maternal, fetal, and environmental factors. Factors such as maternal age, health, genetics, or stress certainly play a role in influencing the ultimate development of the newborn. Fetal physiology and genetics, as well as environmental exposure to elements such as radiation, drugs, or other dangerous chemicals, can all cause an abnormal fetal development.

It is very difficult to isolate a single drug's effect from a variety of other factors when explaining a complication in fetal development. Certainly, polydrug exposure can further complicate the picture.

The period of maximum fetal vulnerability is the first twelve weeks. During this first trimester, development and differentiation of cells into fetal limbs and organs take place. This is when drugs pose the greatest risk to organ development.

The brain and nervous system develop throughout the entire pregnancy and beyond. Thus, the fetal nervous system is vulnerable to damage no matter when a woman uses drugs.

The second trimester involves further maturation of the already developed body parts. Drug exposure at this stage in pregnancy creates a risk of abnormal bleeding or spontaneous abortion.

The third trimester involves maturation of the fetus and preparation for birth. Dangerous drugs such as heroin or cocaine can cause severe withdrawal in the fetus and perhaps premature birth.

Since drugs can have such a magnified effect on the fetus throughout pregnancy, it is crucial that a pregnant woman abstain from all unnecessary drug exposure.

An additional complication happens because the fetal metabolism is very immature compared to that of the mother. As a result, drugs can persist in the fetus for a longer period of time and in higher concentrations than in the adult. Drugs like Valium or cocaine and their metabolites may remain in the fetus's or newborn's system for days or even weeks longer than in the mother. Withdrawal or intoxication in a baby born exposed to PCP may last for days, weeks, or even months after birth.

The problems of fetal drug exposure extend beyond the period of pregnancy. Definite syndromes of neonatal withdrawal, intoxication, and developmental or learning delays have been attributed to a variety of drugs, including alcohol.

Long-term Effects

Research is still being done on the long-term effects in drug-exposed children when they enter school. Symptoms range from mental retardation and convulsions in the most extreme cases, to poor muscular control and cognitive skills, hyperactivity, difficulty concentrating or remembering, violence, apathy and lack of emotion. Many of the effects are reversible, but the cost of the intensive care that is needed is high. In Los Angeles which has special educational programs for drug affected babies, the cost to educate one student is $15,000 per year compared to $4,000 per year to educate an average child.

SPECIFIC DRUG EFFECTS

Despite the difficulties with scientific research on the fetal effects of drug use during pregnancy, medical scientists have identified a variety of specific prenatal and postnatal symptoms and conditions due to alcohol and other psychoactive drugs.

Alcohol

Fetal Alcohol Syndrome (FAS) and Fetal Alcohol Effects (FAE) are well documented in the literature. Fetal Alcohol Syndrome is the third most common cause of mental retardation in the United States.

The Fetal Alcohol Syndrome produces a number of well-defined abnormalities and occurs in the babies of chronic alcoholic women who drink heavily during pregnancy. FAS abnormalities occur in three categories:

- Growth retardation in almost 50% of all FAS cases;

- Central nervous system abnormalities, including developmental and mental retardation in all cases;

- Structural abnormalities consisting of characteristic facial, skeletal, and organ defects.

Growth defects have been seen in infants of mothers who drank even moderately during pregnancy. Significantly decreased birth weights have been observed among infants born to women who averaged only one ounce of alcohol per day during pregnancy.

Neurological damage and mental retardation are permanent, and average IQ's are in the low 60's. Structural abnormalities consist of smaller head size, short eyelids, defective midfacial tissue, abnormal creases in the palms of the hand, and defects in the walls separating the heart chambers.

Five to forty-one percent of FAS infants also have minor abnormalities of the joints, benign tumors of blood vessels, ear defects, drooping eyelids, cleft palates, and smaller eyes and fingernails.

FAS children have a growth rate about two-thirds of the norm, though this may even out as they approach adolescence.

Fetal Alcohol Effects (FAE) refers to the occurrence of negative effects on the fetus but not necessarily all the characteristics described in FAS.

To answer the question of how much alcohol intake is required to produce FAE or FAS, several studies have attempted to define a safe level of alcohol intake during pregnancy. Some recent studies indicate that alcohol use greater than nine shots per day of 100 proof whiskey, or about one and a half bottles of wine per day, increases the frequency of all ab-

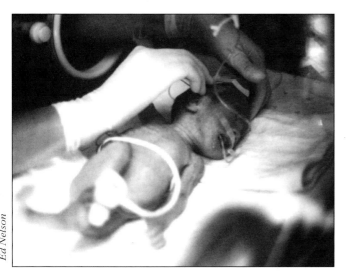

Ed Nelson

....

When babies are born prematurely, whether due to drugs or natural forces, the cost of intensive neonatal care is thousands of dollars a day (often paid for by the government).

....

In 1988, Federal legislation mandated the posting of alcohol warning labels in restaurants and stores that sell liquor, cautioning pregnant women of the dangers of drinking during pregnancy.

normalities associated with fetal alcohol syndrome. Alcohol consumption of as little as one ounce twice a week has been associated with a significant increase in spontaneous abortions.

Alcohol withdrawal in the mother may cause premature labor, whereas alcohol consumption up to and even during labor has resulted in increased nausea and vomiting, low blood pressure and blood sugar, and depression in both mother and newborn.

Alcohol withdrawal can also occur in the addicted newborn resulting in irritability, restlessness, agitation, and increased chance of neonatal mortality. Nursing mothers also pass alcohol to their babies in their breast milk which can result in sedation and lethargy in the infant.

Despite an array of research studies, the exact relationship between alcohol dose and fetal outcome is unknown. However, most physicians now agree that there is no known safe amount of alcohol use during pregnancy. Abstinence is considered the only safe approach.

Cocaine and Amphetamines

With the increasing, widespread use of cocaine, particularly smokable cocaine (crack, free base), and now intravenous use, there has been a dramatic increase in cocaine-affected newborns. In the United States, there are 600,000 regular cocaine users. One third are women (and the number is increasing yearly) with an average

age in the early twenties, the most fertile childbearing years. One can only assume that a large number of these women use cocaine during pregnancy.

> *"My one-year-old was born toxic. She had crack in her system and the hospital called CPS (Child Protective Services), and they kept her, and then I figured it was time for me to stop this. I went into recovery a month after that." 24-year-old recovering crack user*

Currently, in some parts of the country, up to 60% of substance-exposed newborns are born to cocaine or amphetamine-abusing mothers. Even more alarming is the recent disclosure that as many as 20% to 25% of babies born in county hospitals of large metropolitan areas are born cocaine affected. In Hawaii, 20% of the delivering mothers use "ice," smokable methamphetamine. Research on the effects of cocaine and amphetamines during pregnancy is limited. Nevertheless, some definite conclusions can already be drawn.

Cocaine and amphetamines are both strong stimulants. They result in markedly increased heart rates and constriction of blood vessels. These effects, in turn, cause dramatic elevations in blood pressure in both mother and fetus. Rapid fluctuations in both maternal and fetal blood pressure can have serious consequences.

Constriction of blood vessels will result in a decreased blood and oxygen supply to the placenta and fetus. An impaired blood and oxygen supply can result in retarded fetal development. Increased maternal and placental blood pressure can result in a premature separation of the placenta from the wall of the uterus. This abnormal separation, or *abruptio placenta,* has been reported several times, presumably as a result of the acute hypertension associated with cocaine use. An *abruptio placenta* will result in an acutely critical situation, usually resulting in spontaneous abortion or premature delivery. *Abruptio placenta* can be a life-threatening situation for both mother and fetus.

Acutely elevated blood pressure in the fetus can cause a stroke in the brain of the fetus even before it is born. Fetal blood vessels in the brain are very fragile and may be easily damaged as a result of exposure to cocaine. In fact, cases of *in-utero* stroke and postnatal seizures have been reported with cocaine use during pregnancy.

Third trimester use of cocaine can induce sudden fetal activity and uterine contractions within minutes after ingestion. Women have been rushed to the hospital in premature labor shortly after using cocaine.

New research suggests that cocaine exposure during the first trimester only may be as harmful as cocaine exposure throughout pregnancy.

Infants who have been exposed to cocaine during pregnancy often go through a withdrawal syn-

Cocaine Use Linked To Infant Defects

New York

Animal experiments suggest that cocaine use during pregnancy can produce infants with long-term abnormalities in the brain systems that control sensation, movement and emotions, a researcher said yesterday.

This occurs despite the frequent absence of physical defects in the offspring, said Diana Dow-Edwards, a researcher at the State University of New York Health Science Center in Brooklyn.

ing in the infants of cocaine-using mothers.

For example, Chasnoff said, "it appears that these infants are probably having an increased rate of seizures in the neonatal (newborn) period." That could be due to a hypersensitivity in the brain similar to what Dow-Edwards has observed in rats, he said.

Chasnoff also reported that infants of cocaine-using mothers have a significantly smaller head size than normal infants, suggesting a retardation in brain growth.

1988

drome characterized by extreme agitation, increased respiratory rates, hyperactivity, and occasional seizures. These babies are tremulous and deficient in their ability to interact with their environment. They are highly irritable and difficult to console. These effects may be due to drug withdrawal, intoxication, or both.

Cocaine and amphetamine-exposed babies are often growth retarded and may have smaller heads. There are reports of cocaine babies born with abnormalities of the genito-urinary tract and with severe intestinal disease. Studies are currently under way to investigate abnormal sleep and breathing patterns in these high-risk newborns.

The cost of caring for a cocaine exposed baby is over $11,000, almost 4 times the cost of caring for a normal baby.

Current research with cocaine-exposed newborns indicates that many of these infants show typical patterns of neurobehavioral

disorganization, irritability, and poor language development. Many of these abnormal neurobehavioral effects improve over the first three years of life. Studies suggest that 60% to 70% of children prenatally exposed to cocaine will have normal behavior by the age of three.

Opiates & Opioids

Opiate and opioid drugs such as heroin, morphine, codeine, Demerol, Dilaudid, Percodan, methadone, etc. and others have been shown to have negative impacts on pregnant women and their babies. For example, pregnant heroin addicts have greater risk for miscarriages, *abruptio placenta*, still-births, and severe infections from intravenous needle use such as endocarditis, septicemia, hepatitis, and, of course, AIDS.

Babies born to heroin-addicted mothers are often born prematurely and are smaller and weaker than normal. Heroin addicted newborns often go through a period of withdrawal sickness referred to as the Neonatal Narcotic Withdrawal Syndrome. Prenatal exposure to heroin has also been associated with abnormal neurobehavioral development. These infants have abnormal sleep patterns and are also at greater risk for Sudden Infant Death Syndrome (SIDS).

Pregnant women addicted to opiates will go through several periods of drug withdrawal each day. These withdrawal periods alternate with "rushes" following each drug injection. These dramatic fluctuations are believed to be harmful to the fetus and contribute to the variety of maternal/fetal complications.

If a mother becomes truly addicted to opiates, so does the fetus. After birth, and depending on a variety of factors such as the mother's daily dose of drugs, other drug use, and other narcotic use, opiate exposed infants may exhibit the Neonatal Withdrawal Syndrome. Narcotic withdrawal in a newborn may appear shortly after birth or take 7 to 10 days to develop.

Manifestations of the Neonatal Narcotic Withdrawal Syndrome include hyperactivity, irritability, incessant high-pitched crying, increased muscle tone, hyperactive reflexes, sweating, tremors, irregular sleep patterns, increased respiration, uncoordinated and ineffectual sucking and swallowing, sneezing, vomiting, diarrhea, and other symptoms. In severe cases, failure to thrive, seizures or even death may occur. These withdrawal effects may be mild or severe and may last from days in mild cases to months in severe instances.

Most cases of neonatal narcotic withdrawal can be treated with good nursing care, swaddling, and normal maternal/infant bonding behaviors. Only in severe cases is medication for the infant required. Opiates have been found in breast milk in sufficient concentration to expose newborns.

PCP

As with other psychoactive drugs, PCP (phencyclidine) readily crosses the placental barrier and exposes the developing fetus to its effects. Worse, PCP seems to concentrate in amniotic fluid (the fluid that surrounds the fetus in the womb) and may actually expose the fetus to greater concentrations of the drug than those in the rest of the mother's body.

Some people store PCP in fat tissue which can release the drug days, months, and even years later, causing an actual chemical "flashback" and toxic effects. Thus, a mother who may have given up the drug before getting pregnant, still bears a small risk of passing the drug on to her baby during pregnancy.

Very little is known at this time of the effects of PCP on a developing or newborn infant. This is partially because PCP is a relatively new drug (significant abuse dates only to the 1970's). Additionally, PCP is often misrepresented as other drugs. The mother may not even be aware of her PCP use. It has been sold as THC, mescaline, psilocybin, Quaalude, and cocaine as well as many other substances with exotic nicknames, making it difficult to recognize.

Finally, PCP-using mothers are often polydrug users, making it difficult to isolate the effects of PCP alone.

The characteristics of PCP-exposed babies include intense irritability, emotional liability with inconsolability, abnormal muscle tone, tremors, inability to coordinate simple motor tasks, and abnormal response to stimuli. Follow-up studies of these children show continued irritability, difficulty with motor coordination, and, occasionally, slow development. Long-term studies of older PCP exposed children suggest abnormalities in attention span, organizational abilities, and learning abilities. Most studies, however, are only preliminary. Some infants have been born with extremely toxic levels of PCP in their blood and have had major developmental and behavioral disorders through early childhood.

Marijuana

Research into the effects of marijuana on pregnancy is severely lacking, and it is assumed that the incidence of marijuana use by pregnant women is grossly underestimated. In fact, most marijuana-exposed newborns go undetected.

Studies have reported reduced fetal weight gain, shorter gestations, and some congenital anomalies. In fact, women who use marijuana and drink heavily were found to be five times more likely than marijuana non-users to deliver babies with features similar to those identified as part of the Fetal Alcohol Syndrome.

Marijuana use can cause a more difficult labor and delivery compared to the labor and delivery of non-using mothers. Studies of marijuana use by pregnant women have demonstrated increased incidence of premature labor, prolonged or arrested deliveries, abnormal bleeding, increased Caesarean deliveries, abnormal fetal tests, meconium staining (fecal release by the fetus in the womb), and the need for manual removal of the placenta.

Researchers have also found neurological abnormalities, indicating nervous system immaturity in the newborns of regular marijuana users. These babies had abnormal responses to light and visual stimuli, increased tremulousness, "startles," and a high-pitched cry typically associated with drug withdrawal. However, unlike infants undergoing narcotic withdrawal, marijuana babies were not excessively irritable.

Further, one must remember that marijuana today much more potent, by THC concentration, than marijuana of the early 1970's. The research data available at this time has been based upon a high daily marijuana THC dosage of 20 mgs. per joint. The usual street joint of high-grade marijuana today contains 40 mgs of THC, twice the concentration of the test dose. New research using higher concentrations is needed to reevaluate the risk of marijuana on pregnancy and the fetus.

Prescription Drugs

Over-the-counter and prescribed medications are clearly the most common drugs used by pregnant women. It has been estimated that at least two thirds of all pregnant women take at least one drug during pregnancy, usually vitamins or simple analgesics such as aspirin.

Physicians must be especially careful when prescribing medications to treat conditions such as maternal discomfort, anxiety, pain, or infection. Studies have shown a variety of prescription drugs to be harmful to the human fetus. Sedatives-hypnotics are among the most studied of these drugs.

Drugs such as Valium or Xanax (benzodiazepines) freely cross the placental barrier and because of the immature fetal metabolism, accumulate in the fetal blood at levels much greater than in maternal blood. This phenomenon will occur at dosages that are normally safe for the mother alone. Besides high fetal concentrations of the drug, excretion is also slower. The drugs and their metabolites will remain in the fetal and newborn systems days or even weeks longer than in the mother, resulting in dangerously high concentrations of the drug leading to fetal depression, abnormal heart patterns, or even death.

Studies have indicated an increased risk of cleft lip and/or cleft palate when Valium was used in the first 6 months of pregnancy. Other, less common anomalies have also been noted. Of special interest is the fact that some researchers have found that women who combined cigarette smoking with sedative use had a 3- to 7-fold increased risk of delivering a malformed infant compared to those who smoked but did not use sedatives.

A newborn addicted to benzodiazepines may exhibit a variety of neonatal complications. Infants may be "floppy" and have poor muscle tone, or they can be lethargic and have sucking difficulties. A withdrawal syndrome, similar to narcotic withdrawal, may also result. These manifestations of withdrawal may persist for weeks.

Because Valium and its active metabolites are excreted into breast milk, it has been implicated as a cause of lethargy, mental sedation/depression, and weight loss in nursing infants. Since Valium can accumulate in breast-fed babies, its use in lactating women is ill-advised.

Certain anticonvulsants such as Dilantin are now believed to markedly increase a pregnant woman's chance of delivering a child with congenital defects. Antibiotics such as the tetracyclines can cause a variety of adverse effects on fetal teeth and bones and can result in other congenital anomalies.

Nicotine

Smoking during pregnancy is particularly dangerous because tobacco smoke contains more than 2,000 different compounds including nicotine and carbon monoxide. Both have been shown to cross the placental barrier and reduce the fetal supply of oxygen.

The percentage of female smokers in the overall population has steadily increased from 5% in the 1920's to about 35% in the 1980's. By comparison, smoking by males has decreased from 50% to about 35% during the same period of time.

Since the 1930's, it has been known that nicotine and its major metabolite, cotinine, can cross the placental barrier and show up in the amniotic fluid. Further, cotinine has also been detected in the amniotic fluid of non-smoking women (although in much smaller amounts) as a result of their passive exposure to smoking by others.

Recent studies now indicate that women smokers with a heavy habit are about twice as likely to miscarry and have spontaneous abortions as non-smokers. Nicotine damages the placenta and has adverse effects on the developing fetus as well. Stillbirth rates are also higher among smoking mothers.

As with many other psychoactive substances, smoking decreases newborn birthweights. Babies born to mothers who smoke heavily weigh on the average 200 grams (7 oz) less, are 1.4 centimeters shorter, and have a smaller head circumference compared to babies from non-smoking or non-drug-abusing mothers. **It is estimated that if cigarette smoking during pregnancy were eliminated, the infant mortality rate in the U.S.A. would decrease by 30%.**

Although the incidence of physical birth defects is very low in babies born to smoking mothers, there is still a significant increase in some birth defects. Specifically, cleft palate and congenital heart defects occur more frequently with smoking mothers. Smoking results in increased carbon monoxide and carboxyhemoglobin in the mother's blood. This decreases the oxygen capacity of blood and can potentially result in some minor brain and nerve defects which may be hard to detect. Several studies have shown that nicotine is toxic and creates lesions in that part of animal brains which controls breathing. This has been suggested as a possible reason for the increase in "Sudden Infant Death Syndrome" (crib death) seen in babies born to mothers who smoke heavily.

Babies born to heavy smokers have been shown to have increased nervous nursing (weaker sucking reflex) and possibly a depressed immune system at birth resulting in more pneumonia and bronchitis, sleep problems, and less alertness than other infants.

Long-lasting effects of smoking exposure before birth can be retarded development and slowed maturation. Reading, math comprehension, language skills, psychomotor tasks, and IQ test scores of these children lag behind those skills in other children even up to the age of one. There has also been some research that links mothers who smoke excessively to an increased incidence of hyperactive offspring.

Treatment Issues

Clearly, the potential problems of alcohol, tobacco, and drug use during pregnancy suggest that women with a drug problem should ask advice and seek professional help as soon as possible.

The numerous problems facing these women must all be dealt with to insure a healthy outcome for both mother and infant. The proper treatment of substance abuse in pregnant women requires a comprehensive approach from a variety of health care and social service providers as well as a desire on the woman's part to become drug free, begin recovery, and to protect her baby.

> *"I ended up getting pregnant, but into my pregnancy I started using, and it brought me to the hospital with false labor and from there they told be about the MAMA project (Moving Addicted Mothers Ahead) for mothers that have a problem. That was me. I came, and I've been here ever since. And it's been a great help." Recovering crack user*

Intervention is necessary to reduce alcohol and drug related birth defects. Providing specific services (e.g., methadone treatment for pregnant heroin addicts) attracts the pregnant woman to treatment early in pregnancy, thus providing access to essential medical care, parenting training, drug abuse counseling, and referral to other services. Abstinence from all mood-altering chemicals is viewed as an integral part of recovery.

As a result of a heightened awareness of the problem of drug abuse in pregnant women, various programs are now emerging in the United States that specifically treat the pregnant drug user/addict. Unfortunately there are still inadequate resources to help treat all women in need. It is hoped that in the years to come, more private and public funding will be made available to help this population of mothers and infants.

1989

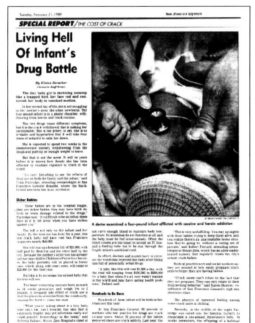

Fig. 8-3
MATERNAL/FETAL/NEONATAL EFFECTS OF DRUGS
COMMONLY ABUSED BY PREGNANT WOMEN

UPPERS

AMPHETAMINES/METHAMPHETAMINES, AMPHETAMINE CONGENERS, DIET PILLS
Mother: Central nervous system (CNS) stimulation, i.e increased heart rate, blood pressure, respiration, anorexia, weight loss, insomnia. Decreased blood flow to placenta. Risk of AIDS with I.V. use.
Fetus: Possible growth retardation and fetal hypoxia.
Neonate/infant: Possible withdrawal or intoxication; low birth weight; increased rate of Sudden Infant Death Syndrome (SIDS). (Adequate studies are lacking.)
Long-term: Long-term effects not known.

COCAINE (crack, freebase, etc.)
Mother: CNS and cardiovascular stimulation: increased heart rate and blood pressure, vascular constrictions; decreased blood flow to placenta; possible placental abruption and bleeding, premature labor.
Fetus: Possible retardation, fetal hypertension and distress; risk for intra-uterine stroke, possible genito-urinary abnormalities, necrotizing enterocolitis.
Neonate/infant: Intoxication and or withdrawal symptoms: irritability/agitation, increased tone, tremors, jitters, inconsolability, increased respiration, risk for seizures; slower drug excretion in newborn; abnormal sleep and ventilatory patterns; increased rate of SIDS.
Long-term: Possible developmental delays; possible long-term neuro-behavioral deficits.

CIGARETTES, SNUFF, CHEWING TOBACCO (nicotine and other compounds in smoke)
Mother: CNS stimulation, respiratory, cardiovascular damage; cancer.
Fetus: Reduced fetal oxygen supply; impaired fetal growth, increased risk for fetal distress and fetal demise, increased risk for spontaneous abortion and premature labor.
Neonate/infant: Growth retardation, smaller head circumference; risk for congenital palate and heart defects; abnormal nursing; increased risk of SIDS.
Long-term: Long-term effects not clear.

CAFFEINE (Coffee, tea, colas, over-the-counter medications)
Mother: Nervousness, irritability.
Fetus: Slight chance of spontaneous abortion, still birth.
Neonate/infant: Decreased birthweight.
Long-term: Long-term effects are not known.

DOWNERS

OPIATES & OPIOIDS (opium, codeine, morphine, heroin, Dilaudid, Percodan, methadone, Darvon, Demerol, Talwin)
Mother: Tolerance, CNS depression; risk for AIDS and other infections with I.V. drug use; acute withdrawal and risk for spontaneous abortion or premature labor.
Fetus: Intra-uterine growth retardation; risk of AIDS and other infections from mother.
Neonate/infant: Addiction and neonatal narcotic withdrawal syndrome including hyperactivity, irritability/agitation, high pitched cry, increased tone, tremors, seizure risk; poor feeding; abnormal sleep and ventilatory patterns; increased risk of SIDS; AIDS risk.
Long-term: Possible long-term neuro-behavioral deficits.

SEDATIVE-HYPNOTICS - BENZODIAZEPINES, BARBITURATES
Mother: Tolerance, CNS depression; respiratory depression; acute withdrawal with risk of premature labor.
Fetus: Drug accumulates in fetus at levels greater than in mother; fetal depression, abnormal heart rhythm, or even death; increased risk for cleft lip/palate.
Neonate/infant: Drug and metabolites may remain in newborn for days or weeks longer than in mother; may result in lethargy, poor muscle tone, sucking difficulties, or even CNS depression; withdrawal may occur.
Long-term: Long-term effects are still under study.

ALCOHOL (beer, wine, hard liquor)
Mother: Tolerance; CNS and respiratory depression; risk for seizures; organ damage to liver, heart, nerve cells/CNS, stomach, etc.; alcohol withdrawal may cause hypertension, tachycardia, premature labor.
Fetus: Possible abnormalities in growth and development. May result in FAS ("fetal alcohol syndrome") or FAE, ("fetal alcohol effects").
Neonate/infant: FAE and FAS symptoms: growth retardation, CNS abnormalities including developmental and mental retardation, and structural abnormalities including characteristic facial, skeletal, and organ defects; possible CNS depression and withdrawal with irritability, restlessness, agitation, and increased risk of neonatal mortality.
Long-term: Mental retardation, developmental delay, low IQ.

ALL AROUNDERS

MARIJUANA (THC)
Mother: CNS depression, but can act as a stimulant; toxic to respiratory system and immune system; increased heart rate, hypotension; may cause more complicated labor and delivery including prolonged or arrested deliveries, abnormal bleeding, meconium staining, etc.
Fetus: Reduced fetal weight gain, shorter gestation, come congenital anomalies.
Neonate/infant: Some neurological abnormalities because of CNS immaturity i.e., abnormal responses to visual stimuli, tremulousness, high pitched cry.
Long-term: Long-term effects are not known.

PCP (phencyclidine)
Mother: Hallucinations, CNS depression (some stimulation); agitation; may complicate labor and delivery.
Fetus: Likely damage to CNS development.
Neonate/infant: Intoxication and/or withdrawal; serious neurological and behavioral defects such as inconsolability, intense irritability, abnormal state control, abnormal muscle tone, tremors, inability to coordinate simple motor tasks, sensory input problems; microcephaly.
Long-term: Developmental delays; abnormalities in attention span and organizational abilities; possible learning problems; studies are preliminary.

LSD
Mother: Hallucinatory and stimulatory effects; may complicate labor and delivery.
Fetus: Likely damage to CNS development.
Neonate/infant: Effects not clearly known yet.
Long-term: Long-term effects not clearly known.

Fig. 8.4   1992 Drug Use in the U.S.

There are 21 million 12- to 17-year-olds
There are 28 million 18- to 25-year-olds

DRUG	Age	Ever Used	Past Year	Past 30 Days
Legal Drugs				
Alcohol	12-17	39%	33%	16%
	18-25	86%	78%	59%
Cigarettes	12-17	34%	18%	10%
	18-25	69%	41%	32%
Smokeless	12-17	10%	5%	3%
Tobacco	18-25	22%	9%	6%
Illicit Drugs				
Any Illicit	12-17	17%	12%	6%
Drug	18-25	52%	26%	13%
Marijuana	12-17	11%	8%	4%
	18-25	48%	23%	11%
Presc. Drug	12-17	6%	4%	1%
incl. stim.	18-25	15%	8%	2%
(illicit use)				
Inhalants	12-17	6%	3%	2%
	18-25	10%	2%	1%
Hallucinogens				
	12-17	3%	2%	1%
	18-25	13%	5%	1%
Cocaine	12-17	2%	1%	.3%
	18-25	16%	6%	2%
Stimulants	12-17	2%	1%	.2%
	18-25	7%	2%	1%
Heroin	12-17	.2%	.1%	.1%
	18-25	1%	.5%	.2%
Anabolic	12-17	.3%	.2%	.1%
Steroids	18-25	.7	n.a.	n.a

National Institute of Drug Abuse Household Survey

YOUTH AND SCHOOL

In spite of all the headlines about "crack," LSD, and MDMA ("ecstasy") use among adolescents, the most serious drug problem by far is still alcohol. Tobacco is a close second, and marijuana third, followed by prescription drugs, inhalants, hallucinogens, cocaine, heroin, and steroids.

"In high school we'd have 'keggers.' We found out whose parents wouldn't be home, have a keg delivered, and have the party there. In college, the drug scene was a little different; besides the alcohol, you could get a better selection of drugs: opium, hashish, mescaline, peyote, LSD, but mostly just marijuana. We were too poor in high school for those." 19-year-old college sophomore

A 1992 survey of college students found that their use of drugs almost coincided with the 18- to- 25-year olds with most percentages only slightly lower. A problem with surveys about illicit drugs is that many users lie about their use even when assured that the survey is confidential particularly if the survey is taken in front of parents. What has been found is that most figures on current or frequent use of illicit drugs in high schools and colleges are underreported.

"We were supposed to put on a skit about drugs, and the minute we sat down we said, 'Now what do the parents want to hear about that?' That's the general attitude all my friends have in dealing with these programs, 'What do the parents want to hear from us?' And a lot of the people teaching these drug programs are also telling us what the parents what us to hear. It's all very stereotypical." 15-year-old high-school student

How Serious Is the Problem

Several ideas present themselves when we look at the figures about drug use in young people. First, of course, is the prevalence of alcohol and tobacco with all their attendant health consequences. The second thought is that, "Gee, these other figures don't seem too high." That's true if 900,000 12- to- 17-year-olds currently using marijuana is not significant. And although the use of alcohol and tobacco far outweighs the use of the other drugs by 2, 5, or even 10 to one, the social, emotional, legal, and financial consequences of illicit drug use can be quite disruptive or destructive.

"A kid we knew stuck a gun in his mouth, maybe to show off, and blew his brains out. There was a question as to whether he was just fooling around or really meant it. We know he was using alcohol, crank, and marijuana, but it wasn't as if the drugs made him a homicidal or suicidal maniac. They just nudged him enough so he just didn't give a damn;

so his common sense was buried. It was like, 'Well, why not blow my brains out.'" 18-year-old high-school senior

The problem is that much drug use in high schools and colleges is experimental. The kids are curious, or bored, or goaded by their friends, or wanting to forget trouble at home, and they just don't look on drug use as this overwhelmingly evil thing.

"There is no way that you are going to get a majority of teenagers to say alcohol is an evil substance. That's because it's legal to buy. And how can you say that cigarettes are evil or awful things when everyone over 18 can buy them." 17-year old high-school student

While the majority of kids that experiment with drugs will not become addicted, the transitory effects of psychoactive drugs can cause problems that could follow the student for many years.

Crime

In some cities, the youth guidance centers or juvenile halls are clogged because of drugs. For example, as many as 85% of the juveniles in the San Francisco Youth Guidance Center are there because of drugs, either using, under the influence, dealing, or committing another crime while loaded. Anywhere from 30% to 62% of all juveniles arrested while committing a felony tested positive for illicit drugs, and over 50% self-reported they had used alcohol in the 72 hours before their arrest.

As to legal drugs:

- 88% of high school seniors had tried alcohol; about one in twenty were drinking daily; and 39% had ingested 5 or more drinks in a row at least once in the past two weeks;

- 27% used cigarettes; 17% were daily smokers.

"Once I started to smoke marijuana and drink, everyone I hung around with liked to get high too. I couldn't imagine not having a friend that didn't get loaded." Ex-high school drug user

The Effect of Drugs on Maturation

In the United States, levels of substance abuse are estimated to be the highest found in any developed country in the world. This is particularly alarming from two perspectives: first, drug use among our youth gives us a preview of future levels of drug abuse in our society; and drugs are generally more potent and toxic in youth due to physiologic and emotional immaturity.

Chemical differences, different hormonal levels, decreased blood elements, immature kidney and liver function, as well as incomplete development of the blood-brain barrier, all contribute to greater effects and toxicity in young users from a typical adult dose of psychoactive drugs. It is for this reason that pediatric doses of drugs are based upon body weight or surface area measure-

Arrest Rate For Youths Doubles

But reports of adult crime are down so far in 1993

By Maitland Zane and Susan Sward
Chronicle Staff Writers

Arrests for juvenile homicide

"We're not immortal. We know that we can die, but life for us is not as meaningful as for adults who have kids and responsibilities. If I die only my friends and my family would be sad, but it's not like I'm skipping out on anyone as if I were a parent or had a big position in a company." 16-year-old high school student

High School Seniors

A 1992 study of high school seniors showed that

- 8% used an illicit drug within the past 30 days;

- 47% had used alcohol and 3.3% drank daily;

- 36% had tried marijuana; 14 currently used it; and 2% to 3% smoked it on a daily basis;

- 10% had tried a psychedelic;

- And only 4% had used cocaine or an amphetamine in the past 30 days.

ments. Thus, youth are more susceptible to the toxic and adverse side effects of drugs and can more readily progress to substance abuse problems.

Further, adolescents have immature levels of sex hormones which are also quite susceptible to drug disruption. Many current drugs of abuse like marijuana, the opiates/opioids, and anabolic steroids ("rhoids") can potentially alter sexual development or function.

The psychological and emotional growth of youth can also be affected by psychoactive drugs during the critical years of maturation. All psychoactive substances alter or distort moods, feelings, emotions, and thought patterns.

The adolescent years are critical to the development of learning and the acquisition of academic skills. Depressant drugs, marijuana, and psychedelics all impair learning, psychological development, and coping skills to some degree. Stimulants have the transient effect of increasing short-term memory, motivation, and learning. Continued or high-dose use, however, greatly impairs the educational process.

These are just some of the considerations which raise great concern over the continued high level of drug abuse by American youth. Nowhere does prevention play a more important role than in addressing drug abuse problems in young people.

"When they start these programs while we're in high school or college, it's usually too late. We are what we are by this time. They have to start when we're young. Clear all us dopers out." 19-year-old college sophomore

PREVENTION

In a good program, there are three levels of drug-abuse prevention based on the students experience with drugs.

Primary Prevention

This program (for drug-naive students who are not even experimenting with drugs), should start even in kindergarten with parent-educator programs and the incorporation of established drug prevention lesson plans within the school's overall curriculum. The most effective prevention programs seem to be where the students are taught self-esteem and confidence and where they are taught not to be afraid of their feelings.

Secondary Prevention

This program (for drug-aware individuals or drug experimenters who do not have a problem with drugs) has found peer educator programs, prevention curriculum, Students Against Drunk Driving, positive role models, and health fairs to be effective in minimizing experimentation with drugs.

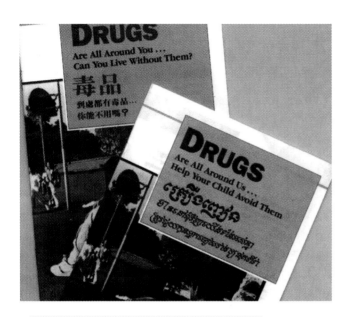

Education should be culture specific. Prevention book-
lets in Chinese and Cambodian by the Oakland Asian
Community Mental Health Services.

*"When I was going through
my wild stage I think what
changed my mind was seeing
someone who went through
their wild days and never
stopped. So I think that there
is a point when you cross
over from experimentation
and go on to abusing." 22-
year-old ex-college student*

Tertiary Prevention

This program (for students who
have had a problem with drugs)
uses student assistance programs,
teenage Narcotics / Cocaine /
Alcohol / Addictions Anonymous
Meetings, peer-intervention
teams, and other activities geared
at getting drug abusers into early
treatment to limit abuse. The hon-
esty of peers seems most effective in reaching students who are
in trouble.

*"If one of my close friends
said to me 'Hey, this drug
thing is a little too far. You
have to think about this,' I
wouldn't laugh at him. I
would think about it. It would
be in my head, and I would
actually think about what he
was saying." 19-year-old
college student*

Predictors of Drug Use

Important work in preventing
substance abuse in youth continues to be developed by researchers
like Steven Glenn, Ph.D., in South
Carolina and Richard Jessor, Ph.D.,
in Colorado. They present four
antecedents or "predictors" of future drug use in children. These
four antecedents do offer many
suggestions for the development
of a comprehensive youth drug
abuse prevention program. The
four antecedent factors which, by
age 12, seem to differentiate future drug abusers from future non
drug abusers are

1. **Strong sense of family participation and involvement.**
By age 12, those children who feel
that they are significant contribut-
ing members of their family unit,
that their participation is important
to and valued by their families,
seem to be less prone towards substance abuse in the future.

*"I was told when I was a kid
to stay away from the
fireplace, 'If you touch it you
are going to burn your hands
off,' 'Don't play with the ax
and be careful to protect your
face so a chip won't hit you.' I
think that this made me
afraid. I felt as if I was too
dumb to learn what to do.
But, I had a friend who, when*

he was little, his parents made him chop wood and build fires. I think what happened to me was counter productive. You don't want your kids to be burned but maybe there is a point in letting them get slightly burned. 'Ouch, that hurts.' That's OK. And then you don't have to be afraid for the rest of your life." 18-year-old college freshman

2. **Established personal position about drugs, alcohol, and sex by age 12.** Children who had a position on these issues, whatever that position may be, and who could articulate how they arrived at their position, how they would act on that position, and what effect their position would have on their lives seem less likely to develop drug or alcohol problems.

3. **Strong "spiritual" sense of community involvement by age 12.** Youth who feel that they are significant to and contribute to their community and the greater society around them, that they are individuals with a role and purpose in society, also seemed less likely to develop significant drug or alcohol problems.

4. **Attachment to a clean and sober adult role model other than one's parents by age 12.** Children who can list one or more non drug-using adults for whom they have esteem and to whom they can turn for information or advice seem less prone to develop drug abuse problems. These positive role models play a critical role in the formative years of a child's development and are often persons like a coach, a teacher, activities leader, minister, relative, neighbor, or family friend.

These factors underscore the need to develop a drug abuse prevention program early and continue such programs through the school years and even into adulthood.

"There is stuff around you in your life, even if you are just bored, that makes you want to experience the effect of a drug. You can change that, if you can make people and yourself happy. If you can be with stable friends, doing something that's important, then you won't abuse drugs." 16-year-old student

COSTS

Detailed analysis of these substance abuse related costs reveals not only an impact on industry but also an impact on the substance abusers themselves.

Loss of productivity

A substance abuser compared to a non drug-abusing employee is

- Late 3 to 14 times more often;

- Absent 5 to 7 times more often and 3 to 4 times more likely to be absent for longer than 8 consecutive days;

- Involved in many more job mistakes;

- Likely to have lower output, make a weaker salesperson, experience "work shrinkage," that is, less productivity despite more hours put forth;

- Likely to appear in a greater number of grievance hearings.

Medical Cost Increases

Substance abusers, as compared to non drug-abusing employees,

- Experience 3 to 4 times more on-the-job accidents;

- Use 3 times more sick leave;

- Overutilize health insurance for themselves and for their families;

- File 5 times more workman's compensation claims;

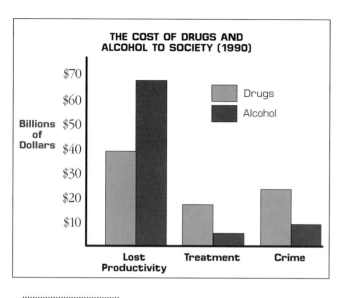

THE COST OF DRUGS AND ALCOHOL TO SOCIETY (1990)

Drugs
Alcohol

Billions of Dollars

$70
$60
$50
$40
$30
$20
$10

Lost Productivity   Treatment   Crime

Fig. 8-5 Approximate cost of drugs and alcohol to society — 1990.

DRUGS AT WORK

Studies on the impact of drug abuse in the American workplace have resulted in estimates that substance abuse cost our industries in lost productivity about $43 billion in 1979, $60 billion in 1983, and 100 billion in 1992.

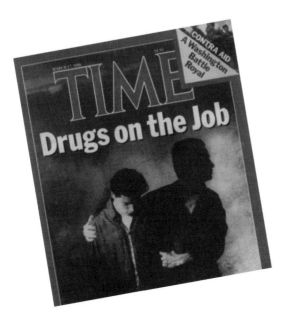

- Increase premiums for the entire company for medical and psychological insurance;

- Endanger the health and well being of co-workers.

Legal cost increases

As tolerance and addiction develop, a drug-abusing employee often enters into some form of criminal activity. Crime at the workplace brought about by drug abuse results in

- Direct and massive losses from embezzlement, pilferage, sales of corporate secrets; and property damaged during commitment of a crime;

- Increased cost of improved company security: more personnel; urine testing costs; product monitoring; quality assurance; intensified employee testing and screening;

- More lawsuits, both internal and external;

- Expanded legal fees, court costs, and attorney expenses;

- Loss of "good will" and negative publicity from drug use and trafficking at the workplace; employee arrests; the perception that there are more substance abusers than just those arrested; and manipulation of client contracts or goods.

EMPLOYEE ASSISTANCE PROGRAMS (EAP)

In response to the increased problem of drugs in the workplace and the resultant drain on profits and productivity, many employers have instituted the mutually beneficial and extremely effective Employee Assistance Programs, or EAP. Those EAP programs which enjoy the greatest success are ones that strike a balance between the legitimate and immediate needs of management to minimize the negative impact drug abuse has on their business with a genuine and sincere concern for the better health of the company's employees.

The EAP is designed to be an additional resource for employees. It is a benefit to them which, if effectively organized and utilized, can assist with a wide range of life and health issues and not just substance abuse problems. Many models for these programs exist which can be both a self-referral resource for the employee or an alternative to more stringent discipline by a supervisor for poor work performance.

Placed into the concept of a full prevention program, the successful EAP can effectively bring to the American workplace a broad-based strategy to address the full spectrum of substance abuse prevention needs.

Many different EAP models have been created, and those with the greatest success share two overall design features:

They "frame" the EAP drug abuse services in a full spectrum prevention program with efforts focused at minimizing employee attraction to drugs as well as helping those with problems to get into treatment.

They utilize an approach in which drug abuse problems are addressed in the context of a diverse range of services provided for a wide spectrum of employee problems (emotional, relationship, financial, wage garnishment, and "burnout").

These two design features have the distinct advantage of lessening the apprehension of employees about taking advantage of the available services for fear of being labeled as a drug abuser; preventing drug problems before they start; and identifying drug problems in employees who are in "denial" (they don't accept the fact that they have a problem) and who at first utilize the EAP for another problem.

The EAP is comprised of six basic components:

(1) Prevention / education / training;

(2) Identification and confidential outreach;

(3) Diagnosis and referral;

(4) Treatment, counseling and a good monitoring system;

(5) Follow-up and focus on aftercare (relapse prevention);

(6) Confidential record system and effectiveness evaluation.

Placing these components in a full spectrum prevention program, the EAP could provide the following services:

Primary Prevention

In the most effective EAP programs both corporate and individual denial are addressed with a systems-oriented approach to prevention. Education and training about the impact of substance abuse are provided at all levels in the corporation: to the administration, unions, and line staff. These segments should all agree on a single corporate policy on drugs and alcohol abuse.

An EAP program exists as an employee benefit designed to assist in a broad range of employee problems. Informational materials about alcohol and drug abuse, the EAP itself, and referral resources are readily available to the employees. Routine health fairs or union meeting presentations are available with curricula and lesson plans developed to help prevent drug abuse.

Secondary Prevention

Both education and training need to be focused on identification and early intervention. Drug identification and information about the major effects of drugs on behavior should be incorporated into the prevention curriculum. The corporation's legal, grievance and escalating discipline policies need to be scrutinized and possibly reworked in regards to the EAP. Security measures (urinalysis, staff review, monitoring, etc.) need to be established in a manner which is both appropriate and humane. These measures could operate both as deterrents to use as well as methods of identifying the abusers.

Tertiary Prevention

The EAP will need to formalize its intervention approach allowing for confidential self referral, peer referral, and supervisor-initiated referral to the EAP. A diagnostic process should be established along with a number of appropriate treatment referrals. Treatment should be confidential, but the EAP should have access to treatment records and an ability to monitor the treatment to insure proper follow-up aftercare and continued recovery efforts. It is important, however, that the employment status of workers be evaluated on work performance and not on their participatory effort in the EAP.

Effectiveness

These programs which are well conceived and which strike a balance between the corporation's security needs and a genuine concern for the better health and welfare of each individual employee have demonstrated not only great effectiveness but also tremendous cost savings to the corporation. Several studies in major corporations such as Southern Pacific, General Motors, Alcoa Aluminum, Eastman-Kodak, and others, have documented a 60% to 85% decrease in absenteeism; 40% to 65% decrease in sick time utilization and personal/family health insurance usage; 45% to 75% decrease in on-the-job accidents; as well as other cost savings once the EAP system was put into operation.

DRUG TESTING

Along with the national concern about drug abuse, there has been an increasing call for the use of drug testing in all walks of life. The Federal Government has even issued a mandate for a drug free workplace. Drug testing has been used for years to determine the blood or breath alcohol level of drivers suspected of drunk driving, of ex-convicts or felons on probation, and of others suspected of a crime. Recently though, some laws have been proposed and even enacted,

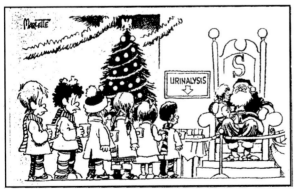

© 1988, Marlette-The Atlanta Constitution-Permission of Creators Syndicate, Inc.
'So this is how he knows if we've been bad or good!...'

calling for random testing of special groups, testing of job applicants, testing of all federal employees, and even random testing of teachers and students. The legal, moral, and ethical debate will continue for years.

In this section we will examine

- The different tests used to determine the presence of drugs in the body;

- The length of time it takes for certain drugs to leave the body;

- The accuracy of the various methods of testing;

- The consequences of false positives and false negatives in drug testing.

THE TESTS

First, it is important for everyone to know that there are many different laboratory procedures used to test for drugs. One can test for drugs in the urine, blood, hair, saliva, sweat and even different tissues of the body. Each test possesses inherent differences in sensitivity, specificity, and accuracy as well as other potential problems. The more common methods are

Chromatography, especially Thin Layer Chromatography or TLC

This method is practical, able to search for a wide variety of drugs at the same time, and fairly sensitive to the presence of even minute amounts of chemicals. The major drawback is its inability to accurately differentiate drugs that may have similar chemical properties. For example, ephedrine, a drug used legally in over-the-counter cold medicines, may be misidentified as an illegal amphetamine.

Enzyme Multiplied Immuno-Assay Techniques or EMIT

These tests are extremely sensitive, very rapidly performed, and fairly easy to operate. However, they cannot usually distinguish the concentration of the drug present and may show positive tests results to environmental traces of a drug; e.g., the presence of marijuana caused by breathing in the air at a rock concert. Also, a separate test must usually be run for each specific suspected drug. Thus, an EMIT test run for only heroin and cocaine, would miss the presence of marijuana, PCP, or any other non-tested drug. EMIT tests can also mistake non-abused chemicals for abused drugs. For example, the presence of opiate alkaloids in the poppy seeds of cakes and pastries can cause a false positive test for opiates. The chemical in Advil or Motrin may be mistaken for marijuana.

Chromatography/Mass Spectrometry Combined or GC/MS

This method is currently the most accurate, sensitive, and reliable method of testing for drugs in the body. However, it is very expensive, requires highly trained operators, and is a very lengthy and tedious process in comparison to other methods. Being very sensitive, it can detect even trace amounts of drugs in the urine and therefore requires skilled interpretation to differentiate environmental exposure from actual use.

Hair Analysis

Researched by Dr. Werner Baumgartner at the Janus Institute in Los Angeles, analysis of hair samples for drugs of abuse may prove to be more practical and even more accurate than other methods. The chemical properties of most psychoactive drugs are such that they are absorbed and stored in human hair cells, so the drugs can be detected almost as long as the hair stays intact, even many decades after the drug is been taken. Further, hair grows at a fairly constant rate for most people, so hair cut close to the scalp may be able to give an accurate six month history of drug use. This could give a better picture of the degree of drug use (to differentiate occasional use from addictive use) and decrease the frequency of testing.

About 40 strands of hair are needed for accurate testing since each individual strand can be tested for the presence of only one drug. Shampoo, excessive sun, and bleach do not seem to affect the results. Recently, a second technique of hair analysis has been developed. Since good detection procedures call for a second test unrelated to the first test to confirm a positive reaction, there will probably be an increase in drug testing by hair analysis in the future.

Currently, some two dozen methods are used to analyze body samples for the presence of drugs. None of these methods is totally foolproof.

DETECTION PERIOD

A great number of factors influence the length of time that a drug can be detected in someone's blood, urine, saliva, or other body tissues. These include an individual's drug absorption rate, metabolism rate, distribution in the body, excretion rate, and the specific testing method employed. With a wide variation of these and other factors, a predictable drug detection period would be, at best, an educated guess. Despite this, the public interest requires that some specific estimates be adopted. For urine testing, these estimates can be divided into three broad periods: latency, detection period range, and redistribution.

Latency

Drugs must be absorbed, circulated by the blood, and finally concentrated in the urine in sufficient quantity before they can be detected. This process generally takes about 2 to 3 hours for most drugs except alcohol which takes about 30 minutes. Thus, someone tested just 30 minutes after using a drug, would probably (but not always) test negative for that drug. A chronic user or addict, however, should have enough chemicals already present to test positive within that time frame.

Alcohol	1/2 to 1 days
Amphetamines (crank, speed, ice)	2-4 days
Barbiturates	
Amobarbital, Pentobarbital	2-4 days
Phenobarbital	up to 30 days
Secobarbital (reds)	2-4 days
Benzodiazepines	
(Valium, Xanax, etc.)	up to 30 days
Cocaine (coke, crack)	12-72 hours
Doriden (loads)	2-4 days
Marijuana	
Casual use to 4 joints per week	5-7 days
Daily use	10-15 days
Chronic, heavy use	1-2 months
Opiates/Opioids	
Dilaudid	2-4 days
Darvon	6-48 hours
Heroin (morphine measured)	2-4 days
Methadone	2-3 days
PCP	
Casual use	2-7 days
Chronic, heavy use	several months
Quaalude	2-4 days

Fig. 8-6 Detection Period Range Chart

Fig. 8-7 compares the length of time cocaine, marijuana, and alcohol remain in the blood. For purposes of testing, there is a cutoff level when testing for certain drugs, so even when there is still some of the drug in someone's blood or urine, it will not be detected by the standard test.

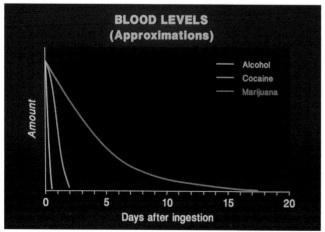

Detection Period Range

Once sufficient amounts of a drug enter the urine, the drug can be detected for a certain length of time by urinalysis. The rough estimates for the more common drugs of abuse are shown in Fig. 8-6.

Again, these are merely rough estimates with wide individual variations. Thus, an individual delaying a urine test 5 days because of cocaine abuse will probably, but not definitely, test negative for cocaine.

Redistribution, Recirculation, Sequestration and Other Variables

Long-acting drugs like PCP, marijuana, and the benzodiazepines can be distributed to certain body tissues or fluids, concentrated and sequestered there, then be recirculated and concentrated back into the urine. This can result in a positive test following negative tests and several months of abstinence. PCP, the most studied drug in this situation, has been found concentrated back into stomach acids or body fat, then rereleased, resulting in a positive urine test. Additionally, there are a few reports of infants and youths testing positive for PCP many years after their intra-uterine exposure to the drug.

ACCURACY OF DRUG TESTING

Despite many claims of confidence in the reliability of drug testing, independent, blind testing of laboratory results continues to document high error rates for many testing programs.

Technological Problems

The discussion of different tests and detection periods has already addressed some problems with false positive results. Other false positive tests result from: some herbal teas containing coca leaf, and therefore testing positive for cocaine; phenylpropanolamine and dextromethorphan in many cold products are often misidentified as amphetamines and opiates respectively; Benadryl is mistaken for methadone; Midol, Primatine-M, Elavil, and Tofranil, for opiates; Tegopen (an antibiotic), for benzodiazepines; Novrad (a cough medicine), for Darvon; poppy seed cake, for opiates; Advil and Motrin, for marijuana; and many others, just because of the limitations of the testing technology.

Handling Problems

Errors also result from the mishandling of urine and other specimen samples taken. Tagging the specimen with the wrong label; mixing and preparing the testing solutions incorrectly; calculation errors; coding the samples and solutions; logging and reporting of results; and exposure of samples to destructive conditions or to drugs in the laboratory have all resulted in inaccurate tests.

Specimen Manipulations

Though there is much concern over the possibility of false positive tests, in actuality, false negative results constitute the bulk of urine testing errors. These result from laboratories being overly cautious in reporting positive results and from specimen manipulation by the testee.

Many manipulations, some effective and some just folklore, have been used by drug abusers to prevent the detection of drugs in their urine. These include diluting the urine with water; putting cleanser, vinegar, salt, or baking soda in the urine bottle; drinking vinegar or Golden Seal Tea before testing; taking a dye like Pyridium before testing; taking water pills like Lasix to dilute urine in the bladder; substituting someone else's urine or even synthetic urine for their own; and even catheterizing and substituting urine in their own bladder before testing.

There is a rigid chain-of-custody for urine samples in good drug-testing laboratories. Detailed paperwork follows each sample.

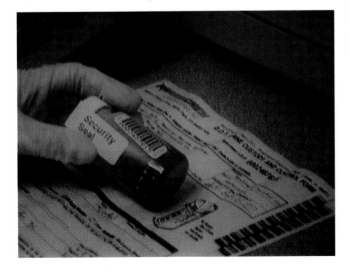

These attempts to manipulate urine testing have grown to such proportions that "clean pee" (drug free urine), has become a profitable black market item. Further, recent designer drugs create a major problem in drug testing. Many have no standard to test against, and some are so potent (the effective dose so small) that they will be impossible to identify in the body.

Inaccurate tests also result from disease states, pregnancy, medical conditions, interference of prescribed drugs, and individual metabolic conditions. We even have a case where a diabetic woman's urine fermented its sugar into alcohol with the yeast present along her genital tract, after the sample was taken and before it was tested. She was inappropriately accused of falling off the wagon.

CONSEQUENCES OF FALSE POSITIVES AND NEGATIVES

Concerns about false positive test results are well publicized, debated, and feared. The prospect that people could lose their jobs, be denied employment, or even lose their freedom over an erroneous positive, certainly underscores such concerns. Even the most accurate testing program cannot, at this time, ensure that false positive tests won't occur.

Less publicized or feared but just as critical are the false negative results. These prevent the discovery of drug abuse and feed the already strong denial process in

the user. They permit the addict to progressively become more impaired and dysfunctional until a major life crisis occurs. False negatives represent a considerable threat to public safety with a train engineer, airline pilot, or even driver who is allowed to function in a diminished capacity. False negatives also present an obstacle to effective treatment and intervention plans.

Extremely potent drugs and designer drugs also present a major problem of false negatives. LSD and fentanyl derivatives cause reactions at the microgram level which make them difficult to locate in any body sample. New designer drugs which have never been analyzed before mean that drug tests have no standards for their identification. These drugs, therefore, go undetected in almost all tests.

Despite the many problems with drug testing, it is still an effective intervention, treatment, and monitoring tool. Addicts who have become totally disabled because of their addiction often state that they wished they had been tested and identified before their lives had been destroyed. Drug abusers in treatment often request increased urine testing to help them focus on their need for confirmed abstinence. It also helps them resist peer pressure. They can say, "Hey, I can't use. I have to be tested." Treatment programs have no better tool to deal with the strong denial and dishonesty in addicts during early treatment than the confrontation of continued positive tests. Continued employment of recovering addicts in jobs that expose the public to high risk would not be acceptable without a reliable drug testing program.

With the technology available at this time, the best chance for a reliable drug testing program would include

- Direct observation of the body specimen being obtained for testing to minimize sample manipulations;

- Established, rigid chain of custody over the sample to minimize recording and mix-up problems;

- Utilization of the most accurate testing methods available (i.e. GC/MS), with a mandatory second, confirmatory test via a different method; testing for a wide range of abused drugs and not just the primary drug of addiction (this is both to both identify the now prevalent pattern of polydrug abuse and to monitor for drug switching or substitution);

- Incorporation of a detailed medical and social history in the interpretation of lab results, e.g., "Is the testee being treated for a medical condition with prescription or over-the-counter drugs which interfere with testing?"

A major controversy in drug testing is the question of mandatory random testing versus probable cause testing. The need for public protection is weighed against civil and individual rights. Given our founding fathers' philosophy and the repulsive element of an observed test, necessary for reliability, testing only when there is probable cause to suspect drug abuse seems the best alternative at this time. But, how many of us would be willing, or would not feel demeaned, to urinate in front of a stranger?

DRUGS AND THE ELDERLY

Overuse (as opposed to occasional use) of psychoactive drugs by the elderly is often overlooked, ignored, or passed off as a minimal health concern of old age. All too often, the attitude is one of "They've lived a full life and made their contribution to society so why disturb their lives now? If they want to abuse drugs at this age, whom will it harm? They deserve to be able to abuse drugs now." This assumes that the unhindered abuse of psychoactive drugs is desirable.

The truth is that addiction is a progressive illness with only a brief initial "honeymoon" phase where psychoactive drugs are exciting and pleasurable. But, continued use leads to progressive physiological, emotional, social, relationship, family, and spiritual consequences that users find intolerable. Oftentimes the elderly abuse psychoactive drugs to deal with their feelings of loneliness, being unwanted, not respected, and rejected by their families and the workplace. The effect of drugs to suppress these feelings and alter states of consciousness is only transitory and ultimately increases problems of low self-esteem and self-worth.

No systematic measure of drug abuse within the elderly has been made as it has within other age groups. Our experience has been that elderly substance abusers are exposed to a wide range of drugs and, as a group, present diverse drug abuse problems, which include the abuse of alcohol, illicit drugs, prescription drugs (which they sometimes share with one another) and even over-the-counter drugs.

Physiological Changes

The human body's physiological functioning and chemistry are very different in the elderly compared to young people and midlife adults. This results in an abnormal response to drugs in the aged as compared to younger adults. Generally, the elderly's enzyme and other bodily functions become less active, conditions which impair their ability to inactivate or excrete drugs. This makes drugs stronger and more toxic in the elderly. For example, Valium is deactivated by liver enzymes but after the age of 30, the liver, little by little, loses its ability to make these deactivation enzymes. Thus, a 10 mg dose of Valium taken by someone age 70 will result in an effect equal to a dose of up to 30 mg taken by someone age 21.

The aged are also more likely to have concurrent illnesses which may greatly alter the effects of drugs in their bodies or make them more sensitive to the toxic and adverse side effects. Conditions like diabetes, liver, heart, and kidney disease all affect or are affected by drug abuse. Further, drugs used to treat these concurrent illnesses along with a greater use of over-the-counter drugs by the aged give rise to a greater potential for drug interactions. Such interactions frequently have synergistic effects on psychoactive drugs (actions which exaggerate their effects). These interactions, combined with a physiological state that also exaggerates the toxic effects, are a prescription for disaster.

Age does not endow a person with immunity to the negative effects of drugs or chemical dependence. In fact, the opposite is closer to reality. Impaired body systems that usually accompany the aging process make the elderly more sensitive to negative drug consequences. Thus prevention, education, and treatment services targeted for the aged are important, unmet needs.

The most commonly abused drugs in the elderly are alcohol; prescription sedatives like Valium; codeine; Darvon and other opioid analgesics; narcotic cough syrups; and over-the-counter sedatives or sleep aids. Note however, that all abused drugs are candidates for abuse by the elderly. Even cocaine and marijuana addiction have been treated in patients 70 years or older.

NEEDLE USE, INFECTION, & AIDS

First, some definitions:

HIV means Human Immuno Deficiency Virus, the virus which causes AIDS; AIDS means Auto Immune Deficiency Syndrome, a group of serious illnesses such as Pneumocystis carinii pneumonia, Kaposi's sarcoma cancer, or tuberculosis, which define when the HIV virus has taken control of the patient's life. However, since 1993, a new definition of AIDS is being used. AIDS is defined by having a T-cell count below 400. T-cell counts measure the level of effectiveness of one's immune system.

Through December 1992 about 60,000 intravenous (I.V.) drug users had full-blown AIDS as a result of injecting themselves with HIV infected needles. This is between 23% and 28% of all cases of AIDS in the United States. With the new definition of AIDS, the real figure is closer to 100,000. In addition, approximately 300,000 more are infected with the HIV virus out of a total of 1,000,000 infected Americans.

What the statistics mean is that in 10 years, barring a dramatic medical breakthrough, most AIDS-infected persons will probably be dead. Some have estimated the infection rate among I.V. drug users to be even higher, approaching 80%. Whatever the exact numbers, the figures are staggering. And these figures don't include all the other diseases that needle use can promote.

NEEDLE USE

The problems with needle use come from several sources. Needle kits are called "outfits," "fits," "rigs," "works," "points," and many other names. Besides putting a large amount of the drug in the blood-stream in a short period of time, needles also inject other substances like powdered milk, procaine, or even Ajax, often used to cut or dilute drugs. They can also inject dangerous bacteria and viruses. Intravenous drug use is also called "mainlining," "geezing," "slamming," or "hitting up."

Fig. 8-8 Number of AIDS cases Reported to the Centers For Disease Control

	1986	1987	1988	1989	1990	1991	1992	1993**
New Cases	13,057	21,273	32,156	38,007	41,000	45,524	47,106	56,000 or *100,000
Cumulative	26,694	50,837	83,123	121,130	162,130	206,342	253,448	309,000 or *409,000

*Figure is based on the new definition of AIDS
**Estimated

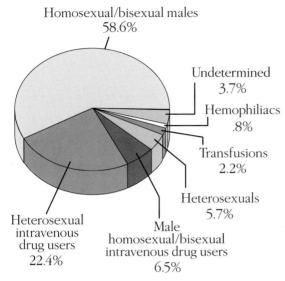

Homosexual/bisexual males
58.6%

Undetermined
3.7%

Hemophiliacs
.8%

Transfusions
2.2%

Heterosexuals
5.7%

Male
homosexual/bisexual
intravenous drug users
6.5%

Heterosexual
intravenous
drug users
22.4%

Fig. 8-9   *Who has Aids?*

Typically, the veins of the arms, wrists, and hands are used first. As these veins become hardened due to the constant sticking, the user will inject into the veins of the neck and the legs. As it becomes difficult to locate usable veins, addicts will also shoot under the skin ("skin popping"). They will also shoot into a muscle in the buttocks, shoulder, or legs ("muscling"). If they become desperate as they run out of places to shoot themselves, they will inject into the neck, foot, and even the dorsal vein in the penis.

Because of the contamination of street drugs, unsafe or non-sterile needle practices, and particularly the sharing of needles, users can contract viral hepatitis, an infection of the liver. Besides AIDS, this is the most common disease in needle users. Another common problem is endocarditis, a sometimes fatal condition caused by certain bacteria that lodge and grow in the valves of the heart.

Needle use can also cause abscesses at a contaminated injection site or they can put bits of foreign matter in the bloodstream which can lodge in the spine, brain, lungs, or eyes and cause an embolism or other problems. Needle users can also contract cotton fever, a very common disease. The symptoms are similar to those of a very bad case of the flu. It is thought to be caused by bits of cotton lodging in various tissues or by infections carried into the body by cotton fibers injected into the blood.

HIV DISEASE AND AIDS

(For more information on AIDS, see Chapter 10 - LOVE, SEX, and DRUGS)

AIDS is a disease that is most often fatal because it destroys the immune system, the body's mechanism that normally fights infection. The affected person becomes susceptible to many infections and diseases such as pneumonia or dozens of others which can prove fatal. Usually, it's a combination of many infections. Many needle users test positive for the HIV (AIDS) virus because they shared a needle used by someone already infected. What happens is that bits of infected blood from an AIDS carrier lodge in the needle. If the needle is dirty and not disinfected, the AIDS virus is passed when the other user sticks the needle into the body.

"At one shooting gallery in New York that I visited, users came in, shoved their money through one hole in the wall, then shoved their arms through another hole in the wall and received an injection. Russian roulette with real bullets seemed safe compared to this practice." Drug education outreach worker

It is impossible to overemphasize the danger of using infected needles because I.V. use of a drug bypasses all the body's natural defenses such as body hairs, mucous membranes, body acids, and enzymes. And the HIV virus itself destroys the body's last line of defense, the immune system.

In fact, recent research shows that in and of themselves, opiates and other drugs of abuse can weaken the immune system. This coupled with the malnutrition and unhealthy habits that compulsive drug use promotes, makes the body unable to fight off any illness.

"I told this guy that was sharing some speed with me that I had AIDS and that he should clean the needle, but

1992

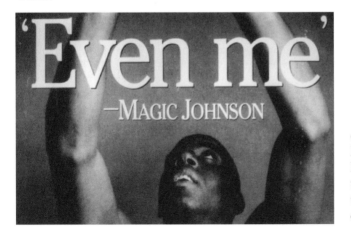

he was so strung out and anxious to shoot up that he pulled a knife on me and made me give him the needle." Intravenous cocaine user

Other HIV Risk Factors

The increased risk of HIV disease in the drug abusing population is much higher because

- Drug abuse requires money, and people will often do anything to raise money to avoid the cocaine crash or heroin withdrawal symptoms;

- Drugs impair judgment leading the user to do things that in a sober light would seem insane;

- Drugs lower inhibitions.

All three effects lead users into high-risk drug and sex practices. Trading sex for drugs is a common practice, and when one is loaded, judgment and common sense are suspended.

"There's this guy I know, really an ugly geek, but he always has a good supply of rocks (crack cocaine). Normally I wouldn't even talk to him, but he knows he's boss. Sometimes I need the drugs so bad and he wants the sex so quickly that we don't use a condom. Real stupid on my part." 22-year-old crack user

The most newsworthy AIDS case since Rock Hudson was Magic Johnson, former star of the Los Angeles Lakers. He contracted the disease from unprotected sex, emphasizing the spread of the disease into the heterosex-

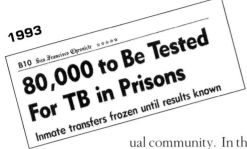

1993

B10 San Francisco Chronicle ★★★★★

80,000 to Be Tested For TB in Prisons

Inmate transfers frozen until results known

ual community. In the rest of the world, spread of the disease through heterosexual contact is much more prevalent than homosexual contact or I.V. drug use.

Tuberculosis

One of the biggest new risks is tuberculosis, a wasting respiratory disease that had become rare in the United States. In recent years, it has become one of the main killers of HIV infected people. It is an airborne infection so it can be spread by being in close (not intimate) contact with someone who's sick with the disease. One form of the disease is very resistant to medication and can cost tens of thousands of dollars to fight, compared to the few thousand that it takes to treat normal TB.

....
Publicity about the dangers of using dirty needles or having unprotected sex is one of the ways to limit the spread of AIDS.

The growing epidemic of TB among people with AIDS or HIV brings up an interesting point about identification of HIV infected people since they are also TB carriers. Identification of TB carriers has been a part of the American Health System for years. However, identification of HIV carriers or those with AIDS is limited by law so, a person's right to privacy and the government's responsibility to protect the public health are in conflict. It will take years to resolve the issue.

Stopping the Spread of AIDS

There are several strategies to stop the spread of AIDS, particularly in the drug-using community. The government can fund a massive education program to teach about the dangers of AIDS. They can try to stop the flow of drugs into the country. They can identify and quarantine those with AIDS. They can try to jail all people involved with drugs. They can hand out free needles to all I.V. drug users. They can encourage all drug abusers to give up I.V. drug use. They can teach drug users how to clean needles with bleach.

In studies by the Center for Disease Control and other agencies, needle exchange along with education seems to be the most effective HIV disease or AIDS prevention strategy. The next most effective method is teaching addicts how to clean their needles with bleach.

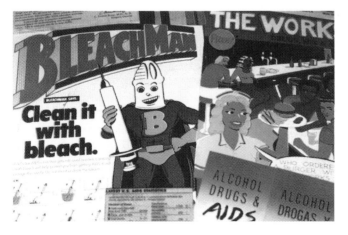

Harm Reduction

In San Francisco, several groups including the Communicable Disease Center of the Haight-Ashbury Free Medical Clinics have outreach programs meant to reach I.V. drug users who are not in treatment. Outreach workers from the Center, armed with AIDS educational materials, free bottles of bleach, and free condoms, go out to the shooting galleries, crack/rock houses, dope pads, and other areas to distribute these materials. Other groups distribute free needles. It's an intervention into behavior without intervening into drug use. The drug use intervention part of the total policy is handled by the other sections of the clinic.

The problem with education about the risks of sharing needles being too closely tied to treatment is that it misses the larger segment of I.V. drug users who are not ready for treatment and therefore at the highest risk for AIDS.

At the Haight-Ashbury Clinic, with a more tolerant policy toward relapses and toward users who can't clean up during their first few tries in the treatment centers, the user is at least in contact on occasion with a treatment facility that can intervene or present important information. Users alienated by the treatment community or in denial are hard to educate.

In just a short period of time, drug users' awareness about the dangers of AIDS and the need to clean needles jumped from a few percent to 85%. The HIV positive segment of the I.V. drug-using population in San Francisco is 15 to 17% compared to 60 to 80% in New York. Part of this HIV infection rate difference between the two coasts is certainly due to the educational effort. Other differences seem to be the greater presence of shooting galleries in New York, the limited number of treatment facilities, the difficulty in obtaining new needles, and language barriers.

Recently, some doubt has been cast on the efficacy of the different medications used (AZT, DDI, and DDC) to treat HIV infection, but studies have shown that people who test positive for HIV who remain clean and sober and maintain a healthy lifestyle with plenty of rest, good food, and exercise will avoid full-blown AIDS for years longer. And those who have an AIDS diagnosis will live months to years longer.

Education, using condoms, and especially needle exchange have been proven to significantly reduce the spread of HIV. A recent study in California showed that 23,500 needles were exchanged during one week in February 1993 at various sites. All studies in the U.S., Canada, Australia, and Europe have shown substantial reductions but not elimination of AIDS risk behavior among participants in a needle-exchange program. **These studies further show that there is no evidence of any increase in I.V. drug use because of needle exchange programs.**

CRADLE TO GRAVE

1. About eleven percent of all pregnant women in America are using psychoactive drugs: alcohol, cocaine, cigarettes, and marijuana.

2. Drugs are particularly dangerous to the fetus because its defense mechanisms such as a drug neutralizing metabolic system, an immune system to fight infections, and well developed organs to handle the effects are not yet developed. For example, each surge of effects from a drug the mother takes gives multiple surges to the defenseless fetus.

3. Major problems from drug use during pregnancy include a higher rate of miscarriage, blood vessel damage, severe withdrawal symptoms, and a much higher risk of SIDS, or "Sudden Infant Death Syndrome."

4. The problems of drug abuse during pregnancy last well beyond the birth of the baby. Withdrawal, intoxication, and developmental delays are commonplace.

5. Fetal alcohol syndrome (FAS) is the third most common cause of mental retardation in the United States.

6. Cocaine and amphetamines are particularly traumatic to the circulatory system of the infant, causing increased blood pressure and heart rate, stroke, and premature placental separation.

7. Besides the danger of miscarriages and placental separation caused by opiates or opioids, particularly heroin, the biggest danger comes from contaminated needles. Eighty percent of children with AIDS are born to addicted mothers who use drugs intravenously.

8. Women who smoke marijuana heavily during pregnancy are five times more likely to deliver babies with features similar to those of fetal alcohol syndrome. Sufficient research into this and other problems associated with marijuana use during pregnancy is lacking.

9. Women who are heavy smokers are twice as likely to miscarry and have spontaneous abortions; they will have smaller babies; and the babies will have a slower maturation rate and a higher risk of SIDS (Sudden Infant Death Syndrome).

10. The majority of teenagers in juvenile detention centers are there because of involvement with drugs—either using, selling, buying, or being under the influence.

11. A well-known study of high school seniors showed that almost a third had used an illegal drug in the past month, mainly marijuana and amphetamines; almost 39% had 5 or more drinks in a row in the past two weeks; 3.3% were drinking every day; and 17% were smoking cigarettes.

12. The levels of substance abuse among youth in the U. S. is among the highest of any developed country.

13. Youths are more likely to experiment with psychoactive drugs; they are more susceptible to peer pressure; their hormonal systems are in the developmental stage so psychological and emotional maturation can be disrupted or delayed by drug use.

14. Drug abuse in the workplace costs American business more than 100 billion dollars a year.

15. Drug abuse in the workplace causes loss of productivity; medical cost increases; and legal cost increases.

16. The most effective answer to drug abuse in the workplace seems to be EAP's (Employee Assistance Programs).

17. Good EAP programs have been documented to decrease absenteeism 60% to 85% and to decrease on the job accidents 45% to 75%.

18. As drug users get older, their bodies become less able to neutralize and metabolize psychoactive drugs.

19. The major types of drug tests are thin layer chromatography (TLC), enzyme multiplied immunoassay technique (EMIT), and gas chromatography/mass spectrometry (GC/MS).

20. The important aspects of testing are the length of time it takes for drugs to leave the body; the accuracy of the various methods; and the consequences of false positives and false negatives.

21. It takes 2 or 3 hours for most drugs to enter the urine and be detectable. Alcohol, the exception, takes 30 minutes.

22. False negative tests can be as damaging as false positives. Failure to recognize a serious addiction can be more serious than damage to one's reputation from a false positive.

23. In New York City, from 60% to 80% of I.V. drug users test positive for the HIV virus.

24. AIDS is a disease which destroys the immune system so the user is susceptible to any infection. Drugs also lower the body's defenses indirectly. In addition, drugs impair judgment and lower inhibitions, so users are more likely to engage in dangerous behavior.

25. The best AIDS prevention program is education on the dangers of sharing dirty needles, and engaging in high-risk sex practices.

26. Other diseases caused by dirty needles include hepatitis, cotton fever, endocarditis, abscesses, malaria, tuberculosis, and syphilis.

QUESTIONS

1. What is the placental barrier?

2. Why are drugs more damaging to the fetus than to the mother?

3. What are two effects to the fetus of alcohol abuse in a pregnant woman?

4. What is FAS and FAE?

5. Why do stimulants cause blood vessel and heart problems to the fetus?

6. What is the relationship between drug use during pregnancy and "Sudden Infant Death Syndrome?"

7. What is the most widely used psychoactive drug in youth?

8. Name three factors that encourage a teenager to use drugs.

9. Name two factors which would help keep a teenager from abusing psychoactive drugs.

10. In what three ways do drugs cost U.S. business?

11. What is an EAP and what are its major functions?

12. What are two common body fluids that can be used to test for drug use and how long does it take for a drug to be detectable?

13. List the most common methods used to detect drugs in the urine.

14. Describe four ways to minimize drug testing errors.

15. Why do drugs affect the elderly more than those in their 20's and 30's?

16. What percentage of I.V. drug users in New York City test positive for the HIV virus?

17. Why is AIDS so deadly?

18. What are two important methods of preventing the spread of AIDS in I.V. drug users?

19. What are two other diseases commonly caused by contaminated needle use in I.V. drug abusers?

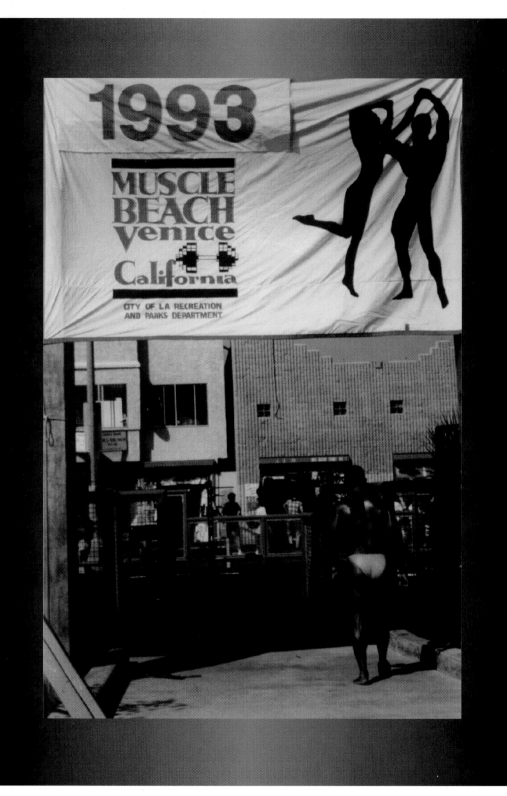

"Muscle Beach," in Venice Beach, California, where the latest body building techniques are discussed. Sometimes the topic of discussion is anabolic-androgenic steroids.

CHAPTER
9

SPORTS
AND DRUGS*

By Michael Holstein, Ph.D.

1984
Steroid Use Rampant

1990
SPORTSTALK
BEHIND THE SCENES IN THE WORLD OF SPORTS
Q & A — SPORTS
Pressure to win
leads to drug abuse

DR. BOB GOLDMAN, LPRC

1992
Alzado Dies of Brain Cancer
At 43 — He Blamed Steroids

"I was so wild about winning. Winning, winning, winning. I never thought about anything else." Lyle Alzado, former NFL star

In a survey a number of years ago, a group of several hundred superior athletes were asked, "If you could take a drug that would guarantee a world record or an Olympic gold medal in your sport, but afterwards, it would kill you within the year, would you take it?"

More than half the athletes said "Yes," they would. That means that more than half the athletes were willing to die just so they could be the best in their chosen sport. Given this overwhelming desire to win at any cost, athletes' continued use and abuse of drugs with long-term, damaging side effects becomes more comprehensible. Add to an athlete's inherent motivation to succeed, the physical and mental dependence that can result from drug abuse, and the scope of the problem becomes clear.

Drugs are perceived by many athletes who abuse them as a short cut to the tedious training and preparation necessary for competition. They are the quick way to put on pounds, to increase stamina, to get up for a game, to relieve pain, or to keep up with other athletes who one suspects of using drugs.

In addition, since many drugs used in sports create a feeling of confidence and excitement, the drugs themselves can become motivators for an athlete to abuse them. Drugs may be used to reward oneself, to cope with pain, to socialize, or for any other number of reasons, many of which mirror the motives for drug abuse in society at large. Psychoactive drugs such as cocaine, marijuana, alcohol, tobacco, and LSD may have no performance-enhancing effects, and many, in fact, diminish performance, but nevertheless, they attract the athlete.

"What you have to understand is that a young man doesn't think past tomorrow. All he is interested in is winning the neighborhood game and having the best looking girl on his arm and looking the best that he possibly can. And these are technically the motivations for him taking the drug. And then he goes to college where peer pressure and the desire not to disappoint the home town folks puts further pressure on the him. Then if he's lucky enough to make it to the pro ranks it becomes a matter of money." High school football coach giving testimony to Congressional panel on drugs and sports

The question coaches, parents, teachers, and particularly the athletes themselves have to ask is, "Are the consequences of drug use and abuse in sports worth it?" In this chapter, the effects of drugs on performance, as well as their side effects and long-term effects will be examined.

BACKGROUND

HISTORY

The use of drugs in sports is not new. History records Greek Olympic athletes in the 3rd century B.C. who ate mushrooms to improve their performance. About the same time, athletes in Macedonia were preparing for their events by drinking ground donkey hooves boiled in oil and garnished with rose petals. Roman gladiators took stimulants (betel nuts or ephedrine) to give them endurance. In 200 A.D. in the work, Gymnastikos, the philosopher Philostratus wrote a handbook on practices for athletes. He urged, "Athletes should be free from the use of clay and mud and other irksome medicines."

By the 1800's more sophisticated substances were being used to improve performance including opium, morphine, cocaine, caffeine, nitroglycerine, sugar cubes soaked in ether, and even strychnine. These substances and others were used by cyclists, swimmers, and other athletes. Boxers, for example, drank water laced with cocaine between rounds. Long-distance runners were followed on bicycles by doctors who gave them a mixture of brandy and strychnine.

By the 1950's and 1960's drug abuse by athletes had become widespread for several reasons:

Social Acceptance

During the 50's, drugs were associated primarily with the avant-garde in music and the arts. In the 60's, the wide availability of drugs as part of the rock scene, the growing counter-culture lifestyle, and the protest movement signaled that the mood of the country was becoming more tolerant of drug use. There was also an attitude that drugs could fix anything.

Availability

A greater variety of drugs was being produced, most notably anabolic steroids (compounds derived from the male hormone testosterone or synthesized versions of it) which increase weight, strength, muscle mass, and aggressiveness. Testosterone had been isolated in the 1930's and used in its pure form or in compounds to help injury victims and survivors of World War II concentration camps gain weight.

By the 50's, synthetic testosterone compounds were used regularly in sports, first by body builders and weight lifters who wanted to increase weight and strength, and later by many athletes to try to accelerate their training and development.

New versions of amphetamines which initially increase alertness and energy were also being used and abused. Amphetamines had been used in World War II by various countries, to delay fatigue and increase endurance of their troops. When veterans returned home to the playing fields, some continued to rely on the drugs to try to give themselves a competitive edge. Some athletes also became convinced that they could increase their endurance with the use of amphetamines.

International Politics

There were also political pressures to improve the collective performance of a country's athletes as a way of demonstrating the superiority of a political system. The 50's and 60's were the Cold War era. The Russians were rumored to be using anabolic steroids during the 1956 Olympics, as were many of the Communist bloc countries, especially East Germany in succeeding Olympics. America wanted its athletes to stay ahead of the Russians and the rest of the Communist bloc, and the use of performance-enhancing drugs was thought to be the only way that Americans could maintain their competitiveness in international athletics.

Commercialization of Sports

Beginning in the 1950's, the excellence of an athlete's performance began to matter less and less. With televised sports events, the explosive growth of professional sports, larger and larger salaries, purses, prizes, and big money for commercial endorsements of products, the public's attitude changed from respect for athletic excellence to envy of athletes' salaries and an expectation that for that kind of money they had better be a winner.

This attitude of winning at any cost was echoed by many coaches.

"Winning is not the most important thing, it's the only thing." Vince Lombard, Green Bay Packers coach, 1956-1964

....

Advertisements that combine sports and alcohol are as plentiful as advertisements that combine sex and alcohol.

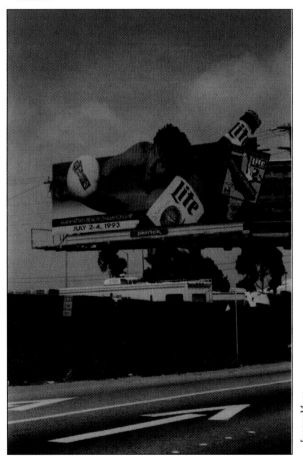

Jason Moss

Over the past 30 years, the financial and social pressures to win have encouraged athletes to try drugs as a way to gain an advantage. "Do what you have to, but just win, Baby" became our society's best advice to athletes.

"The only yardstick for success our society has is being a champion." John Madden, former NFL coach; sportscaster

Many athletes make more from endorsements than from salary, making winning even more crucial in the minds of athletes.

"I hate to lose . . . I only care about winning. Second place means nothing." Ivan Lendl, tennis player

In addition, companies that produce alcohol and tobacco have long been associated with sports. TV beer commercials, tail-gate parties, the sale of beer and wine at sporting events, the "Lite Beer Player of the Game," locker-room dousings with champagne after a championship game, and closeups of baseball players with a wad of chewing tobacco in their cheek seem to make the linkage between alcohol, tobacco, and sports natural and traditional. This mind set encourages the idea that other drugs are also acceptable in sports.

Though our attention during the last decade has been riveted on the deaths and scandals involving cocaine and steroid abuse, in terms of health effects, alcohol and nicotine are still the number one culprits. Nevertheless, in the 90's, athletes continue to abuse substances that cover a very large, diverse group of drugs, chemicals, and other substances, many of which are not psychoactive but most of which are being misused in the context that they are taken.

EXTENT OF ABUSE

The extent of drug use and abuse in sports is difficult to determine. For the common drugs of abuse such as alcohol, marijuana, tobacco, and cocaine the figures are probably comparable to society as a whole. In one month in 1993, approximately 98 million Americans drank alcohol, 54 million used cigarettes, 7 million used smokeless tobacco, 9 million used marijuana, 1.3 million used cocaine, and 1/2 a million used heroin.

The difference in sports comes with performance-enhancing or strength-enhancing drugs. In the 70's, over half of the NFL football players admitted to using amphetamines on a regular basis. One study in 1982 suggested that 70 to 80% of anabolic steroids prescribed in the U.S. were being diverted from medical uses.

A 15-year study published in 1985 reported that 20% of college athletes said they used anabolic steroids compared with 1% of non-athlete students, though anecdotal evidence in football and other strength sports suggests the numbers are much higher.

Athletes in certain sports use more of one drug than another. For example, football players in this survey reported 10% anabolic steroid use.

The figures will vary radically from state to state and from university to university, but the figures give a sense of the scope of the problem. In 1990, steroids were designated a controlled substance so the use has been declining in collegiate and professional sports.

The NCAA has an off season anabolic steroid random testing program. Of 2,000 student-athletes tested under this program, 3.5% tested positive.

Currently, it is estimated that 350,000 junior high and high school students have used or are using anabolic steroids. This is what they admitted to. The real numbers are probably higher. Another report indicates that as collegiate testing for steroids becomes more stringent, young athletes are encouraged to bulk up on steroids during high school and then go clean when they get to college. This is particu-

Fig. 9-1 In 1985 and 1989, Michigan State surveyed student athletes and found the following use of drugs in the previous year.

DRUG	1985	1989
Amphetamines	8%	3%
Anabolic steroids	4%	5%
Barbiturates	2%	2%
Alcohol	88%	89%
Cocaine/crack	17%	5%
Psychedelics	4%	4%
Marijuana/hashish	36%	28%

larly disturbing because an effect of anabolic steroids is to stunt hormonal and bone development in young athletes.

THE DRUGS

To understand the physical, mental, legal, and moral consequences of drug use in sports, it is necessary to examine the drugs themselves. Although there are literally hundreds of drugs and techniques that are used in connection with sports, we have focused on the most used and abused.

The following three categories of drugs used in sports are based on athlete's motives and the context in which use occurs rather than pharmacological properties of the substances. There is some overlap: drugs used to enhance performance might also give a pleasurable high.

- Therapeutic Drugs
- Performance-enhancing drugs (ergogenic drugs)
- Street/Recreational drugs

THERAPEUTIC DRUGS

These are drugs used for specific medical problems, usually in accordance with standards of good medical practice.

Anti-Bacterial Agents

Examples include antibiotics (penicillin, tetracycline, etc.) used to cure systemic infections, or disinfectants and antiseptics used to kill skin bacteria. With these drugs, there are appropriate medical indications for use and no risk of abuse.

Analgesics (pain-killers)

These drugs are normally used to deaden pain. They include both topical analgesics which desensitize nerve endings on the skin (alcohol and menthol, or local anesthetics such as procaine and lidocaine), and systemic analgesics such as aspirin, and Tylenol for mild to moderate pain or narcotic (opiate and opioid) analgesics for moderate to severe pain. The opiates and opioids inhibit the transmission of pain signals in the central nervous system.

The most common opiates used in sports are meperidine (Demerol, the most widely prescribed), morphine, codeine, and propoxyphene (Darvon). These drugs are either ingested or injected.

Besides the pain-killing effects, opiates can cause sedation, drowsiness, dulling of the senses, mood changes, nausea, and euphoria. Opiates are usually not performance enhancers; they just allow users to play through the pain and perform at or near their previous levels.

The biggest danger from these drugs results from their ability to block pain without repairing the damage. Normally, pain is the body's warning signal that some muscle, organ, or tissue is damaged and that it should be protected. If those signals are constantly short-circuited, the user becomes confused about what the body is saying.

Pain-killing drugs present some of the most difficult ethical questions about the use of drugs in sports. The dividing line between responsible use of the analgesics (as well as the muscle relaxants and the antihistamines) and abuse is crossed when they are employed to allow an injured player to continue performing when that activity could aggravate the injury or lead to a permanent disability, i.e., an athlete who may be playing on an anesthetized sprain or broken bone.

In addition, since tolerance develops so rapidly with opiates, increasing amounts become necessary to achieve pain relief. The problem is that tissue dependence can develop along with the analgesic effects, making it easier for the user to slip into compulsive use of the drug.

Muscle Relaxants

There are several classes of muscle relaxants, drugs that are used to treat muscle strains, ligament sprains, and the resultant severe spasms. They are also used to control tremors or shaking. Some athletes also use them to control performance anxiety.

The classes are

• Skeletal muscle relaxants such as Soma and Robaxin;

• Benzodiazepines such as Valium and Dalmane;

• Barbiturates such as Tuinal and Amytal.

These drugs are used to treat muscle strains and ligament sprains and the resultant severe spasms that accompany them.

The skeletal muscle relaxants are actually central nervous system depressants aimed at areas of the brain responsible for muscular coordination and activity. The abuse of these drugs for their mental effects is rare.

As with analgesics, the performance enhancement of these drugs is minimal because the drugs are depressants and can also cause sedation, blurred vision, decreased concentration, impaired memory, respiratory depression, and mild euphoria.

The benzodiazepines and barbiturates in particular also have a dependence liability since accelerating use causes tolerance and tissue dependence. The benzodiazepines also stay in the body for a long period of time, causing delayed effects when they're not wanted.

"I couldn't imagine anyone performing under the influence of alcohol or a barbiturate. If they got to that point they would probably hurt themselves. Occasionally some competed with a stimulant." Former college diving champion

Anti-inflammatory Drugs

When injuries occur to ligaments, tendons, and muscles, the soft tissue adjacent to the injury experiences pain and swelling. This inflammation begins the healing process, largely by increasing the blood supply to the area. These drugs control the inflammation and lessen pain.

Anti-inflammatory drugs come in two classes. NSAID's or non-steroidal anti-inflammatory drugs (typically Motrin or Advil, Indocin, Butazoliden, or Clinoril), and corticosteroids such as cortisone and Prednisone (corticosteroids are different than androgenic-anabolic steroids). The physical side effects of the NSAID's are relatively minor; gastric irritability, possible gastrointestinal bleeding, and hypertension.

But with the corticosteroids, side effects are a significant consideration. Prolonged use can cause water retention, bone thinning, muscle and tendon weakness, skin problems such as delayed wound healing, vertigo, headaches, and glaucoma. Psychoactive effects are minimal.

One other drug used for its anti-inflammatory effects is DMSO (dimethylsulfoxide). It is used topically to decrease inflammation and promote healing. DMSO at 80% to 100% concentration is effective in decreasing inflammation. This concentration will also burn the skin unless sufficient tolerance has been achieved. In high concentrations, DMSO is toxic to the liver and has been associated with cataract formation in the eye.

As with analgesics and skeletal muscle relaxants, when athletes are using anti-inflammatory drugs, a careful examination must be done to ensure that the injury is not serious and that practice or play can continue without risk of aggravating the injury. There is the risk that these drugs will be used as a "cure" for the injury. They should not be used solely to enable the athlete to resume activity, but should be part of the overall healing process. Ice, elevation, rest, physical therapy, and other treatment measures must accompany pharmacological relief of pain.

Where possible, over-the-counter remedies should take precedence over prescription and/or banned substances. Drugs used to provide pain relief or promote healing do not generally excite controversy and are not construed as providing an unfair advantage. Care must be taken to inform the athlete of the kind of drug being used and possible side effects. For their part, athletes should be sure that where possible they avoid substances banned by the International Olympic Committee (IOC) when they consult medical practitioners for treatment of their injuries.

PERFORMANCE-ENHANCING (ERGOGENIC) or APPEARANCE-ENHANCING DRUGS

This is a very broad and very general category of drugs, to which we will add other substances and even techniques used to enhance performance. Many of the drugs are illegal without a prescription, and most of the drugs, substances, and techniques, are banned by various sport governing bodies such as the International Olympic Committee and the NCAA. These ergogenic or energy producing drugs, substances, and techniques possess

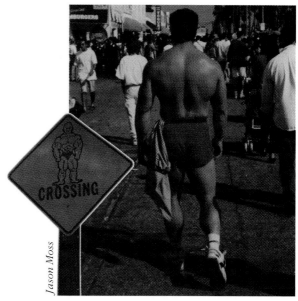

Jason Moss

various capabilities for boosting an athlete's performance by giving a temporary competitive edge.

Anabolic-Androgenic Steroids (AAS) or "Rhoids":

This group of drugs, derived from the male hormone testosterone or synthesized versions of it, have replaced amphetamines as the most abused performance-enhancing drugs today. Controversy surrounds the widespread use of anabolic steroids because they have marked benefits along with toxic side effects.

The benefits athletes look for in "rhoids" are increases in body weight, lean muscle mass, and increased muscular strength, but evidence suggests that such gains must be accompanied by weight training and a high-protein diet. Many students use AAS's strictly to enhance personal appearance.

"The men I knew who used steroids the most were 5'8" and under, and they talked about how they were the runts of the class and the 98 pound weakling at the beach. Steroids is one way they felt they could overcome that." Ex-weightlifter.

The drugs also increase aggressiveness and confidence, traits that are of value in many sports.

Patterns of Use —
Cycling and Stacking

Anabolic steroid users may take from 20 to 200 times the usually prescribed daily dosage. Some athletes practice "steroid stacking" by using three or more kinds of oral or injectable steroids, and alternating between "cycles" of use and non-use.

Cycling means taking the drugs for a 4- to 18-week period during intensive training and then stopping the drugs for a period of several weeks to several months to give the body a pharmacological rest. Some studies have reported that 82% of those using rhoids during a training cycle combined three or more different anabolic steroids in that time, and 30% used seven or more.

"As I progressed, I changed steroids whenever I felt my body building a tolerance to what I was taking. I mixed combinations like a chemist." NFL lineman

Of special concern is the fact that up to 99% of "rhoid" users have injected the drug, and most increase their dosage during the course of their training.

Physical Side Effects

"Androgenic" means producing masculine characteristics; "anabolic" means muscle-building; and "steroids" is the chemical classification of the natural and synthetic compounds resembling bodily hormones like testosterone. So far no pharmacological process has been able to separate the desirable muscle-building properties of AAS from their dangerous hormonal side effects. Although an athlete may want only anabolic effects, he or she will also have to accept the androgenic consequences.

In men, these drugs can result in an initial masculinization effect which includes an increase in muscle mass and muscle tone. Most users also report an initial bloated appearance. However, long-term use results in suppression of the body's own natural production of testosterone. As a consequence, men develop more feminine characteristics, decreased size of sexual organs, and an impairment of sexual functioning.

In women, similar gains in muscular development may be considered beautiful to some, but long-term use results in masculinizing effects such as increased facial hair, decreased breast size, lowered voice, and clitoral enlargement.

"This woman friend of mine walked in to the gym after being gone for 3 weeks. Her face was square and had unusual amounts of blond hair all over it. Her voice was really deep, and her back had cystic acne on it which she never had before. Even her skin was as tight as a drum. I found out later that she had shot up straight testosterone. She was fine with it because she 'wasn't going to have kids anyway.' That was just one more reason for me to stop competing. She went from beauty to freak in 3 weeks." Former body builder

Mental and Emotional Effects

Anabolic steroids also have a dramatic effect on emotions. Users feel more confident and aggressive while using these substances. Some researchers think that the confidence that "rhoids" can induce is sought after as much as the physical effects.

As use continues, the emotional balance of many users starts to swing from confidence to aggressiveness, to emotional instability, to rage and back to depression or to psychosis. This "rhoid rage" can lead to irrational behavior.

> *"After a dinner date this guy attacked me in my apartment. He was in the middle of a "rhoid" cycle. I put up a great fight and he gave up, but if he was determined, there was no way I could have overpowered him. I don't know if it was the drugs or he was just crazy." College coed*

Compulsive Use and Addiction

About a third of the users experience a sense of euphoria or well-being (at least initially) which contributes to their continued and compulsive abuse of "rhoids."

In a survey of hard-core AAS users in their senior year in high school, 25% said they wouldn't stop using even if it were proven beyond a doubt that AAS's cause permanent sterility, liver cancer, or heart attacks.

In a college survey of 45 weight lifters who were regular AAS users, half reported 3 or more symptoms of addiction, particularly withdrawal symptoms. Withdrawal symptoms include fatigue, depressed mood, restlessness, insomnia, no desire to eat, and lack of sexual desire. Even between cycles users will continue with low doses to avoid withdrawal.

Fig. 9-2 Physical and mental effects on male and female users of anabolic-androgenic steroids.

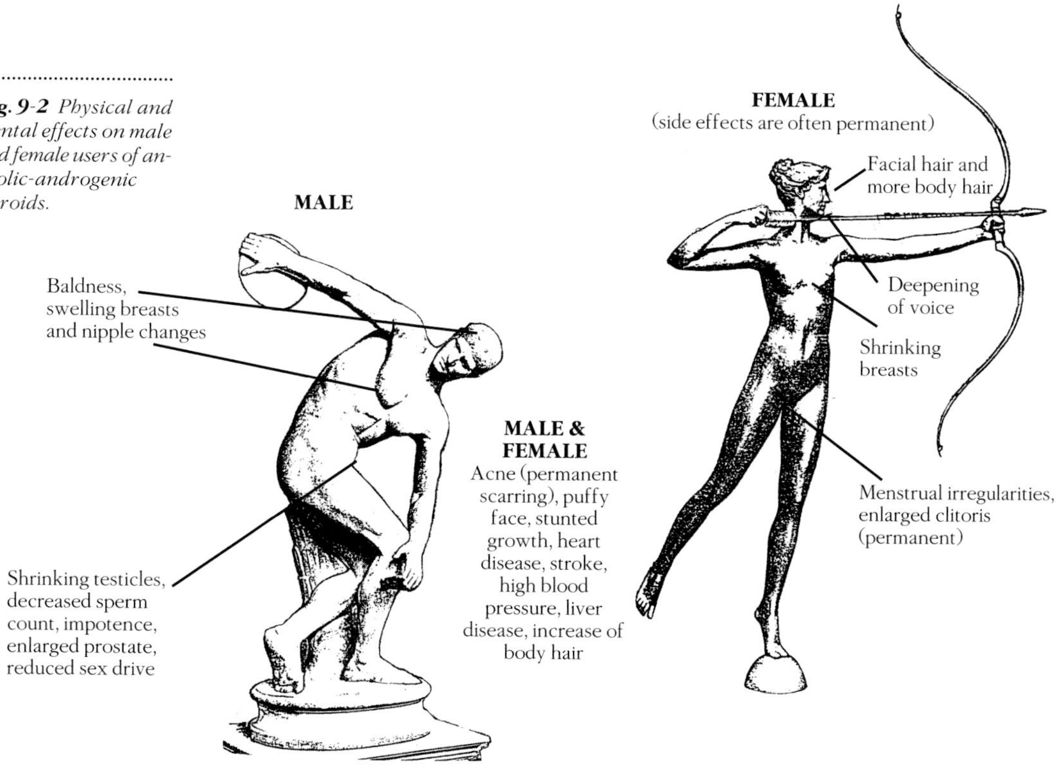

MALE

Baldness, swelling breasts and nipple changes

Shrinking testicles, decreased sperm count, impotence, enlarged prostate, reduced sex drive

MALE & FEMALE
Acne (permanent scarring), puffy face, stunted growth, heart disease, stroke, high blood pressure, liver disease, increase of body hair

FEMALE
(side effects are often permanent)

Facial hair and more body hair

Deepening of voice

Shrinking breasts

Menstrual irregularities, enlarged clitoris (permanent)

"It was addicting, mentally addicting. I just didn't feel strong unless I was taking something. When I retired I kept taking the stuff. I couldn't stand the thought of being weak." Lyle Alzado, former NFL star

Do Steroids Work?

The medical establishment finally admitted that AAS's did increase mass and muscle strength and did increase aggressiveness. The question though is *"Are the side effects worth the performance improvement?"*

"I took steroids from 1976 to 1983. In the middle of 1979, my body began turning a yellowish color, I was very aggressive and combative, had high blood pressure, and testicular atrophy. I was hospitalized twice with near kidney failure, liver tumors, and severe personality disorders. During my second hospital stay, the doctors found I had become sterile. Two years after I quit using and started training without drugs, I set 6 new world records in power lifting, something I thought was impossible without the steroids." Richard L. Sandlin, Former Assistant Coach, University of Alabama, before U.S. House of Representatives subcommittee on Crime, 1990

Supply and Cost

"We all knew who was using. We exchanged information on any new drugs that were on the market. We got our steroids through the gym owner. In fact, he would inject them for us, in the rear." Weight lifter

Athletes obtain steroids in different ways: from the black market (at gyms, from mail order companies, or friends), or from unscrupulous doctors, veterinarians, or pharmacists. Serious users spend 200 to 400 dollars per week on anabolic steroids and other strength drugs, so a single cycle can cost thousands of dollars. Some professional athletes spend 20,000 to 30,000 dollars a year. At a conservative estimate, the black market for steroids grosses 200 to 400 million dollars a year. Most of the product comes from up to 20 underground laboratories in the U.S. and foreign countries.

HCG or Human Chorionic Gonadotropin

This drug (isolated from placenta) and clomiphene or tamoxifen (synthetic drugs used to induce fertility and treat breast cancer) are occasionally used after anabolic steroid treatment to restart the body's own testosterone production. Toxic effects on the liver and reproductive system have been reported from the use of these substances to deal with the testosterone suppression caused by "rhoid" abuse.

Amphetamines

These constitute a class of more than 30 related stimulant drugs. They work by releasing "energy" chemicals in the brain and from the adrenal glands which cause blood vessel constriction and increased heart rate and blood pressure. The user feels energetic, alert, and confident. Athletes take (or are given) amphetamines to make themselves more aggressive, alert and to reduce fatigue. Athletes take them before an athletic event: football players to become more aggressive; runners to increase speed and energy; tennis players to improve concentration and reaction time.

Virtually all amphetamines and methamphetamines ("crank," methadrine), and amphetamine congeners (Tepanil, Ritalin, Ionamin, Cylert), are banned by the International Olympic Committee.

Negative effects include anxiety, restlessness, and impaired judgment. Heavy use sometimes brings on paranoia, heart and blood pressure problems, and convulsions. Chronic use can result in psychosis, paranoid delusions, and repetitive, compulsive behavior, as well as addiction. There have been reports of fatal heat stroke among athletes using amphetamines since the drug redistributes blood away from the skin thereby impairing the body's cooling system. The elevated mood (feeling "up") from the drug has sometimes led to errors and misjudgments.

Caffeine

It can increase performance slightly at blood levels of 10mg/ml. The Olympic committee puts a limit on caffeine which is the equivalent of about 3 strong cups of coffee just before competition.

Human Growth Hormone (HGH)

This was a fad drug during the 80's chiefly among football players who thought that HGH increased muscles, bone growth, and connective tissue strength. Before 1985 the drug could only be collected from the pituitary glands of infants and growing children; since then, synthetic versions have been developed. Its popularity rests on the hope that it will cause fewer side effects than "rhoids" and that it will continue to be undetectable. Also, unlike "rhoids" which only increase muscle strength without affecting tendon or ligament strength, HGH increases connective tissue as well as muscle strength. Thus, HGH users hope to avoid the frequent tendon, ligament, and bone damage which occurs with "rhoid" use.

Some of the negative effects of use include increased growth of body hair, cardiovascular disease, hypertension, thickened skin, soft tissue swelling, and diabetes.

Few reliable studies exist, and there are no documented performance-enhancing effects as yet. Long-term effects of use are similarly unknown at this time, although gigantism and unusual development of the hands, feet, and limbs have been noted in children given the drug to stimulate growth.

Periactin

This is an antihistamine used for colds and allergic reactions. Periactin is believed to increase strength and cause weight gain. Its side effects include decreased performance, sweating, and sedation.

Adrenalin & Amyl or Isobutyl Nitrite

This combination is taken by weight lifters just prior to their performance to increase strength. The down side is dizziness (a dangerous side effect with a 400 pound barbell over one's head) and rapid heart beat and hypertension.

Blood Doping

Blood doping, the practice of injecting extra blood, either one's own or someone else's, is used to increase endurance by increasing the number of red blood cells available to carry oxygen. Blood doping is used by athletes in such sports as cycling, long-distance running, cross-country skiing, and other events that require endurance. Because doping involves blood transfusion, dangers include poor storage, viral or bacterial infections, and even fatal reactions due to mislabeling. No test yet exists to accurately detect blood doping, so athletes have a clear-cut decision to make: to cheat or not to cheat.

Beta-Blockers propranolol (Inderol), atenolol (Tenormin)

These constitute a class of IOC-banned drugs which block nerve cell activity at the heart, kidney, and blood vessels and are therefore often prescribed for heart disease in order to lower blood pressure, lessen the heart rate, and block stimulatory responses. They block adrenalin from binding onto beta-receptors on the heart. They also block nerve cell activity in the brain and are used to calm and steady the body. They are also used to control migraine headaches and the symptoms of a panic attack or "performance fright." Because of their ability to calm the brain and tremors, they are sought by some athletes involved in riflery, archery, diving, ski-jumping, and biathlon and pentathlon.

Beta blockers are dangerous in those with hypertension or heart problems. They can also cause fatigue, lethargy, dreams, occasional nausea, vomiting, and temporary impotence. Another negative effect of these drugs is interference with production of the liver enzyme needed to eliminate wastes.

Diuretics

These are drugs that increase the rate of urine formation thus speeding the elimination of water from the body. Athletes use these drugs for 2 reasons.

• To lose weight rapidly. This is important in sports where people compete in certain weight classes.

• To avoid detection of illegal drugs during testing by increasing urination.

"I was given a diuretic a week before I was to compete with instructions not to drink more than a half cup of water per day. I probably lost 12 pounds of water that week. I left the dorm the morning of my competition and my neighbor across the hall didn't recognize me because my face was so drawn. I wouldn't have placed second if the gym owner hadn't given me the diuretic." Competitive wrestler

Athletes trying to make their weight will use diuretics, exercise, self-induced vomiting, excess sweating in a sauna, and fasting. This is done in spite of the evidence that dehydration significantly diminishes performance. Some athletes will lose 3 to 5% of their weight in a couple of days.

Erythropoietin (EPO)

EPO has been termed one of the most dangerous drugs abused by athletes. It appeared in the late 1980's and is a synthetic version of the human hormone that stimulates the production of oxygen-laden red blood cells. It is used as a substitute for blood doping, and there is evidence that it increases performance in endurance sports.

The dangers from unsupervised EPO administration result from the thickening of the blood which can lead to clots that might cause stroke or heart attack. Sweating and the accompanying increase in blood viscosity magnifies this potential danger of blood clots even more. A number of deaths among European cyclists from this kind of blood doping has been reported.

STREET/RECREATIONAL DRUGS

The term "recreational," which has been used to describe drug use in social contexts, for pleasure, reward, or compensation, is misleading, because it conveys the idea of legitimate pleasure or fun and the sense that drug use can be controlled. But health hazards and liability to addiction are just as great for drugs that are used for

enjoyment as those that are used for their pain-killing or performance-enhancing effects. When drug use goes beyond occasional or experimental use, it will become habitual and compulsive. Frequency of use, quantity of intake, and the amount of harm caused to the user will determine when use becomes abuse. Frequency, quantity, and harm vary for each individual. A drug doesn't know or care that it's being used "just for fun," and a user has great difficulty in recognizing when use becomes abuse.

"I think once you really get the first rush from cocaine, no other one is really like that one. And so you continue to chase that one feeling that you got the first time. We used to say, 'We were chasing the little green man.'"
Recovering pro athlete

Athletes take drugs to adjust their moods for a number of reasons. Some use stimulants such as amphetamines ("crank," "whites," "black beauties") as a way of getting "up" for competition. Or they will use drugs such as alcohol, Xanax, Valium, barbiturates, opiates, and even marijuana as self-rewards for enduring the stress they experience while performing before so many people or as a tranquilizer to calm down after the excitement of competition or to counteract the effects of stimulants used to enhance their performance.

Or they will use drugs in order to conform, to fit into social situations where drug use is encouraged as they comply with peer pressure, imitate the behavior of older role models, or shape behavior to conform to their image of an athlete.

Finally, athletes may turn to drugs for many of the same reasons as non-athletes: to help cope with the demands of a heavy schedule (practice, travel time, course work); to reduce stress; to compensate for loneliness; to fill up time on long road trips.

Alcohol

It is generally recognized that in small to moderate amounts, alcohol is usually not addicting. It must be kept in mind that about 10% of drinkers will become alcoholic, and thus, up to one in ten players will have difficulty moderating alcohol use. Use among athletes is widespread. In one study, 65% of over 2000 athletes questioned in Division I, II, and III college institutions said they had consumed alcohol during the previous month, about a quarter of whom began drinking by junior high school.

Research demonstrates that alcohol is not an ergogenic drug, except in sports like riflery where the calming and sedating effects of alcohol can steady the hand. In general, alcohol consumption negatively affects reaction time, coordination, and balance, although studies suggest that low-dose alcohol consumption does not produce impaired performance in all people. The NFL "Drug Policy" statement calls alcohol "without question the most abused drug in our sport." The problem is how to alert athletes to the health and performance consequences of a drug

that has general social, legal, and moral acceptance in society. Early education, recognition and treatment seem the answer.

Marijuana

This all arounder can either stimulate or depress user depending on the strength of the drug and the mood of the smoker. Tolerance to the drug develops, and so more is used, which can lead to impaired performance.

In a sport like competitive diving where coordination, timing, and poise are crucial, marijuana has little value.

> *"My sport was so oriented to space and time that we did drugs more for recreation, not to perform better. Using marijuana affected my ambition in a major way. It clouded my realistic image of how I was performing. I would tend to settle for a lower level of performance. I couldn't see the bigger picture."* Competitive spring board diver

Further, marijuana lowers blood pressure which has caused fainting spells in football linemen who have to go from a down position to a standing one quickly and often during a game. It inhibits sweating which has caused heat prostration and strokes in athletes, and it impairs the ability of users to follow a moving object like a ball in play (decreased tracking ability).

In a study at a major university, researchers studied a group of football players over a period of 4 years. The athletes admitted who was using marijuana and who wasn't. All the athletes thought they were doing well and performing well, but when an objective study was made of their performance, those that smoked marijuana did much more poorly: they dropped more passes, committed more errors, and suffered more injuries during their college career.

Athletes will use marijuana to let down from the pressures of competition and to relax. Some will use it to relax the night before competition, although hangover-like effects might impair performance the next day. The most controversial aspects of use for athletes surrounds the claims that its use leads to apathy and impaired motivation. It seems safe to say that these effects depend on the individual athlete.

"Over time, the grass would slow down my reaction time so subtly that I wasn't readily aware of it as I would have been with a sedative or a pain killer. Slowly the cumulative effects of the grass affected my performance." Ex-college baseball player

Interestingly, marijuana is not prohibited by the International Olympic Committee because they know that there are no performance-enhancing effects from the drug. Any prohibition is usually done by the Olympic Committee of each country.

Cocaine

Like other stimulants, cocaine may be used to intensify sensory stimulation and increase energy. Athletes also use cocaine to capture the natural high they experienced during competition.

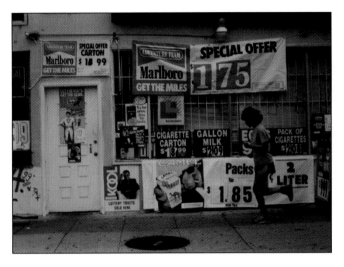

"When you have played before seventy thousand people and come off the field, you're back down to normal, so to speak. You want to get back up there with cocaine. It replaces that high with an artificial stimulation. But the comedown from cocaine is very, very draining, emotionally, physically, and nutritionally. It's totally different than coming down from the natural high."
Former NFL rushing back

In spite of its high cost, cocaine is abused by athletes who can afford the expense, usually by professional athletes who have both the money and free time. Cocaine is also used both for its pain-killing properties and as an ergogenic drug, giving them a boost of thirty minutes on average compared with hours for amphetamines. Some football players refer to it as the "second-half drug," and use has been reported among baseball players at the end of a long, arduous season.

The adverse effects of cocaine have less to do with physical dependence than psychological addiction. Use reinforces continued use. Because of the intense euphoria of a cocaine high, athletes come to depend on it after competition to keep them feeling like heroes.

Risks of use include sudden cardiac collapse (Len Bias died at the age of 22 of "cocaine intoxication"), convulsions, seizure, heat stroke, hemorrhage, and delirium. It can also lead to behavioral and personality changes.

Amphetamines

Besides being used as performance-enhancing drugs, amphetamines are used "recreationally." These drugs produce effects and problems similar to cocaine. Since their effects last longer, amphetamines are more often used to try to enhance performance, whereas cocaine is used to reward it.

Cigarettes

The active ingredient in cigarettes is nicotine, a mild stimulant. The performance-enhancing effects of this mild stimulant are minimal compared to the performance-diminishing side effects. Smoking reduces the ability of the blood to transport oxygen to the body's tissues. Smoking significantly decreases lung capacity in heavy smokers. As few as 10 puffs of a cigarette in a casual smoker will reduce airway conductance. And finally, smoking aggravates the cardiovascular system through constriction of blood vessels and stimulation of the sympathetic nervous system.

Smokeless Tobacco

One of television images of baseball is that of the baseball player with a large wad of chewing tobacco in his cheek. Many players feel that they can receive the performance-enhancing stimulatory effects of nicotine without the performance-diminishing respiratory side effects. While respiratory problems are avoided, cardiovascular problems remain along with bad breath, stained teeth, tooth loss, and an increased risk of oral lesions or cancers. Research has shown that smokeless tobacco does not increase reaction time or movement time but that it does speed up the heart rate and raise the blood pressure.

CONCLUSIONS

Summary

Drug abuse in sports has many ramifications. Society's win-at-any-cost attitude that is passed to athletes by management, coaches, trainers, fans, and the media has inadvertently encouraged drug abuse by professional athletes to a much greater degree than it tolerates drug abuse by pilots, truck drivers, or even employees in the work place. Yet, athletes face the same health risks, and when they are using drugs, they too endanger others.

Anabolic steroids induce aggressiveness, hostility, and anger in the users often detached from any compassion or concern for anybody else. The wrestlers or football players under its influence often compete beyond the goal of just winning and may be bent upon injuring or maiming their opponents. Increased violence in sports, involving athletes, spouses, and fans, may be a direct result of the increasing abuse of drugs by athletes.

Under the influence of amphetamines or other stimulants which increase endurance, motor sport athletes and others also experience increased confidence with feelings of omnipotence and grandeur which impair their judgment and logic. These feelings can influence an athlete to take inappropriate chances or make ill-advised decisions which threaten the safety of both spectators and other competitors.

Analgesics, anesthetics, and anti-inflammatory steroids (cortisone) all diminish or block pain in an injured athlete. This allows them to continue to perform despite serious injury. An all-too-common situation in sports, this practice gravely threatens the safety of injured athletes as well as that of their competitors and team members who are relying on an expected level of performance and interaction.

POLICY RECOMMENDATIONS

If we believe that athletic competition should be a measure of individual excellence unaided by performance-enhancing drugs, then attitudes towards drug use and abuse by athletes need to change.

Any plan to change these attitudes and stop the abuse of drugs in sports must include policy creation and dissemination, identification of users, intervention, treatment, and above all, prevention education.

Policy Formation

A definite drug policy should be formulated. It exists in many organizations, but it must be extended to all levels of society.

There should be clearly formulated, well-illustrated guidelines that spell out the differences between acceptable drug use and unacceptable drug abuse. No drugs should be administered before they have been tested safe for use.

The policy should be fair. It should be formulated beforehand, and the consequences of abuse of alcohol, steroids, or other drugs explained to everyone in pre-season meetings. It should apply consistently to all involved ("stars" as well as "subs"). All those responsible should be willing to enforce the policy.

A case can be made for a series of graduated penalties for first and subsequent violations, later violations involving counseling and then treatment. There is reason to believe that first violations should be addressed with fairly lenient penalties to increase the likelihood that more athletes will be reported and that the policy will be enforced.

An athlete should be confronted immediately if substance abuse is suspected and given explanations of why the rules have been broken and what the consequences are. Denial and fear are usual defense responses by drug abusers. Discipline should be firm, but it should be accompanied by understanding and suggestions about additional assistance.

In these matters and at all stages of drug abuse prevention, role models should be provided by coaches, staff, and team captains.

> *"You have to get them down at the high school level, and the responsibility falls on the coach. This is where the morals and the standards are formed for these students. Everyone remembers their high school coach, whether good or bad. They are the ones that get the kid when he really has no idea what the hazards are. All the kid cares about is tomorrow."*
> High school coach

Identification and Referral

Awareness training for coaches, administrators, and support staff about drug use and abuse is essential as well as effective intervention methods. Self-identification and referral of users should also be encouraged.

Coaches, trainers, and staff should be alerted to specific signs of drug abuse by athletes. The following symptoms are indications of problems, not necessarily of substance abuse and should be followed by further investigation.

1) Diminished interest in the sport;
2) Lowered level of performance; less energy;
3) Decreased motivation;
4) Late attendance at practice; missed practices;
5) Changes in personality; mood swings;
6) Hyperactivity;
7) Inattentiveness; wandering looks;
8) Change in peer group;
9) Isolation.

Coaches, trainers, and staff should also be alerted to signs of steroid use and abuse:

1) Quick weight gain;
2) Increased aggressiveness or violence;
3) Sudden and dramatic increase muscular definition;
4) Severe acne;
5) Breast development in males;
6) Menstrual problems in females;
7) Loss of hair in males; growth of facial and bodily hair in females;
8) Ultra definition or change in shape of face;
9) Deepening of voice.

"No matter what an athlete tells you, I don't care who, don't believe them if they tell you these substances aren't widely used. We're not born to be 280 or 300 pounds or jump 30 feet. Some people are born that way, but not many. I think the coaches knew guys were built certain ways, and they knew those guys couldn't look the way they did without taking stuff. But the coaches just coached and looked the other way." Lyle Alzado

Drug Testing

Drug testing has become an integral part of many prevention and treatment programs. Since denial is so prevalent with drug use, only testing in many cases can break through the athlete's defenses. The problem with drug testing is that it is expensive, it doesn't test for all drugs, and it is very invasive of a person's privacy. The advantages are that given the danger of drugs to athletes and to the concept of sports itself, drug testing would seem to make sense. The question is, "does it work?"

Many drug testing policies are handed down by the IOC, the NCAA, or local athletic groups. The problem is that those who use know many of the tricks of avoiding detection. In addition, the cost of a single test is about $100. Few sports programs can afford random or mandatory testing at a level where it would truly be effective. On the other hand, sometimes just the threat is enough to cut down on abuse so there is real value there. In the end, peer support, effective treatment programs, and especially prevention education targeted for athletes, are the best hope for sports.

Peer Support

Peer monitoring and support groups should be formed, particularly at the high school and college level. Unfortunately, the identification, intervention, and treatment of athletes is coming from outside sources such as management, a conference, or a committee. The more that can be done to stimulate internal monitoring so that athletes deal with athletes (like physicians dealing with physicians, college professors with college professors), the more effective the system will be. Respect, caring, and treatment are more important than attack.

TREATMENT

For student-athletes who are abusing drugs, a user-friendly counseling system should also be in place, one that guarantees confidentiality. The attitude should be directed to aiding the person who happens to be an athlete to recognize patterns of abuse. The wrong approach is to treat the problem as one involving an athlete who happens to be a person. The focus should be on recovery which is a long-term, often lifelong process during which one deals with all aspects of his or her life, especially those that threaten to pull the person back into drug abuse. There should be easy access to local rehabilitation programs and a promotion of participation in available support groups.

There should be, for example, specific alternatives to drugs for someone who says, "I can't take the pressure of playing in front of all those people." The treatment should focus on that fear, rather than saying, "Well that's your job. Get out there and play." The program should help focus people on their recovery.

A peer group can also be used in recovery. Among people with similar backgrounds, goals, and values, recovering athletes can relate to others, feel more comfortable facing their problems and talking about them among other athletes. They don't feel threatened or diminished, and the support from other athletes lessens the denial.

Prevention-Education Programs

Drug abuse prevention programs should be incorporated into a training system, a continuous, longitudinal model that goes from beginning to end of an athlete's career and one that includes family members. This means a four-year educational model for both high-school and college. This is an educational challenge, and it needs to be met by a well-defined curriculum.

Ideally, athletics should be put in the context of personal development and life-long wellness. The problems that athletes face in preparing for competition, maintaining an academic schedule, developing a social life, and preparing for a career should be discussed, and ways of coping with the stresses and challenges other than with drugs should be explored.

Stress reduction exercises, meditation, prayer, and discussion groups can all be helpful in assisting athletes to deal with stress. They also need to appreciate the highs and lows experienced from competition. They need to learn how to appreciate their performance and have pride in the work they put into training.

Experience has found that in general, rational people who have enough information about the consequences of drug abuse will avoid drugs. They will not be willing to trade the short-term effect for the severe physiological stress on the body, the impaired responses, the delayed reaction time, the higher doses, the potential for permanent physical and mental damage and even life-threatening consequences of drug abuse.

....

Lyle Alzado was one of the few professional athletes to publicly speak out against performance-enhancing drugs, particularly steroids and human growth hormone. The magazine appeared in 1991.

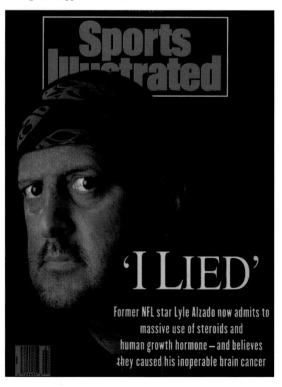

ETHICS

Taking drugs violates the assumption of fair competition on which sports rest. It is a kind of cheating that can go on before the game begins, while it is being played, and after its conclusion. Drugs violate the very nature of sport which since the time of the Greeks was a measure of personal excellence, the result of a sound mind in a healthy body. The outcome of athletic contests was to be determined by discipline, training, and effort. There is a real threat that the public will walk away from sports if they perceive that winning is based on access to the latest pharmacology and schemes to evade urine testing. Drugs also rob the athlete of feelings of self accomplishment and tarnish the pride of winning. And because our society treats sports figures as heroes and role models, drug abusing athletes diminish all of us.

"If I had known I would be this sick now, I would have tried to make it in football on my own, naturally. Whoever is doing this stuff, if you stay on it too long, or maybe if you get on it at all, you're going to get something bad from it." Lyle Alzado, former NFL star (Alzado died in 1992 at the age of 42 from brain cancer which he felt was caused by his 20 year use of steroids and human growth hormone.)

SPORTS AND DRUGS

1. Athletes use drugs as a short-cut means of preparing for competition, as a reward, to lessen pain, and to socialize.

2. Drug use among athletes dates from the time of the early Greeks. Drug use continues through the present because of increased availability of drugs, new drugs, a "win at any cost" attitude in international competitions, and increased financial incentives to succeed.

3. Steroids represent a particular problem in athletics because, although use among collegiate and professional athletes is decreasing (possibly because of increased testing), use continues among high-school athletes.

4. Three classes of drugs available to athletes are therapeutic drugs, performance or appearance-enhancing drugs, and recreational drugs.

5. Undesirable effects of opiates include mood changes, nausea, and tissue dependence. A danger of various pain-killing drugs is that athletes will aggravate injuries while playing injured.

6. The two kinds of anti-inflammatory drugs are NSAID's and corticosteroids. Side effects of the latter are more serious than those of the former.

7. Androgenic anabolic steroids are derived from or imitate the male hormone testosterone. Athletes use them to increase weight, strength, and/or muscle mass and definition.

8. The side effects of anabolic steroid abuse are acne, lowered sexdrive, shrinking of testicles in men, breast reduction in women, bloated appearance, anger, and aggressiveness.

9. Amphetamines are used to "boost" the athlete, to increase energy, alertness, aggression, and reaction time. The negative effects from occasional use of amphetamines include irritability, restlessness, anxiety, and heart or blood pressure problems. Chronic to heavy use of the drug can result in psychosis, paranoia, and addiction.

10. Blood doping involves injecting extra blood into an athlete to increase the oxygen content of the blood. Because of the risk of infection, it is considered dangerous.

11. Marijuana acts either as a stimulant or depressant, and it is the most widely abused illegal drug. Athletes turn to marijuana to relax or calm down.

12. Cocaine may be used by athletes for its stimulant effects. Psychological addiction is more usual than physical dependence.

13. Drug abuse by athletes involves dangers to athletes, opponents, family, friends, and fans. Anabolic steroids promote increased violence. Amphetamines and other stimulants impair reason. Pain medications encourage athletes to play while injured.

14. Policies on drug use in sports should be fair and compassionate. They should involve identification and referral, testing, treatment, and extensive, career-long education for athletes.

15. Drug use in sports risks loss of fan support. It imperils the notion of fair competition, and it robs athletes who abuse drugs of a sense of self-worth and personal achievement.

QUESTIONS

1. Why do some athletes use drugs?

2. Why did anabolic steroids and amphetamines begin to be abused by athletes during the 1950's?

3. Which are the two drugs most widely abused by athletes?

4. Name two muscle relaxants that stay in the body for an extended period and involve both tolerance and tissue dependence.

5. What are "cycling" and "stacking"?

6. What is "rhoid rage"?

7. List negative effects of anabolic steroids on females and males.

8. Why do some athletes choose human growth hormone (HGH) rather than steroids? What are some of the negative effects of HGH?

9. Why is the ethical issue so clear-cut for blood doping?

10. In which sports are beta-blockers found and why?

11. Why can the term "recreational drugs" be misleading?

12. What are the major differences between cocaine and amphetamine effects?

13. What are the risks to athletes of inappropriate use of analgesics, anesthetics, and anti-inflammatory steroids?

14. Name several signs of substance abuse by athletes.

15. Name several signs of abuse of anabolic steroids by athletes.

16. List several alternatives to drugs for stress control.

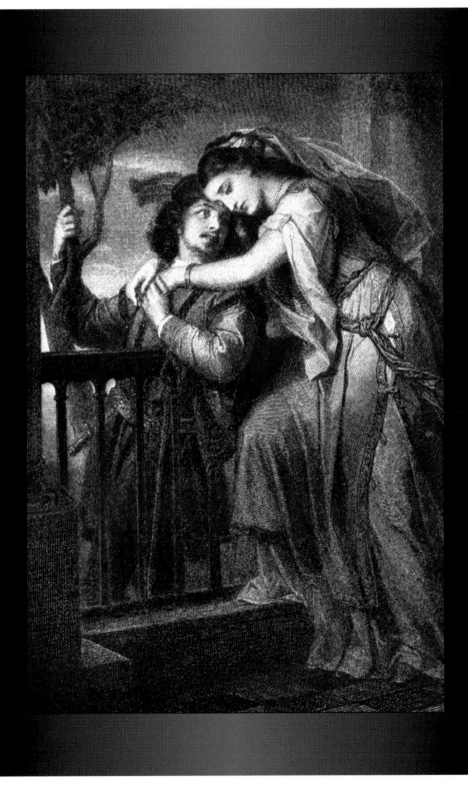

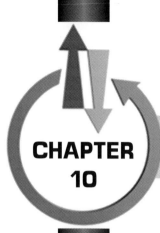

CHAPTER 10

SEX, LOVE, AND DRUGS

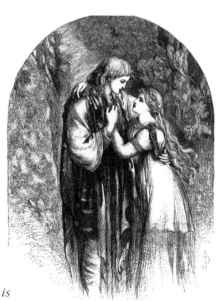

*The deepest human need is
the need to overcome the
prison of our aloneness.
  —Erich Fromm*

Our desire for friendship, affection, love, intimacy, and sex is crucial to our functioning as human beings. That functioning is affected by drugs in many different and complicated ways. For example, some drugs such as alcohol, marijuana, and "ecstasy" lower inhibitions. Others including cocaine, amphetamines, and some inhalants alter the physical sensations of sexuality and counter low self-esteem or shyness.

*"It felt real ecstatic, very euphoric. My mind had a great deal
of pleasure. I felt like somebody." Cocaine user*

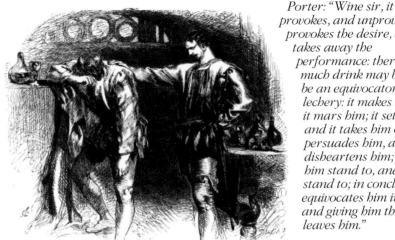

Porter: "Wine sir, it provokes, and unprovokes: it provokes the desire, but it takes away the performance: therefore, much drink may be said to be an equivocator with lechery: it makes him, and it mars him; it sets him on, and it takes him off; it persuades him, and disheartens him; makes him stand to, and not stand to; in conclusion, equivocates him in a sleep, and giving him the lie, leaves him."

Macbeth, William Shakespeare

Drugs generally substitute a simple physical sensation or the illusion of one, for the more complex (yet more rewarding) true emotion such as desire for intimacy, comfort, love of children, satisfaction, or release from anxiety.

What psychoactive drugs do is artificially manipulate natural biochemicals, thereby counterfeiting, stimulating, blocking, or confusing true emotions and sensations about romance, love, and sex.

"I'm usually tense around people. With alcohol I feel looser. I feel friendlier. I start conversations, and I get pretty amorous." 16-year-old alcohol user

Because the emotional makeup of human beings is so complex, this chapter will focus more on drugs and sexual activity rather than drugs and the full spectrum of human emotion. However, it is important to remember that drug use and abuse have as much to do with motivation and emotions as they do with physical sensations.

DESIRE, EXCITATION, AND ORGASM

Contradictions are the rule when sex and drugs are combined because sexual behavior involves desire, excitation, and orgasm, and as Shakespeare pointed out, drugs affect each part differently and, at time,s in opposite ways.

Desire is the most complex of the stages. Does desire mean the desire to be close or the desire to have sex? Will a person use drugs for lust or love? Is there a difference between a man's and a woman's view of desire? Is desire a method our body created to perpetuate the species? These are all important considerations, but for our purposes, "desire" means the desire to have sexual intimacies. (The moral questions about if and when to have sex are beyond the scope of this chapter.)

Excitation on the other hand is more clear cut than sexual desire. It can be defined by physical changes that occur as a result of

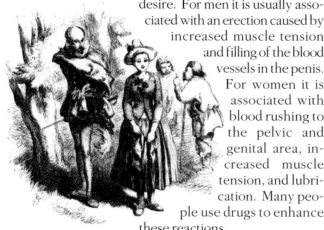

desire. For men it is usually associated with an erection caused by increased muscle tension and filling of the blood vessels in the penis. For women it is associated with blood rushing to the pelvic and genital area, increased muscle tension, and lubrication. Many people use drugs to enhance these reactions.

Orgasm in men is signaled by ejaculation, release of muscular tension and release of excess blood from the genital area. In women it is signaled by rhythmic contractions of vaginal muscles, release of muscular tension, and release of excess blood from the pelvic area. People use drugs to enhance, intensify, or delay orgasm.

When drugs are used to affect sexual behavior, such factors as the dosage, route of administration, mood, mental health, physi-

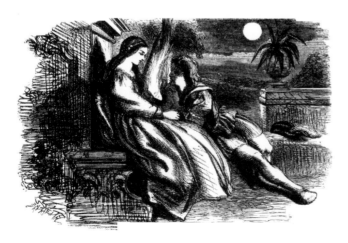

cal condition, and level of use of the user, and particularly the setting in which the drug is used, all have an influence on sexual behavior. A recent divorcé drinking alone at home will have quite a different reaction to 3 shots of scotch than he would in a singles bar talking to a woman.

SOCIAL IMPACT

"There's something about a scotch on ice that gives me the courage to try to pick up a woman. I think I look cool with a shot glass in my hand." 22-year-old social drinker

Drugs not only have an impact on all phases of sexual behavior from puberty, to dating, to marital relations, but also on sexual violence i.e., sexual harassment, rape (including date rape), and child molestation. The violence occurs because drugs decrease inhibitions, increase aggressiveness and disrupt judgment. Drugs also encourage high-risk sexual behavior like prostitution, group sex and anonymous sex which spread sexually transmitted diseases like syphilis, gonorrhea, hepatitis B, and AIDS.

"I'm monogamous. I'm with just one boyfriend at a time. I've been with him for 2 months now. The one before I was with for 4 months." Teenage crack user

The 60's and 70's signaled an increase in the use and availability of marijuana in high schools and colleges along with increased sexual activity. In addition, the onset of the "crack" epidemic in the 80's that continued into the 90's made a low-cost, ultra-compulsive, "fast-food drug" available to a younger population, causing an increase in regular and especially high-risk sexual activity.

"These were women that otherwise I would never even have the nerve to approach. Once I've got crack, then I'm someone who's desirable, and I can do with these women anything that I want to. And, that's what got me involved with crack cocaine." Crack user

GENERAL EFFECTS

Physically, psychoactive drugs affect hormonal release (testosterone, estrogen, adrenaline, etc.), blood flow, blood pressure, nerve sensitivity, and muscle tension which in turn affect excitation (erectile ability) and orgasm. For example, heroin desensitizes penile and vaginal nerve endings.

Alcohol dilates blood vessels making it harder for excess blood to stay in the genital area thereby making it difficult to maintain an erection. Steroids increase testosterone which stimulates the fight center of the brain making a user more sexually aggressive.

Mentally, drugs affect self-confidence, inhibition, judgment, and ultimately desire. Many of the mental effects are a result of drugs' manipulation of neurotransmitters in the central nervous system particularly serotonin, dopamine, endorphin, and norepinephrine (noradrenaline). The neurotransmitters, in turn, can stimulate our pleasure, reward, and satiation centers.

For example, cocaine releases dopamine which stimulates our pleasure center in the limbic system, the same system stimulated during excitation and orgasm. In addition, drugs affect the hypothalamus which can trigger hormonal changes.

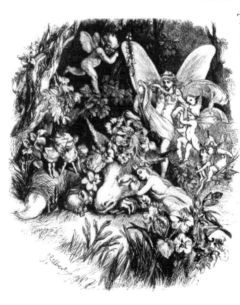

The actual effect of drugs and what the user hopes they will do can vary radically. In a survey at the Haight-Ashbury Clinic, regular drug users said they combined sex and drugs in order to

1. lower their inhibitions,

2. try to make themselves perform better,

3. increase their fantasies.

"I was sort of shy and it made me feel I was super smart, super pretty, a super person. Being at that age, I felt very awkward and uncomfortable." Teenage crack user

"It's a very euphoric, satisfying kind of effect, and it's similar to sex . . . but different." Heroin user

These are some of the reasons people combine sex and drugs, often searching for a shortcut to complex emotions, but the reaction to psychoactive drugs is so variable, often escalating into compulsive and addictive behavior, that many of the initial, desired effects on sexuality and performance change with time.

"When you take a large number of pills, you're less able to perform, to the point of impotence. As I got up to 5 or 10 crosstops a day, I couldn't get an erection." Speed user

"Lots of times, I don't want to be bothered by anybody or anyone touching me like my boyfriend; if he wants to hug me or kiss me, I just say, 'Don't touch me.'" Heroin user

In addition, compulsion and addiction can force many users to do almost anything for their drug.

"It's two types of women using drugs. One's a 'tossup,' who'll do anything for a rock. They've lost everything they have. They have no self-respect. They have nothing. Me and my sister on the other hand, we'd work a dude in a minute to get his dope. Once we got his dope it's, 'Go on, get outta my house.'" Crack user

Sex and love are such complicated processes and so tied in with our mental state that people use drugs not only to enhance their sexuality but also to shield themselves from their sexuality and even from any emotional involvement.

SIDE EFFECTS

"When I started taking drugs, it helped me suppress my emotions. The only unfortunate thing was that when the drugs would wear off, the emotions would be unleashed, no control of them, using the wrong emotion at the wrong time." Heroin user

Early drug experimentation disturbs, arrests, and even reverses emotional growth.

"When you begin to use drugs around twelve or thirteen, you never have rites of passage. You never get indoctrinated into the 'adulthood' of society. Many people we treat actually began using substances at that age, so their rites of passage haven't occurred when we see them at thirty, or thirty five." Drug counselor

Since those extra years of emotional growth that have been lost are so crucial to a woman's and a man's maturation, the results can cause huge changes in the fabric of society. For example, 28% of all children born in the United States in 1992 were born out of wedlock, up from 17 % in 1980.

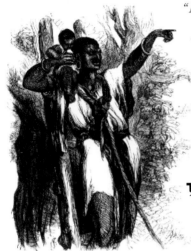

"My baby was born with a positive drug screen, so child protective services took him away. Later they took my other two kids away until I cleaned up my act." 19-year-old crack user

THE DRUGS

Drug using behavior takes on a life of its own as tolerance, withdrawal, and side effects overwhelm the original intentions of the user. Since each drug is different, it is necessary to examine each separately.

One problem in examining each separately is that most drug use and abuse involves more than one drug, most notably alcohol and another substance, so the interactions cause contradictory effects. If alcohol and cocaine are ingested, the contraction of blood vessels by the cocaine fights the dilation by the alcohol, and the lowering of inhibitions by the alcohol is exaggerated by the increased aggression caused by the cocaine.

Finally, the expectations (personal and cultural) of what a drug is supposed to do sexually can have a greater impact than the drug's real effects. Therefore, studies on the impact of individual drugs contain a certain amount of generalization and even guesswork.

UPPERS

The two strongest stimulants, cocaine and amphetamines, are sometimes called love drugs because they force the release of the neurotransmitters dopamine and norepinephrine, body chemicals closely associated with natural sexual and romantic reactions. In fact some popular magazines called these neurotransmitters natural amphetamines because they can produce elation and euphoria. But stimulating these neurotransmitters artificially with drugs can cause harmful side effects and disrupt natural sexual reactions.

Cocaine

Effects: Although the effects on sexual activity can vary from user to user, the most commonly reported reactions are

Low-dose use: Males: usually stimulates desire and erectile ability while delaying ejaculation.

Females: decreases/increases desire, increases intensity of orgasm.

High-dose use: Males: Prolongs erection and delays ejaculation; strong tendency to atypical and high-risk sexual practices such as multiple partners.

Females: Usually decreases desire, increases/decreases orgasmic ability; tendency to atypical and high-risk sexual practices.

Prolonged use: Males: Reduces sexual desire; reduces erectile and ejaculatory ability;

increases high-risk sexual activity and trading sex for drugs.

Females: Reduces desire and orgasmic ability; encourages high-risk sexual activity and trading sex for drugs.

> *"The kind of feeling you get when you inject it . . . it's sort of like the feeling when you're making love with your wife, when you climax. You know, that feeling that you get inside you; and it builds up your sex drive."* Cocaine user

> *"After a while, when you keep doing it, you're impotent, and it doesn't have any effect. The opposite sex can do anything they want to you and you won't react. Your body doesn't react to any kind of touch or emotion."* Same cocaine user after one month of daily use

Cocaine, a central nervous system stimulant, initially augments men's orgasmic feeling, and men use it as an adjunct to sexual practices. Many male users' street names for cocaine reflect their view of the drug: "girl," "lady," "dama blanca." But, cocaine loans people a good feeling at a cost. It gets people high through their own dopamine and norepinephrine release, and as they continue to use, their natural stores of these neurotransmitters become depleted. Their ability to enjoy sex and reach orgasm becomes more difficult.

As the neurotransmitter depletion escalates, impotence and the lack of desire for anything but the cocaine become more common. This loss of the ability to react naturally leads many users into very strange sexual practices in an effort to recapture the initial sensations.

In major cities, there's been a dramatic increase in the number of all sexually transmitted diseases because of increased high-risk behaviors such as intercourse without condoms. This occurs despite the continued concern about AIDS.

In fact, 5-6% of non-I.V., non-anal receptive, heterosexual cocaine users are HIV positive.

> *"Have you noticed that since crack came in, nobody lays down where you have one on top and one on the bottom. The woman's got to be on her knees. This is because you're incapable of having an erection. You're also incapable of being able to climax."* Crack user

Since the effects of cocaine on sexual activity are closely tied to the dose and frequency of use, the method of ingestion has much to do with the drug's effect on sexuality.

Chewing coca leaves: puts small amounts into the system over a long period of time.

Snorting cocaine: puts modest amounts into the brain in 5 to 10 minutes.

I.V. use: puts a large amount directly in the blood stream and into the brain in 10 to 15 seconds.

Smoking crack or freebase: puts a small but purified amount into the brain in 7 to 10 seconds.

What this means is that the more intense forms of cocaine use, such as smoking, lead to compulsive use sooner, so the negative side effects in relation to sexuality occur more quickly. Five to 20 minutes after smoking, the rush turns into a restless irritability and loss of the feeling of pleasure (dysphoria) so another rock of crack is needed. Compulsive users will use anywhere from 3 to 50 rocks per day.

"Crack feels like more, that's all I can say. You take one hit and that one hit is not enough. A thousand hits is not enough. You just want to keep going because it's like a ten-second head rush, and you don't get that effect again unless you take another hit." Crack user

Since the cost rises so swiftly, sex often becomes a way to get money for drugs, a means to an end. This is particularly true with female crack users.

"There's no such thing as a functional addict. I was stealing to get it, doing anything I had to get it, lying to my family, selling my body. And since rocks were about $10 each, I became a $10 whore." 22-year-old crack addict

At many crack houses and crack "parties," frequent sexual activity is common. One of the effects of cocaine use is delayed ejaculation along with an anesthetic effect on the genitals. Therefore, repeated intercourse leads to abrasions and lesions, making sexually transmitted diseases and infections more common, primarily because bacteria and viruses can enter more readily through the damaged skin. These effects also occur with amphetamine use.

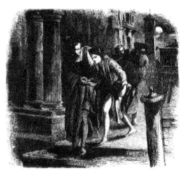

Amphetamine

Mentally and physically, amphetamine stimulates the user over a longer period of time than cocaine. It is popular with heterosexuals and particularly male homosexuals because it can prolong an erection, increase endurance, and intensify an orgasm during initial low-dose use. High-dose and prolonged use, however, have quite the opposite effect on human sexuality.

Effects:

Low-dose use: Male: Increases/decreases desire, prolongs erection, and delays ejaculation (varies with user).

Female: Usually increases desire and delays orgasm.

High-dose use: Male: Decreases/increases desire, decreases/ increases erectile ability, delays ejaculation, increases atypical behavior.

Female: Decreases desire, decreases or halts orgasm, increases atypical behavior.

Prolonged Use: Male: Decreases desire and erectile ability; delays or stops ejaculation. Some impotence. Increases atypical behavior.

Female: Decreases desire and orgasm; increases atypical behavior.

"I wasn't a whole person without it. I needed the drug to become myself, especially dealing with my peers. When I had the drug, I'd be really outgoing with girls." 19-year-old speed user

The popularity of amphetamines (speed, diet pills) rose to new levels during the "Summer of Love" in 1967 in San Francisco when the concept of "free love" and uninhibited sexual activities became fashionable. The increase in confidence plus some enhancement of desire, erectile ability, and delay in orgasm made it a "love drug." Unfortunately, since tolerance develops so rapidly, the side effects overwhelmed the benefits fairly quickly leading to prolonged high-dose use, mental and physical exhaustion, increased paranoia, and intensified aggression and violence, so the "Summer of Love" produced a large number of clients for the newly formed Haight-Ashbury clinics (and emergency rooms throughout the country).

With some users, the desire for sex increases when they start coming down off amphetamines. Many users get initially too wired for sex. They just talk, or dance, or engage in a variety of nervous activities.

"I'd love to be rushing any time of the day. It's the best part of speeding. I could do some and go dancing, and it would be just like if I was in bed with sex, the most fascinating ...whatever you might choose to experience. Or it might just be to go to bed behind it. I do things and I don't know who I'm doing them with." Intravenous methamphetamine user

Intravenous use of amphetamine is more intense than swallowing "cross tops," or snorting "crank." Many male I.V. users have an erection simultaneously with injection. I.V. use leads more readily to sexual aggressiveness which, in turn, helps spread various diseases.

"Ice," a smokable methamphetamine, seems to lead to sexual dysfunction more rapidly than snorting because it lasts longer and the high is more intense.

"When I was high there were a couple of times when I seriously considered passing the disease on to those I didn't like, and I know a couple of people who've done it on purpose. 'I'll fix his wagon, he won't rip me off. If he does, he'll be dead.' That's real sick, that's just real sick." HIV positive methamphetamine user

Tobacco

Tobacco, more than any of the psychoactive drugs connected with sexual activity, has been culturally rather than physiologically tied to romance and sex: initially the mysterious stranger who offers to light a woman's cigarette and then the image of a couple smoking after sex. In the romantic 1944 movie, "To Have and Have Not," Humphrey Bogart and Lauren Bacall managed to smoke 21 cigarettes in 90 minutes of film.

The connection between tobacco and sex has not been lost on the tobacco industry. A tobacco company paid $350,000 to have James Bond (the suave ladies' man) smoke in his last film. The character hadn't smoked in films in 17 years. (Incidentally, many leading men like Steve McQueen [50], Humphrey Bogart [57], and Gary Cooper [60] all died of lung cancer caused by smoking.)

Physically, nicotine is a mild stimulant with minimal effects on sexual functioning. Men who smoke have a lower sperm count, abnormal sperm, and dose-related chromosome damage. Women are more likely to have a spontaneous abortion from smoking during pregnancy. The long-term illnesses caused by smoking, such as emphysema and lung cancer, have much more of an impact on sexual functioning than the short-term effects.

DOWNERS, OPIATES, AND OPIOIDS

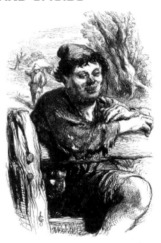

"If all pleasure is relief from tension, junk affords relief from this whole life process. Junk suspends the whole cycle of tension."

— *William Burroughs*

HEROIN

The effects may vary from user to user, but in general,

Low-dose use: Males: Decreases desire and erectile ability; delays ejaculation.

Females: Decreases desire and the strength of orgasm.

High-dose use: Males: Replaces desire, greatly decreases erectile and ejaculation ability.

Females: Greatly decreases desire and orgasm.

Prolonged use: Males: Greatly decreases desire except during withdrawal from the opiate; decreases erectile and ejaculation ability.

Females: Irregular menstruation; greatly decreases desire and both the quality and strength of orgasm; promotes sex for drugs behavior and prostitution.

Drug researchers describe the relief from tension through heroin use that William Burroughs wrote about as a "reduction in aggression, a feeling of warmth, a sense of fullness in the stomach, a desire to sleep, dreaming with some fantasies, and a slowing down of time."

Many addicts during detoxification report an increase in desire, erectile ability, and orgasm. This seems to confirm that the use of heroin will suppress sexual activities.

The effects users report have more to do with their individual makeup. Some "nod out" when using, some feel "up." These differences can be explained by selective tolerance of different functions of the body. For example, with prolonged use, the user's pupils will still be pinned, but the depression of emotions will not be as severe.

"I was kind of shy when I wasn't high. And the only way I can compare how I was when I was high is, I was like one helluva vacuum cleaner salesman." Ex-heroin user

"Heroin made me so mellow. I didn't think about nothin', I didn't care about nothin', I didn't feel nothin.'" Heroin user

As the habit increases and many users go on the "nod, " interest in sex continues to decline.

"All I could think about was the need to get high, and I lived to use and I used to live. There was no in-between. The only thing I could think about was the obsession to shoot dope." Recovering heroin user

In one study, 60% of heroin addicts reported an overall decrease in desire (impaired sexual desire or libido). While they were high on heroin, that figure jumped to 90%. In another study, 70% reported delayed ejaculation when using which is why some users self-medicate to cure premature ejaculation. Further, the overall rate of impotence (inability to become sexually aroused) in one study of male addicts was 39% jumping to 53% when they were actually high.

One explanation for the decrease in desire and erectile ability is that heroin blocks adrenaline release (decreasing energy) and dilates blood vessels (shunting blood away from the penis and clitoris). As a painkiller, it also decreases sensitivity.

A study of female heroin addicts showed 60% reported decreased desire (libido) while using. Also, 1/3 of female addicts in another study had excess pain during intercourse before using heroin, but only 6% had pain during intercourse after using heroin (again, the painkiller effect).

"You feel less like a woman. You start to look more masculine. You feel out of your skin. The same sort of people you really loved aren't attracted to you anymore. Your period stops." Heroin user

It's important to understand that pre-drug functioning has a lot to do with users' reactions while under the influence. People with preexisting problems are more likely to be drawn to drug use for self-medication whether it's to avoid sex, augment sensations, or treat oneself for a specific problem.

Methadone

Whether methadone or heroin causes more sexual dysfunction depends on which study is read. Methadone's effect on sexual function is similar to that of heroin except that Methadone is longer acting and so affects sexual functioning longer. Testosterone levels in methadone users were found to be lower than in a number of heroin addicts (probably because of the continuous use). On the other hand, much of the anxiety associated with hustling for heroin is eliminated when a user connects with a methadone

clinic. Women also report a decrease in sexual desire and menstrual dysfunction while on methadone.

SEDATIVE-HYPNOTICS

Many sedative-hypnotics such as the benzodiazepines, barbiturates and the street Quaaludes have been called alcohol in pill form and touted as sexual enhancers or "love drugs" at one time or another.

As with alcohol, it is a case of lowered inhibitions and relaxation versus physical depression that makes one unable to perform or respond sexually. Along with the disinhibition, sedative-hypnotics also impair judgment making the user more susceptible to unwanted sexual advances.

Benzodiazepines

Normal low-dose use of the benzodiazepines such as Klonopin, Xanax, Halcion, Valium, etc. have a minimal effect on sexual functioning although as an anti-anxiety agent, they can help relax the user. As the dose grows though, the sedative effects take over, making the user unable to ward off unwanted sexual advances. The user becomes lethargic and sleepy and experiences extensive muscle relaxation. With abuse comes sexual dysfunction and total apathy towards sexual stimulation.

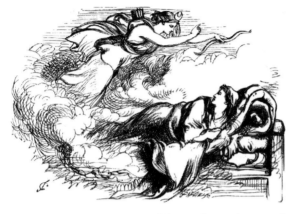

"Sexually and mentally, everything is so down. If I were a man, I couldn't have a hard-on. As a woman, I don't have an orgasm. Sexually and the same mentally; your mind is just mush; but you don't care. The last thing you worry about is sex." Valium addict

The use of benzodiazepines during conception and the early months of pregnancy increases the number of birth defects. (In fact, the infamous Thalidomide which caused so many birth defects in the 60's was a sedative-hypnotic though not a benzodiazepine.) Like Thalidomide, a specific birth defect, cleft palate syndrome, is definitely associated with the use of benzodiazepines during pregnancy.

Barbiturates

For women and for men, barbiturates act very much like alcohol, i.e., they lower inhibitions initially, but as use increases, they impair performance. They work on the central nervous system rather than directly on the genitals.

"I'd go into a bar, and my rap was pretty good. I thought I was Rudolph Valentino. And a few times, I picked up a couple girls, and brought them home to my house, and it was a big disappointment. To them I mean. I couldn't do anything. I was on Tuinals, Seconals. They couldn't excite me. I wasn't able to perform anything. And then I'd try to turn them onto the pills. It was a sad scene." Recovered barbiturate user

Quaaludes

Only street Quaaludes are available now. They were popular because of

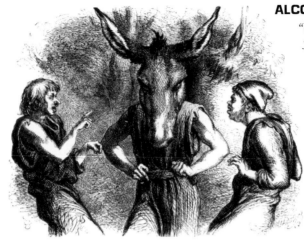

ALCOHOL

*"One drink of wine, and
you act like a monkey;
two drinks, and you
strut like a peacock;
three drinks, and
you roar like a lion;
and four drinks-you
behave like a pig.*

*—Henry Vollam
Morton 1936*

More than any other psychoactive drug, alcohol has insinuated itself in the lore, culture, and mythology of sexual and romantic behavior: champagne to celebrate an anniversary, the cocktail before sex, or beer swilled before a date rape.

Alcohol's physical effects on sexual functioning are closely related to blood alcohol levels. Its mental effects, however, are less strictly dose related and have more to do with the psychological makeup of the user and the setting in which used.

Effects vary from user to user.

Low-dose use: Males: Usually increases desire (lowered inhibitions, relaxation); slightly decreases erectile ability; delays ejaculation.

Females: Usually increases desire and intensity of orgasm.

High-dose use: Males: Increases/decreases desire; greatly decreases erectile and ejaculatory ability; causes some impotence.

the belief that they helped sexually by relaxing and disinhibiting the user. Increased or high-dose use generally brought dysfunction and impairment of erection. Despite this problem, "Ludes" so effectively lowered inhibitions and resistance to sexual advances that they too were called the "love drug" (one of many so-called "love drugs" that have appeared throughout history).

SOMA (Carisopodal)

This sedative has recently become a popular abuse item. It is sold as a skeletal muscle relaxant and is not classified or controlled as an abusable substance. As with all sedatives, it lowers inhibitions. Users take 3 to 5 tabs at one time to mimic the effects of Quaaludes or barbiturates. Since it is not controlled and comes from a variety of generic drug houses (notable "DANS," from Danberry Labs), it is readily available and rarely comes under legal scrutiny, unlike controlled sedatives.

Females: Greatly lowers desire and intensity of orgasm; (lowered inhibitions make a woman more susceptible to coercion and rape).

Prolonged Use: Males: Decreases desire, erectile ability, and ejaculatory ability; causes some impotence.

Females: Decreases desire; decreases intensity of orgasm; or blocks orgasm completely.

"Sure I can have sex without alcohol. I've just never had occasion to do it."
Problem drinker

Men and Alcohol

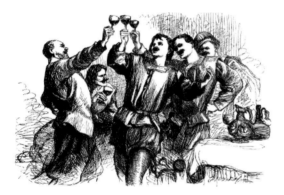

The familiar release of inhibitions both in words and deeds is the key to alcohol's dual effect on a man's sexual activity, i.e., more desire/less performance.

"At a party, at a friend's house, it's usually a race between scoring and snoring." *College drinker*

In men, a blood alcohol level of .05 (about 3 beers in one hour) has a very measurable physical effect on erectile ability, and yet legal intoxication in most states is

twice that amount. On the other hand, mentally, even one drink can loosen the tongue.

"One of the good things about alcohol is it numbs the ugly part of your brain … at one o'clock in the morning, everyone looks beautiful."
Alcohol abuser

Magazines, movies and television promote a close relationship between a drink and sex: the meeting at the bar or the offer of a drink at someone's apartment.

Candy
is Dandy
But Liquor
Is Quicker.
　　—Odgen Nash 1940

Physically, alcohol diminishes spinal reflexes (thus decreasing sensitivity and erectile ability) and dilates blood vessels (interfering with the ability to have an erection or ejaculation). Even a few drinks lower testosterone levels. Low testosterone is often coupled with diminished sexual desire and lowered levels of aggression (a certain amount of aggressiveness is required for many sexual encounters and performance). Initially, however, alcohol seems to give men more power because it acts on the area of the brain that regulates fear and anxiety thereby promoting not decreasing aggressiveness. It also seems to be a way for men to obtain a satisfying feeling about themselves and their masculinity which society ties to sexual prowess. As alcoholism progresses, many men feel less powerful and tend to shy away from the bedroom and even become asexual.

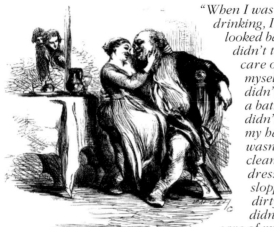

"When I was drinking, I looked bad. I didn't take care of myself, I didn't take a bath, I didn't comb my hair. I wasn't clean, and dressed sloppily, dirty. I didn't take care of my house; I'd leave bottles all over." Alcoholic

Long-term alcohol abuse greatly lowers testosterone levels, a reaction to the toxic effects of alcohol on the liver causing impaired liver function. Decreased testosterone (male hormone) in turn causes an increase in estrogen (female hormone) which causes male breast enlargement, testicular atrophy, low sperm count, and loss of body hair, in addition to loss of libido (desire).

Severe liver damage is generally not reversible, so long-term sexual problems in alcoholics are common. About 8% of alcoholics are impotent and only half will recover function during sobriety. Since alcohol is a protoplasmic poison, secondary nerve damage to genital nerves can also occur. And finally, when returning to sexual activity, a recovering alcoholic has excessive anxiety, so dysfunction can be intensified by one or two bad performances.

Women and Alcohol

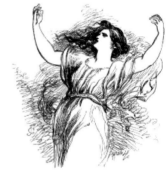

Alcohol's depressant effects on the fear and anxiety center of the brain have the greatest effect on a woman's sexual functioning. In most societies, more taboos and restrictions are placed on a woman's sexuality than on a man's. In one study, 65% of the women polled said alcohol improved their sexual functioning mostly in regard to the quality of their orgasm. Since women can passively engage in intercourse, or fake orgasm, or might not even be sure what an orgasm should be, the relationship between women's sexual functioning and alcohol is much harder to measure.

Many alcoholic females seem to to associate their identity as a woman with their sexual activity. Inevitably, because alcohol diminishes sexual arousal, women suffer lowered self esteem and feelings of inadequacy. Typically, the alcoholic denies that what is happening to her sexuality is related to what is happening with her progressive alcohol use.

"When I drank it was like, 'I feel fine, like I'm in control.' But, I'm really not. I stumble, get loud, lose some inhibitions. I didn't know what I was doing and I really didn't care." Alcoholic

In one study of chronic female alcoholics, 36% said they had orgasms less than 5% of the time. In both men and women, as the drinking progresses, no matter what the results in the bedroom, the alcoholic behavior is reinforced, and as the drinking progresses, it is difficult for the alcoholic to do anything but drink. Sex is merely something to do while drinking.

"We had separated twice before. I'm on my third separation from him right now. It was just...we stopped making love. You know, we would hardly talk." Alcoholic

When one partner in a marriage is an alcoholic or has a drinking problem, the man is much more likely to leave. Because of financial and emotional considerations and the presence of children, the woman will usually stay much longer in an alcoholically dysfunctional marriage.

ALL AROUNDERS

Marijuana

"Sometimes you can't let out feelings just when you're straight; you won't let it out. But if you're with your girlfriend and someone close, you can let out your feelings a lot better. And the way you feel about things." Teenage marijuana smoker

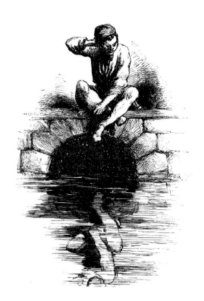

Marijuana has been called "the mirror that magnifies" because many of its effects—sensory enhancement, prolongation of time sense, increased affectional bonding, disinhibition, diffusion of ego, and sexualized fantasy —suggest a preexisting desire for these sensations.

Effects vary from user to user and depend heavily on the setting.

Low-dose use: Male: Increases physical sensitivity; increases desire; lowers inhibitions especially if used with alcohol.

Female: Increases desire; increases physical sensitivity.

High-dose use: Male: Decreases inhibitions; effects vary depending on THC content of marijuana.

Female: Decreases inhibitions; varies depending on THC content.

Prolonged use: Male: Lowers desire; decreases erectile and ejaculatory ability; lowers testosterone levels.

Female: Decreases desire and ability to have an orgasm.

In a survey, adults and teenagers were asked whether marijuana enhanced sexual pleasure. About a quarter believed that it did, half were uncertain, and the remainder either did not respond or said it did not. Women were more likely to report heightened sexual desire than men. In a survey at the Haight-Ashbury Clinic of regular users, 80% described marijuana as a sexual enhancer, but only 10% of those polled described it as a strong sexual enhancer.

Many regular users report that marijuana increases the quality of the orgasm.

"It's great though, when you have it and you're with your girlfriend and you know, when you make love, it's always better and lasts longer and everything."
Marijuana user

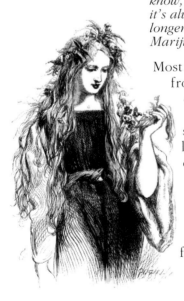

Most of the reported effects from marijuana were general comments such as "feelings of sexual pleasure" rather than specifics like prolonged excitation or delayed orgasm.

Marijuana, more than any psychoactive drug, shows the difficulty in separating the actual effects from the influence of the set and setting where the drug is used. If the drug is used in a social setting, at a party, or on a date, the expectation is that it will make both parties more relaxed, less inhibited, and more likely to do things they wouldn't normally do.

The social turmoil in the 60's created a mind set that expanded the use of marijuana. It was supposed to free users from the Victorian attitudes of the 50's. And, just as alcohol creates expectations in certain social situations, so does marijuana. Marijuana makes smokers more of what they are or want to be. If users smoke by themselves, then their expectations are probably to remain alone.

There are also many users who smoke to excess, 3 to 10 joints a day, so the marijuana can cause hangovers, lethargy, sexual dysfunction, and lowered desire. The secondary or psychological impotence rate among daily users is twice that (19%) of non-users. Also in the study, the daily users had sex 80% less often than non-users, and orgasm occurred 40% less frequently.

The other problem with excess smoking and sexual functioning is that the user often forgets how to have relations without being high, and so the cycle of excessive use is perpetuated. (The loss of sexual interest in other cultures from hashish use is well known.)

LSD

"Compared with sex under LSD, the way you've been making love, no matter how ecstatic the pleasure you think you get from it . . . is like making love to a department store window dummy." Timothy Leary

"Its hard to imagine LSD and sex in the same breath. As you approach vegetable how can you think about being an animal." Former acid head

As the above quotations show, the effects of LSD on sexual activity can vary greatly. Since so much of the effect of a psychedelic like LSD depends on the mood of the user and the setting where it is used (as well as the dosage and a half dozen other factors), most data are anecdotal. Since LSD use triggers so much distortion of the senses, a trip becomes very internalized for many users, and intercourse can become a very narcissistic experience. For others, it becomes a very complex and unpredictable experience. As with marijuana, the expectations of the user are crucial to the effect.

MDA and MDMA ("ecstasy," "rave")

These drugs are related to amphetamines but are classified as psychedelics. The effects of MDA and MDMA ("Ecstasy," "rave") last about 4 to 8 hours.

Both are known as "love drugs." On the street however, it's almost impossible for users to know which drug they are buying. MDA, MDMA, speed, or meth are often misrepresented by street dealers to unsuspecting consumers.

Users say MDMA and MDA (at moderate doses), unlike a regular methamphetamine, calm them, and give them warm feelings toward others and a heightened sensual awareness. The warm feelings supposedly make closer relations with those around them possible. However, only 25% to 50% of the users report these reactions. And most novice users, 90% in one study, said they would not try the drug again.

The most common side effects (muscle tension, jaw clenching, nausea, sweating, blurred vision, ataxia, and anxiety) and the residual effects (exhaustion, depression, occasional flashbacks and numbness) are often ignored in the party atmosphere of "rave clubs." Further, heat prostration, dehydration, and even death from high body temperature have resulted from abuse of MDMA.

"Rave Clubs" became popular in England and the United States in the 90's. These are either dance clubs which cater to the "Rave scene" or warehouses and buildings temporarily converted to a dance club (often created for the weekend on the spur of the moment) where drug use, particularly MDMA, speed, and alcohol, is widespread. MDMA is also used at smaller parties and on college campuses.

People are stacking doses, taking several doses several hours apart at these parties, so by the end of the evening they are getting a "speed" effect. Some of the more psychedelic effects fade very quickly if MDMA is taken too often.

Most of the reports about the sexual effects of MDMA and MDA are anecdotal, and since polydrug use is quite widespread (especially involving amphetamine and alcohol), accurate data is lacking.

PCP

PCP doesn't seem to have any particular sexual enhancement for desire, erection, or orgasm and so, except for disinhibition, is rarely used as a sexual enhancer. In a few cases, the anesthetic properties of PCP (an animal tranquilizer) are used to deaden pain for unusual or even bizarre sexual practices.

INHALANTS

Poppers: amyl and butyl nitrite

The volatile nitrites, which are vasodilators and muscle relaxants and are sold over the counter as Bolt, Rush, and Locker Room, gained fame in the 80's because of the suspicion that their use aggravated the HIV virus. Although no proof was found for this theory, their use, particularly by the gay community, was widely publicized. If inhaled just prior to orgasm, they prolong and seem to enhance the sensation. Abused as orgasm intensifiers by both the gay and straight communities in the 1960's, they too gained the reputation of being yet another "love drug." It is interesting to note, however, that the vasodilating effects of these drugs also act on blood vessels of the penis, resulting in loss of erection if used too early in sexual activity.

Nitrous oxide

Nitrous oxide, also known as laughing gas, is used in dentistry. One study of 15 dental personnel (Layzer 1978), found that long-term exposure had caused impotence in 7 cases. The impotence was slowly reversed when exposure to the gas was discontinued. More often than not, nitrous oxide is used in combination with a wide range of drugs (alcohol, grass, cocaine, etc.) and is not in itself looked upon as a sexually-enhancing substance.

PSYCHIATRIC MEDICATIONS

"As a general rule, depressed patients usually lose their interest in sex, anxious patients have a sex drive but cannot calm down long enough to have sex, and manic patients want to have sex all day long."

Jack Gorman, M.D. (The Essential Guide to Psychiatric Drugs)

Psychiatric medications, medications to treat existing mental disorders such as depression, anxiety, psychoses, mania, and obsessive-compulsive disorders, differ from street drugs in several ways when it comes to sexual functioning. First, the medications are generally non-addicting (except for the benzodiazepines), so misuse of these medications by addicts is limited. Second, the medications are medically supervised, so patients know exactly what they are getting. Third, most psychotropic medications produce undesirable mental effects and are unpopular as street drugs. Finally, most patients who use these medications have preexisting emotional problems which can impair sexual functioning. By treating the mental condition, the drugs can also affect the sexual problems of the user. For example, an antidepressant can make a patient more able to engage in intimate relations and sexual appreciation, capabilities which were impaired by the depression.

Antidepressants

Various studies involving tricyclic antidepressants such as desipramine (Norpramine), imipramine (Tofranil), amitriptyline (Elavil), and amoxapine (Asendin) have been linked to decreased desire with long-term use, and some problems with erection and a delay in orgasm. Initially, however, in many cases, the relief from depression makes the user more able to participate in sexual activities. Many of the MAO

inhibitors, such as Prozac, Nardil, and Parnate, cause delay or inhibition of orgasm. Delayed orgasm often goes away with time. In contrast, trazodone (Desyrel) has caused painful and prolonged erections which could only be reversed by surgery.

Antipsychotics

Mellaril (Thioridazine) inhibits erectile function and ejaculation, Thorazine (chlorpromazine) and Haldol (haloperidol) can inhibit desire, erectile function, and ejaculation. Impaired ejaculation appears to be the most common side effect of the major tranquilizers (antipsychotics). All of these effects were greatest when the dosage was highest.

Lithium

There are some reports of decreased desire and difficulty maintaining an erection as the dosage increases.

OTHERS

BuSpar

The antianxiety agent, BuSpar, seems to help sexual functioning by lowering anxiety, but not sedating the patient.

L-Dopa

When used to treat Parkinsonism in the late 1960's, L-Dopa gained notoriety as yet another in a long list of "love drugs." L-Dopa is transformed into dopamine in the brain, one of the brain chemicals responsible for the feelings of orgasm. Its popularity soon dwindled, indicating that its effect on sexuality may have been more from its ability to control the physical problems associated with Parkinsonism than from any real sexual enhancement ability.

Steroids

Anabolic steroids are derivatives of the male hormone, testosterone. Testosterone regulates physical and sexual development in the male. It also seems to increase lean body mass. Medically, they are prescribed to treat men with a low testosterone level or to treat certain types of anemia.

Many teens may take them because they think it helps them increase sexual or athletic performance. The problem is that when one tinkers with the physiology, the side effects can be devastating.

Besides increasing muscle size, steroids increase aggressiveness (called "rhoid rage") and increase libido (sexual appetite), sometimes resulting in aberrant sexual and violent behavior. Repeated use can lead to impotence, reduction in testicle size, reduction of sperm production, breast enlargement, acne, and prostate enlargement.

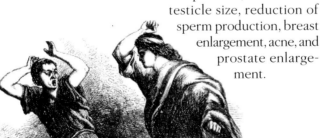

In females steroids cause masculinization, enlargement of the clitoris, excessive hair growth, reduction of breast size, and abnormal menstrual cycles. Many of the effects in women are permanent.

APHRODISIACS

The search for true aphrodisiacs is complicated by the complexity of the sexual response. Are we talking about affection, love, or lust when we discuss drugs that enhance sexuality? Are we talking about drugs that change the mental or the physical aspects of sexuality? Is the drug expected to increase desire, prolong excitation, increase lubrication, delay orgasm or improve its quality? Is a drug that lowers inhibitions an aphrodisiac?

Heroin sometimes delays orgasm; cocaine sometimes increases desire or prolongs an erection; alcohol lowers inhibitions thereby increasing desire; an antidepressant relieves depression thereby increasing desire; Butyl nitrite intensifies orgasm; MDMA (Ecstasy) is touted as an aphrodisiac because it supposedly promotes closeness; marijuana increases the sensitivity to touch.

Some purported aphrodisiacs such as Spanish fly or ground rhinoceros horn work by irritating the urethra and bladder promoting a pseudosexual excitement. But Spanish fly (cantharidin derived from a beetle) is actually toxic.

Pheromones are human hormones, discovered in sweat. The scent or odor of these substances

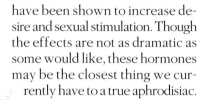

have been shown to increase desire and sexual stimulation. Though the effects are not as dramatic as some would like, these hormones may be the closest thing we currently have to a true aphrodisiac.

Yohimbine is an alkaloid obtained from several plant sources including the yohimbe tree in West Africa. This psychedelic produces some hallucinations and a mild euphoria. It has been used in high doses as a treatment for impotence in men by increasing blood pressure and heart rate thereby increasing penile blood flow. It can produce acute anxiety at low dosages.

Many of the reported effects of psychoactive drugs as aphrodisiacs come about because they help correct an existing deficiency or imbalance in the patient such as low levels of testosterone (anabolic steroids) or low levels of zinc (zinc). One problem is that the body adapts to any drug so that its effectiveness decreases with time. Next, with illegal substances, controlled use is difficult, and side effects start to overwhelm any benefits. Third, and perhaps most significant, the psychological roots of most feelings are quite complex and are generally more important to sexual functioning than mere enhancement of sensations. Drugs can distort, magnify, or eliminate feelings involved with erotic activities.

Research is being conducted on a number of drugs that are anecdotally alleged to enhance sexuality, but most have not shown any real or consistent ability to do this.

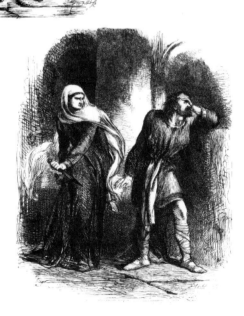

Other Alleged Sexual Enhancers

DRUG/SUBSTANCE	SOURCE	MAJOR PROBLEMS ASSOCIATED WITH USE
Bromocriptine mesylate (Parlodel)	Ergot alkaloid	Amenorrhea, galactorrhea, impotence, loss of libido, oligospermia.
Clomiphene citrate (Clomid)	Synthetic fertility pill	Multiple births, liver toxicity, ovarian cysts, insomnia, depression, fatigue.
Ginseng root	Panax ginseng	Hypertension, wide variation in potency, no impact on sexual enhancement.
Levo tryptophan (L-Tryptophan, Trofan)	Protein found in meat, milk, dairy products	Serious blood and muscle problems, no proven ability to increase libido.
Luteinizing hormone releasing hormone (LHRH, HRF, Gonadorelin)	Human hypothalmic hormone	Only studied in men, no sexual enhancement effect.
Naloxone (Narcan) Naltrexone (Trexan)	Synthetic opiate antagonist	Total lack of human evidence that it affects libido.
Parachlorophenyl-alanine (PCPA)	Synthetic serotonin synthesis inhibitor	Very limited results only with migraine sufferers.
Pheromones (alpha androstenol, et.al.)	Wide variety of human hormone secretions	Limited effectiveness from these scent or odor substances.
Rhinoceros horns	Rhinoceros	No proven effectiveness, rhinoceros extinction.
Yohimbine	Corynanthe yohimbe (African tree)	Hypertension, anxiety, hallucinations.
Zinc	Essential metal element	Gastric ulcers, diarrhea and dehydration at high doses. Limited efficacy in zinc-deficient patients and must be given at high doses.

SUBSTANCE ABUSE AND SEXUAL ASSAULT

One in every three women in this country will be a victim of sexual violence in her lifetime.

In addition, a recent study on college campuses found that about 75% of rapists (including date rapists) and more than half their victims were drinking alcohol or using other drugs before the assault. All of the gang rapes in this study involved alcohol. In another study of 1356 white male convicted sex offenders, two-thirds of the pedophiles (those who sexually assault children) were drunk at the time of the assault, as were half of the heterosexual rapists. The close involvement of psychoactive drugs and sexual assault has much to do with the specific effects of the drugs and the existing tendencies or character traits of the user. Some generalizations can be made:

1) Alcohol lowers inhibitions and muddles rational thought, making the user more likely to act out irrational or unwanted desires;

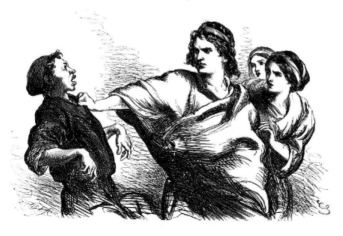

2) Cocaine and amphetamines increase confidence and aggression, making the male user more likely to overpower his date;

3) Marijuana and Quaaludes lower inhibitions, making male users more likely to carry out their desires, wanted or not or making the woman less able to resist;

4) PCP and heroin make the user less sensitive or indifferent to pain, making users more likely to damage their partners;

5) And steroids increase aggression and irrational behavior.

In most cases, the male user already has tendencies that push him towards antisocial behavior, and the alcohol or other drug is the final trigger. The trigger can also be an emotion such as anger, hate, or in some cases lust. For example, with date rape, the man may just intend to have sex, but when he is refused, or doesn't get his way, he becomes angry and takes what he feels is his. In the final analysis, rape is motivated by a need to overpower, humiliate, and dominate a victim, not a desire to have sex.

The limbic system of the older brain which controls sexual desire also controls the other emotions, so anything which short circuits this area of the brain (such as drugs or stress), can trigger other desires or imbalances. For example, if we try to stimulate desire by stimulating the limbic system with cocaine, we also stimulate the food satiation reward center causing some to become malnourished. Cocaine also stimulates the fright center triggering paranoia. In addition, the effect of a psychoactive drug on the victim affects her natural defenses. i.e., alcohol and marijuana lower inhibitions and willpower making the person less able, physically and mentally, to withstand an assault.

Finally, many people use drugs to help them cope with or even forget a sexual assault or sexual abuse.

TREATMENT

Drugs can be used to try to enhance sexual activity or to protect someone from his or her sexual feelings. If the use of drugs has gotten out of hand and/or sexual dysfunction has occurred, treatment is necessary. Because the problems are complex, treatment has to have several components.

First, if the drug abuse has become chronic or if the user can't have sex without drugs, then he or she has to stop using and detoxify. Detoxification must occur before any other problems are tackled.

Next, the reasons for sexual problems have to be addressed while the drug addiction is being treated. Finally, the user has to learn how to function sexually (and emotionally) without drugs.

In many 12-step groups and other drug treatment programs, more than two thirds of the members were sexually or physically abused as children. Since this kind of abuse generally leads to emotional and sexual difficulties in later life, many victims use alcohol, drugs, or food to deal with problems such as fear of touching, premature ejaculation, lack of orgasm, impotence, sexual rage, and fear of intimacy. Treating these problems is a long-term effort, so detoxification is just the beginning. And sometimes, taking away a person's drugs in treatment means taking away the way they function sexually and emotionally. Part of treatment is showing clients alternative ways to function.

In treatment, it is important to see drug/sex behavior as part of the whole person and not mistake a symptom for the disease.

SEXUALLY TRANSMITTED DISEASES

In spite of the fear of sexually transmitted diseases, particularly AIDS but including gonorrhea, syphilis, genital herpes, genital warts, chlamydia, and hepatitis B, and in spite of a dramatic growth in unwanted pregnancies, the practice of unsafe and unprotected sex continues, but there has been a small decrease in some diseases.

The very nature of sexual activity clouds judgment as do most drugs. When drugs are combined, it is no wonder that almost half of all sexually active teenagers have had chlamydia, the fastest growing of all sexually transmitted diseases.

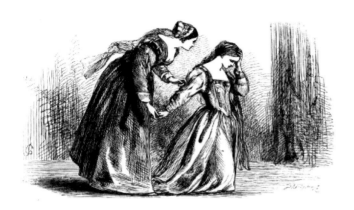

In fact, experts think that as many as 4 million Americans have caught the disease (often without knowing it). Perhaps 20% of all sexually active men and women have genital herpes. Even syphilis, which had diminished dramatically in the last 50 years, has started to climb again. The relationship of crack cocaine to high-risk sexual activity has also fueled the problem.

> *"This woman was pregnant, she was living on the street, she was prostituting, was HIV postive, and had a $250-a-day habit. I mean she's not a bad looking woman, but she was definitely into her smack and her cocaine. She told me she had to sleep with at least 5 guys a day, minimum, to support her habit. I wonder how many people she's given her diseases to."* AIDS patient

In the United States in 1992, the Centers for Disease Control received reports of

- 491,000 new cases of gonorrhea;

- 362,000 new cases of chlamydia;

- 21,000 new cases of hepatitis B;

- 34,179 new cases of primary and secondary syphilis;

- 17,000 new cases of genital herpes;

- 16,600 new cases of genital warts;

- and 47,106 new cases of full blown AIDS. Under the new definition of AIDS, that number would climb to almost 100,000.

One million people or one in every 250 people in the United States is infected with the HIV virus and virtually all of them will develop AIDS.

In 1990, the World Health Organization (WHO) said that

- 6.8 million people worldwide have AIDS and 18 million are HIV positive;

- 60% of all worldwide infections have resulted from **heterosexual** intercourse.

By the year 2,000 WHO predicts that:

- 40 million people will be infected with HIV;

- Up to 70% of all HIV infections will result from heterosexual intercourse.

In contrast, the methods of transmission in the United States are, for the present, somewhat different. Homosexual transmission still accounts for the majority of new cases:

In New York City alone, 60% to 80% of I.V. drugs users are HIV positive.

About 10% of all AIDS cases are women, and, in the past the majority of these got it from I.V. drug use. However, in 1993, heterosexual contact (usually with I.V. drug users) became the more prevalent cause.

As sexual activity increases, often fueled by the lowered inhibitions brought about by drug use, the number of infections of all sexually transmitted diseases continues to climb.

It is important to remember the pattern of the spread of communicable diseases. They start slowly but then rage through the most susceptible groups. In the case of AIDS in the United States, the gay community that practiced unsafe sex was the most vulnerable compared to other countries where heterosexual high-risk sexual activity spread the disease. Once the most vulnerable have been infected, there is usually a lull in the increase of the disease. During such lulls, a false sense of security along with clouded judgment, builds up a new well of infection. As we approach the year 2,000, most experts predict that the majority of new

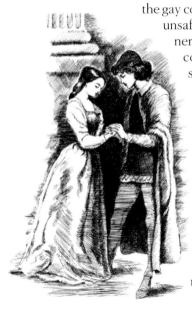

cases of AIDS in the U.S. (as with the rest of the world) will be in the heterosexual and drug-using communities. Continuing public education and public health activities are crucial to stem the spread of AIDS and, for that matter, all sexually transmitted diseases.

SOME FINAL WORDS

People use drugs to try to either enhance their sexual functioning or to protect themselves from emotions. In both cases, the drugs are used as a shortcut, bypassing the real work that needs to be done, i.e., emotional commitment, communication, caring, affection, dealing with childhood traumas, and learning to be an adult.

As with addiction, initial and low-dose use of many psychoactive substances can have a transient, seductively pleasing impact on one's sexuality. Continued high-dose or long-term use, however, greatly impairs one's sexuality and leads to sexual dysfunction. Sex without drugs enables people to have more intense and pleasurable experiences and to develop emotionally. Sex with drugs usually becomes progressively less pleasurable and more dysfunctional.

REVIEW

SEX, LOVE, AND DRUGS

1. Those who use drugs to achieve sexual gratification are usually looking for a quick sensation rather than enduring emotions.

2. Drugs affect desire, excitation, and orgasm, often in diverse and contradictory ways.

3. Desire is more dependent on the basic personality of the user and the set and setting where the drug is used rather than the drug itself.

4. The social effects of combining drugs and sexual activity, usually caused by lowered inhibitions or the need to support a drug habit, are increased sexual activity, high-risk sexual practices, sexual aggression, and an increase in sexually transmitted diseases.

5. Physical effects of drugs include hormonal changes, blood flow and blood pressure changes, nerve stimulation or desensitization, and muscle tension changes, all of which affect sexual response.

6. Cocaine and amphetamines affect males in low doses by stimulating desire, but in high doses, they makes orgasm more difficult. In females, they can either increase or decrease desire and orgasm, but in high doses, a decrease is much more likely.

7. With amphetamines and cocaine, over use can lead to exhaustion, paranoia, and increased sexual aggression and violence.

8. Tobacco has been popularized and sold as a companion to sex. Illnesses associated with smoking have much more of an effect on sexual functioning than any short-term effects.

9. Opiates and opioids generally suppress sexual activity. Sixty percent of addicts report a general decrease of desire; 90% report decreased desire while they were high.

10. Sedative-hypnotics enhance desire by lowering inhibitions and inducing relaxation. But with abuse, sexual dysfunction and apathy have been reported.

11. There has been a cultural link between love, sex, and alcohol. Initially, alcohol lowers inhibitions and often increases aggressiveness. Long-term abuse causes a decrease in performance.

12. Alcohol initially is reported to enhance female orgasm, though long-term use diminishes arousal and self-esteem.

13. Expectations about use, some physical effects, and decreasing inhibitions have popularized the use of marijuana as a sexual enhancer. High-dose or long-term use generally lowers desire and physical response.

14. Because of the distortion of the senses involved with psychedelics, their effect on a sexual experience can be very unpredictable.

15. Psychotropic medications such as antidepressants may enable patients to engage in sexual activities that their depression or psychosis kept them from doing.

16. The search for a true aphrodisiac may be illusive because sexuality is more a matter of mental attitude than physical sensation.

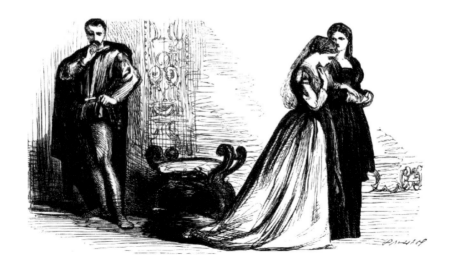

QUESTIONS

1. What are the three phases of sexual activity?

2. Name several social consequences of using drugs to enhance sexuality.

3. List three motives regular drug users give for combining sex and drugs.

4. What are the physical and mental effects of using low to moderate doses of cocaine or amphetamines to enhance a sexual experience?

5. What are the effects of prolonged use of amphetamines or cocaine on a sexual experience?

6. Illustrate several cultural connections between tobacco and sex.

7. Why are sedative-hypnotics used in connection with sex?

8. Illustrate several cultural connections between alcohol and sex.

9. Why are the effects of alcohol on sexual performance sometimes contradictory?

10. How can the setting, in which marijuana is used, influence the effects of a sexual experience?

11. What side effects might have led 90% of first-time MDMA users to say they would not use the drug again?

12. How do antidepressants help people overcome sexual dysfunction?

13. Name five supposed sexual enhancers and the major problem associated with their use.

13. What are the major causes of sexual assault associated with substance abuse?

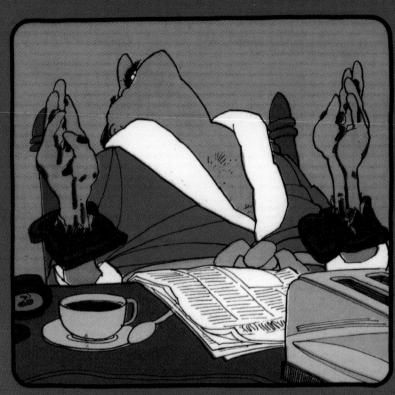

Joseph stumbles across his brain's
pleasure center.

THE NEIGHBORHOOD by JERRY VAN AMERONGEN
Copyright 1986 - Jerry Van Amerongen.
Reprinted with special permission of Cowles Syndicate Inc.

CHAPTER 11

FROM EXPERIMENTATION TO COMPULSION INTO TREATMENT

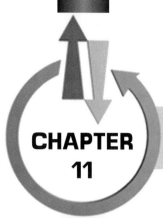

1990

Responding to the Demand

Treatment Programs Multiplying

1915

World.

AS FIFTEEN DRUG SLAVES ARE TAKEN IN FOR CURE, 20 MORE ARE SHUT OUT

Drug Fiends Giving Up Fight;
147 of Them in 3 Hospitals

1988

Scientists Pinpoint Brain Irregularities In Drug Addicts

Researchers seek
treatments to alter
chemical imbalances.

By DANIEL GOLEMAN

THEORIES OF ADDICTION (ADDICTIONIOLOGY)

In the past two decades, a tremendous amount of research and many theories have been generated to help understand the process of drug addiction. These theories govern the way addicts are treated. Traditionally, there have been three separate major schools of thought about addiction. One emphasizes the effects of heredity,another, the effects of environment and behavior, and the last, the physiological effects of psychoactive drugs.

Addictive Disease Model (heredity)

Behavioral/Environmental Model (environment)

Academic Model (psychoactive drugs)

In this chapter we will discuss many of the accepted theories of addiction and then combine those theories in a compulsion curve.

ADDICTIVE DISEASE MODEL (heredity)

This model maintains that the disease of addiction is a chronic, progressive, relapsing, incurable, and potentially fatal condition that is a consequence of genetic defi-

ciencies in brain tissues and/or neurotransmitters. It also maintains that addiction is set into motion by experimentation with the drug by a susceptible host in an environment that is conducive to drug misuse. The susceptible user quickly experiences a compulsion to use, a loss of control, and a determination to continue the use despite negative physical, emotional, or life consequences.

Several studies of twins, along with other human and animal studies, strongly support the addictive disease theory that heredity and not environment is the stronger influence on uncontrolled, compulsive drug use. A number of the studies looked at twins who were separated from their genetic parents and each other at birth and went to live in different households. They found that if one twin of alcoholic parents was raised in a non-drinking household, it still had the same chance of become a problem drinker as the other twin raised in a drinking household.

This and the other studies showed that the children of alcoholics have a much greater risk of becoming alcoholics than the children of non-alcoholics. They seem to metabolize alcohol differently and are born with different levels of certain brain neurotransmitters (met-enkephalin, GABA, serotonin) than those not genetically at risk.

There is reason to hypothesize that similar genetic influences may be found for compulsive use of

Addiction and the tendency to addiction cross all social and racial barriers.

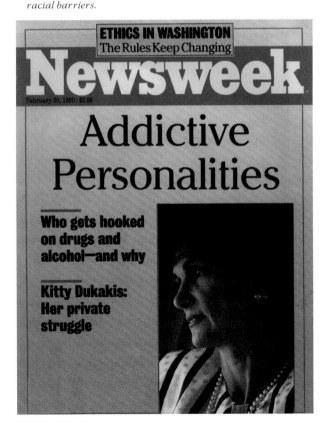

ETHICS IN WASHINGTON
The Rules Keep Changing

Newsweek

February 20, 1989 ; $2.00

Addictive Personalities

Who gets hooked on drugs and alcohol—and why

Kitty Dukakis: Her private struggle

other psychoactive substances, not just alcohol. These alterations in levels of enzymes and other biochemicals cause addicts to react differently from nonaddicts to the same drug or life experience.

Addictive disease, under this definition, is characterized by

- Impulsive drug abuse marked by intoxication throughout the day and an overwhelming need to continue use;

- Loss of control over the use of a drug with an inability to reduce intake or stop use;

- Repeated attempts to control use with periods of temporary abstinence interrupted by relapse into compulsive, continual drug use;

- Continuation of abuse despite the progressive development of serious physical, mental, or social disorders aggravated by the use of the substance;

- Episodes or complications which result from intoxication such as an alcoholic blackout, opiate overdose, loss of job, breakup of a relationship, arrest, heart attack, or any other disabling or impairing condition.

In the new definition of alcoholism, denial has been added as one of the symptoms of addiction.

BEHAVIORAL/ ENVIRONMENTALLY INFLUENCED CHEMICAL DEPENDENCIES (environment)

Environmental and developmental influences can also result in changes in brain hormones as seen in animal studies. Chronic stress, for example, can decrease brain levels of met-enkephalin (a neurotransmitter) in mice, making normal alcohol-avoiding mice more susceptible to alcohol use (see Chapter 5). Many sociologic studies suggest that physical/emotional stress such as caused by abuse, anger, peer pressure, and other environmental factors cause people to seek, use, and sustain their continued dependence on drugs.

In this model, there are five levels of drug use from experimentation to addiction.

Experimentation

The person doesn't seek out the drug. He or she is just curious about it or is influenced by friends or society and may take some, only when it becomes available, to satisfy that curiosity. No patterns of use develop, and it has no negative consequences in the person's life. Drug use is limited to only a few exposures.

"I remember the first time a friend of mine gave me this little yellow popper, and he said, 'Here's a present for you,' and I said, 'Oh, what's this?' And he said, 'Well, it's amyl nitrite, you know, and you take it and you snap it, and hold it up to your nose and inhale it.' And so I said, 'Okay.'" Inhalant user

Social/Recreational

Whether it's a beer at a restaurant, a joint with a friend, or a sniff of cocaine at a party, with recreational/social use, the person does seek out a drug and does want to experience a certain effect, but there is no established pattern. Drug use is infrequent, sporadic, and has little impact on the person's life.

"There's a lot of times you don't get stoned alone. You get stoned with your friends. If you come to school, you say to your friends, 'Hey Johnny, let's get stoned.' Everybody does it." Marijuana smoker

Habituation

With habituation, there is a definite pattern of use: the TGIF high, the five cups of coffee everyday. No matter what happens that day, the person will use that drug. As long as it doesn't affect his or her life in a really negative way, it could be called habituation. This level of use clearly demonstrates that one has lost control of use of the drug. Regardless how frequently or infrequently a drug is used, a definite pattern of use indicates that the drug is now controlling the user.

"You would say that I was a habitual user, but I don't really think that's the case. So, it is a habit. I like a drink. And the question you know ...the question is, 'Could I go a day without having a drink?' I think so but I've never had a reason to try." "Social drinker"

Drug Abuse

Our definition of drug abuse is, **"The continued use of a drug despite negative consequences."** It's the use of "speed" in spite of high blood pressure; the use of LSD though there's a history of mental instability; the alcoholic diabetic; or the two-pack-a-day smoker with emphysema. No matter how often you use a drug, if you develop negative consequences in your relationships, social life, finances, legal status, health, or emotional well being and you still use, then you are a drug abuser.

"I had an EEG and a CAT scan and I was told that I had lowered my seizure threshold by doing so many stimulants. The reason I actually stopped was because I discovered heroin, and I liked it better. I would probably have continued using speed, even with the seizures." "Speed" user

Addiction

The step between abuse and addiction has to do with compulsion. That is, if the person spends most of the time either getting, using or thinking about the drug; when, in spite of negative health consequences, mental or physical, the person continues to use it; after withdrawal, the user still has a strong tendency to start using again—that's addiction. The user has lost control of his or her use of the drug, and it has become the most important thing in life.

> *"I used to walk crooked, my balance was off all the time, my speech got slurred, but I enjoyed it and I liked it, and as many pills as I had, I would take. I didn't really care about overdosing which I did many times. A few times, the police picked me up right off the gutter."*
> Barbiturate user

ACADEMIC MODEL (Psychoactive drugs)

In this model, addiction is brought about by the adaptation of the body to the toxic effects of drugs at the biochemical and cellular level. The idea is that "Given sufficient quantities of drugs for an appropriate duration of time, changes in body/brain cells will occur which will lead to addiction." Four physiological changes characterize this process: tolerance, tissue dependence, withdrawal syndrome, and psychic dependence.

Tolerance

An increased resistance to the drug's euphoric and other effects occurs which necessitates larger and larger doses to maintain a "high." This occurs through several different processes including actual changes in liver cells which help to metabolize drugs more rapidly.

Tissue Dependence

There are actual changes in body cells which occur because of addiction, so the body "needs" the drug to stay in balance. For example, 80 to 120 mg of Valium taken for 42 days causes a buildup of certain chemicals in the brain. The user then has to keep taking Valium to prevent these chemicals from flooding the body, resulting in possible withdrawal convulsions and other adverse reactions.

Withdrawal Syndrome

Physical signs and symptoms of tissue dependence appear when the drug is stopped as the body tries to return to "normal." Abrupt cessation from cocaine abuse will result in depression, sleep disturbances, lethargy, muscle aches, and a tremendous craving for the drug.

Psychic Dependence

This results from the direct influence of drugs on brain chemistry. The drug causes an altered state of consciousness and distorted perceptions pleasurable to the user. These reinforce the continued use of the drug. Psychic dependence can therefore result from the misuse of drugs to deal with life's problems or from their use to compensate for inherited deficiencies in brain-reward hormones. Further, drugs also have the innate ability to mesmerize or hypnotize the user into continual use (called the positive, reinforcing action of drugs).

COMPULSION CURVE

As mentioned previously, there are many models and hypotheses about addiction. Most, however, include factors of genetics, environment, behavior, pharmacology, and psychology. We have tried to unify them in Chapter 5 on Alcohol when we discuss the way different strains of mice react to alcohol and stress, and we will discuss these ideas in Chapter 12 on Dual Diagnosis when we expand on the concept of how heredity, environment, and psychoactive drugs all work together to determine not only addiction but our mental balance as well. In this chapter, we will use a visual set of graphs using the concept of a "compulsion curve" to explore addiction.

First, it's important to remember that all people are born with an inherited sensitivity to specific drugs, with a certain neurochemical balance. Some are more sensitive than others (Fig. 11-1).

Then, someone uses a drug and is possibly subjected to stress and becomes more sensitive as the brain chemistry is disrupted. So as that person moves up on the curve, he or she passes through various use patterns and approaches addiction. Those with a low inherited sensitivity to drugs would have to use a lot of drugs over a longer period of time and are possibly subject to a lot of stress to push themselves along. It might take them 10 years to become an alcoholic (Fig. 11-2).

People in the middle of the scale, with moderate sensitivity, might need 3 or 4 years to slip into addictive behavior. People with a high inherited sensitivity might slip into addiction immediately or after just a couple of weeks of use. Their bodies are primed for addiction. They don't have to induce that deficiency in their brain chemistry. It's already there (Fig. 11-3).

The slope of the compulsion curve is very gradual at the low sensitivity end but dramatically steeper at the high sensitivity end. This demonstrates the accelerating nature of drug abuse.

So what happens if people stop taking the drug? Do they return to their starting point? The answer is unclear. Current evidence clearly suggests that there will be some rebound in the balance of the disrupted neurotransmitters, but those with inherited high sensitivity, in particular, will not return to the balance and sensitivity they started with (Fig. 11-4).

Other evidence suggests that neurotransmitters may rebound almost back to normal levels in those with short-term, non-inherited disruption. When the sensitivity doesn't return to normal, users are more at risk for addiction the next time they start to use. This is due to a process called "sensitization" or "imprinting." The brain remembers the drug using habits and sensations during abuse of the drug.

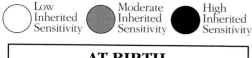

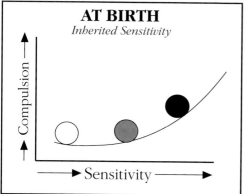

Fig. 11-1

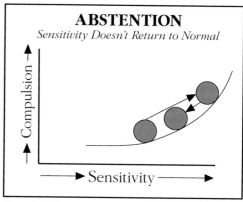

Fig. 11-4

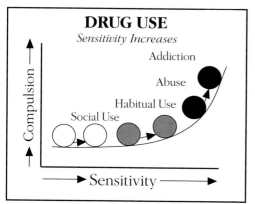

Fig. 11-2

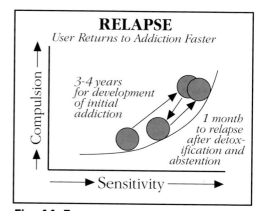

Fig. 11-5

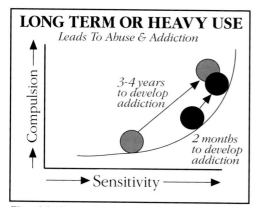

Fig. 11-3

For example, if it took a person three years to develop barbiturate addiction and then that person abstains from use for a while, it might only take one month to relapse back into abuse or addiction. If it took four weeks to become addicted to cigarettes, it might take just one cigarette now to relapse (Fig. 11-5). And regardless of how one gets to the addictive end of the curve, almost everyone agrees that once there, it is virtually impossible to return to controlled experimental, social, or habitual patterns of use. The process leading to addiction can be arrested to minimize the negative impact of drug use, but this cannot be accomplished without abstinence from all psychoactive drugs and utilization of recovery techniques, counseling, 12-step support programs (such as Alcoholics Anonymous) or other treatment modalities.

TREATMENT

INTRODUCTION

Horace B. Day concluded his book on the problems of opium dependence in 1868 with his statement that, "There is no agreement among the medical profession as to the proper treatment of opium disease or morphinism." This statement is still applicable today in a much broader sense to treatment of all chemical dependencies. As we have noted throughout this book, addiction is a complex interaction between biologic, social and toxic factors—heredity, environment and psychoactive drugs. Given these multiple influences, treatment has evolved along various paths, all of which enjoy some success in decreasing the deleterious impact that addiction has on the individual. However, no single treatment has proven to be universally effective for all addicts.

"My old man got off 'smack' through NA [Narcotics Anonymous], but I couldn't get into it. I had to check myself into the hospital program. His program was cheaper." 28-year-old heroin addict

It is also very important to review the physical withdrawal syndrome produced by a drug or a combination of drugs when considering treatment. Withdrawal from alcohol and sedative-hypnotic drugs like Valium or Klonopin may produce life-threatening seizures which require medical and hospital management to treat.

"My mother swore off the booze and Valium for my wedding. She was too good to her word. She started withdrawing and having convulsions at my reception and almost died in the ambulance. Nice honeymoon." 23-year-old bride

Treatment starts with a recognition and acceptance of addiction by the addict. This diagnosis oftentimes requires an intervention and an assessment to support and validate the need for treatment. Only then can an addict be entered into a continuum of lifelong processes to assist her or him in a quest for recovery.

Fig. 11-6 PROTOCOL FOR CLIENT INTAKE

This is the protocol for the Haight-Ashbury Drug Clinic. It emphasizes the complexity of treating a compulsive drug user who comes in for treatment, particularly if other problems such as medical complications, mental problems (dual diagnosis), or HIV disease are involved. The limiting factor for many clinics is their budget.

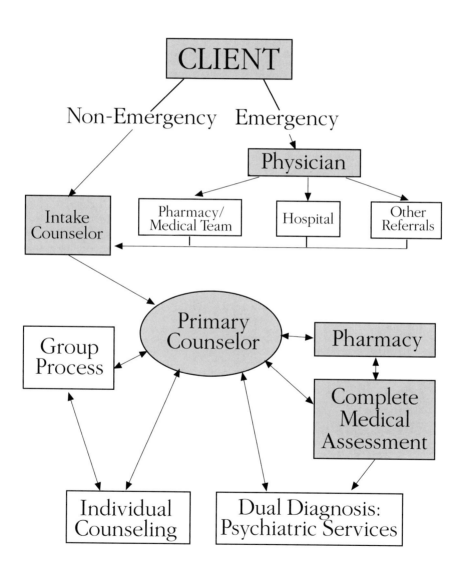

"I thought my luck was the pits: my girl friend split, I got canned, and got thrown out of my apartment. I still had enough for 8 rocks. That cooled the pain. And then I ran out of rocks and my mind returned a little. That's the incredible thing about coke. It never occurred to me, even after all the crap that I'd been through, that the cocaine was the problem, not my luck." Crack addict

It is vital to remember that addiction is a dysfunction of the mind. Brain cells, unlike all other cells, are the only nonreplicated cells of the human body. We are all born with all the brain cells we will ever get, unlike skin cells which are totally replaced every eight days or so. Thus, the brain cell disease of addiction is a chronic process, which can be treated and arrested but not one that can be reversed or cured. Recovery is a lifelong process, not a 30-day wonder. Addicts must refrain from ever abusing psychoactive drugs if they want to avoid relapsing into addiction.

"I'd been in this program for two years. I thought I could have one drink to relax with some friends I ran into. I had about five scotches, and ended up using all night long in a hotel with 2 prostitutes. I went through about $700 and was broke, and then I stole $150 from my roommate." Crack user

RECOGNITION AND ACCEPTANCE

This essential first step in all treatment approaches for chemical dependency is also the most difficult to accomplish. Denial is the universal defense mechanism experienced by addicts, their families and by those in their environment. Denial prevents or delays the proper recognition and acceptance of a chemical dependency problem. Denial is a refusal to acknowledge the negative impact that the addiction is having on one's life. It is also the shifting of responsibility of negative consequences to other causes rather than addiction.

"It seems like every time I would hit the pipe, my daughter would say, 'Mommy, Mommy,' for some reason. And so I would say, 'Why are you bothering me?' It really made me crazy. I mean my son would just pick on things and make noise or something." Crack user

"You'd use drugs too if you had to deal with the problems I have to deal with in my life." 54-year-old surgeon (Demerol addict)

The medical profession also has a tendency to deny or overlook addiction. How often is a caffeine intake history done by physicians who treat anxiety and insomnia in a businessman?

Usually those closest to the addict (his or her family or spouse) have the best chance to make the earliest recognition of addiction. Denial, plus the toxic effects that psychoactive drugs have on judgement and memory, make the addict likely to be the last person to recognize her or his addiction. After close relations, others able to recognize addiction include friends or co-workers, employers, the IRS, the medical professions and the law.

> *"Charlie hit bottom, but the only reason he got into treatment was they busted him for possession and made him go to meetings at the jail. I went to the joint lots of times, but it was always for stealing so I didn't get into treatment. Then the little strokes and the memory gaps started, so even stupid me knew I had a problem." 30-year-old crank (methamphetamine) addict*

Once addiction is suspected, various diagnostic tools can be used to help verify, support or clarify the potential diagnosis of chemical addiction. Several diagnostic criteria have been developed to assist clinicians in making a diagnosis of chemical dependence. Some of the more common ones used are the following:

• The American Psychiatric Association Diagnostic and Statistical Manual of Mental Disorders (DSM-IIIR) relies on the pattern and duration of drug use; the negative impact of drugs on the social or occupational functioning of the user; and the pathological effects (i.e. tolerance or withdrawal symptoms) to confirm a diagnosis of addiction;

• The Selective Severity Assessment (SSA) in the identification or withdrawal status evaluates eleven physiologic signs (pulse, temperature, tremors, etc.) to confirm the severity of the addiction in an addict;

* The National Council on Alcoholism Criteria for Diagnosis of Alcoholism (NCA CRIT) and its Modified Criteria (MODCRIT) outline two bases on which to make the diagnosis of alcoholism:

1) physical and clinical parameters and

2) behavioral, psychological and attitudinal impact;

• The simplest diagnostic aid is the Michigan Alcoholism Screening Test (MAST) which uses just 25 questions which are primarily directed at negative life effects of alcohol on the user. Positive responses to each question are "weighted" with a score reflective of the degree of alcoholism they represent in the respondent;

• The Addiction Severity Index (ASI) represents the most comprehensive and lengthy criteria for the diagnosis of chemical dependency.

There are several more diagnostic tools being used, all of which are helpful to the addict or their loved ones in overcoming the denial of addiction.

> *"The fourth step in Alcoholics Anonymous is making an inventory of your character defects. Well, I'd been a real jerk all my life, but it wasn't until I did my own inventory that I realized the damage I'd done. It made me realize I was a drunk." Recovering alcoholic*

Addiction is a progressive illness which leads to severe life impairment and dysfunction when left to proceed without disruption. The earlier it is recognized, accepted, and treated, the more likely the recovering user will have a rewarding life and good health. All too often, users come in for treatment after they have hit rock bottom leaving their hopes for a quality life handicapped.

"It had gotten to the point where the depression was so great that I didn't want to go to work anymore. I had just neglected all my responsibilities. It was just a lot of depressing days that I couldn't take anymore."
Recovering polydrug abuser

INTERVENTION

Addiction is the only illness which requires a self diagnosis for treatment to be effective. When a physician tells patients that they have high blood pressure, they usually accept that diagnosis without question and make changes in their lives to improve their health. But, when addicts are first confronted with their addiction, they almost always deny any drug problem and continue to abuse drugs. Thus, special strategies have been developed to attack the denial in addicts and help them recognize their dependence on drugs. Generally referred to as intervention, these strategies have been documented since the late 1800's to effectively bring addicts into treatment and hold them there. Further, there are now specialists who help to organize and implement intervention.

"When my dog died, I got a prescription for Xanax to help 'cause I felt so bad. Then I got Dalmane to help me sleep, Valium for my muscle tension, Librax for my upset stomach, Klonopin for my headaches, and even Ativan to help me cut down on my drinking, all on Medicare. And because they were prescribed, I never thought I had a problem until they literally dragged me into the living room for an intervention." Recovering benzodiazepine addict

Most intervention strategies consist of the following elements:

Love

An intervention should always start and end with an expression of love and genuine concern for the well being of the addict. Multiple participants should be recruited from various aspects of the addict's life — all of whom share a sense of true affection for the addict but recognize the progressive impairment of the addiction and are bold enough to commit themselves to participation in the intervention. Generally this intervention team consists of family members, close friends and co-workers, other recovering addicts, a representative of the addict's spiritual community (clergy or community leader) and a lead facilitator.

Facilitator

A professional intervention specialist or a knowledgeable chemical dependency treatment professional is selected to organize the intervention, educate the participants about addiction and treatment options, train and assist team members in the preparation of their statements, and support or confirm the diagnosis of addiction. The team meets and prepares its intervention without revealing their activities to the addict.

Intervention Statements

Each team member prepares a statement that they will make to the addict at the time of the intervention. Each statement consists of four parts:

A. How much they love, care for or respect the addict.

B. Specific evidence they have personally witnessed or experienced related to the addiction and the pain they have personally experienced from the incident(s).

C. Their knowledge that the incidents occurred not because of the addict's intent but because of the effects that the drug has caused on the addict's behavior.

D. Reaffirmation of their love, concern or respect for the addict with a strong request that he or she recognize and accept their illness and enter treatment for it immediately.

Anticipated Defenses and Outcomes

The facilitator prepares the team to deal with expected defense mechanisms like denial, rationalization, minimization, anger, and accusations. The team also prepares for all logistics (reserving a program or hospital admission, packed clothing and toiletries, coverage for work or home duties, etc.) such that the addict will have no excuse or delay in entering treatment immediately should a successful intervention ensue. The team also prepares for contingencies and alternative treatments other than the ones they selected should the addict refuse to accept their recommendations.

Intervention

Timing, location and surprise are imperative components of the actual intervention event. A neutral, non-threatening and private location must be secured for the intervention. It should occur at a time (usually early Sunday mornings) when the addict is most likely to be sober or not to be under the influence of a drug. The evidence presented in statements should include current incidents. A reliable plan should be developed to get the addict to the location which does not cause her or him to suspect what is about to occur. Finally, the facilitator has prepared the order of the statements which has been rehearsed by the team prior to the intervention.

Contingency

Successful or not, it is important for the intervention team members to continue to meet after the intervention to process their experience. This also provides the opportunity for team members (especially family members) to explore their own support or treatment needs for issues like codependency, enabling, or adult children of addicts syndrome.

Despite the inherent risks of anger or rejection which may result from an unsuccessful intervention, the potential benefit from these strategies far outweigh the risks. At a very minimum, the pathological effects of secrecy which pervade an addiction have been brought out to all those who are most affected by it, allowing a chance for successful treatment.

TREATMENT CONTINUUM

"I know it sounds strange, but the best thing that ever happened to me was that I became an addict. That's because my addiction forced me into treatment and the recovery process, and through recovery I found what was missing in my life."
Nurse with 20 years of recovery time

The chronic, progressive and relapsing nature of addiction is a depressing and degrading process. Addicts invariably lose self esteem and a large percentage (34%-38%) develop suicidal depression by the time they enter treatment. Recovery is a spiritually uplifting and motivating process through which individuals gain a sense of purpose, community and meaning for their lives. There are multiple modalities developed to treat addiction ranging from long-term (2 or more years) residential treatment, to short-term (28 days or less) of outpatient medical and nonmedical psycho-social approaches. Whatever the modality used, treatment should address four major phases: detoxification, initial abstinence, sobriety, and continuous recovery. It is necessary for the addict to commit to abstinence from the abused drug through all phases of treatment.

"When I first came into the program, I thought I could just detox and that would be it. It would hold. I've been here for two years now and I'm just beginning to understand that I have barely started on my road towards recovery."
Recovering heroin addict

Detoxification

The first step is to get the drug out of the system. The user's body chemistry has become so unbalanced that only abstinence will give it time to metabolize the drug and begin to normalize neurotransmitter balance. It takes about a week to detoxify from a drug such as cocaine and perhaps another four weeks to ten months until the body chemistry settles down.

Assessment of the severity of addiction is important to determine whether the addict requires hospitalization, residential treatment, or whether the addict can be managed on an outpatient basis. Physical dependence to alcohol or sedatives, major medical or psychiatric complications, pregnancy, or an overdosed addict are all indications for initiating detoxification in a hospital-based program.

A variety of specific medical treatments are used during the detoxification phase to ease the symptoms of withdrawal and minimize the initial drug craving which occur.

• Catapres (Clonodine) dampens the withdrawal symptoms of opiate, alcohol and even nicotine addiction.

• Phenobarbital is used to prevent withdrawal seizures and other symptoms associated with alcohol and sedative-hypnotic dependence.

• Methadone is the federally-approved medication for opiate-addiction treatment while levo alpha acetyl methadol and buprenorphine are being developed as alternatives for methadone in the detoxification or maintenance of opioid addictions.

• Antipsychotic medications like Haldol (haloperidol) and antidepressants like Norpramin (desipramine) and Tofranil (imipramine) have been used in the initial detoxification of cocaine, amphetamine or other stimulant drug addiction.

• Parlodel (bromocriptine), Symmetrel (amantadine), and L-Dopa have been used to treat the craving associated with cocaine and stimulant drug dependence. Similarly, Trexan (naltrexone) and ritanserin have been used to dampen alcohol cravings.

• Nicoderm, Habitrol, or Prostep patches (nicotine) are approved to treat the withdrawal symptoms of tobacco whereas Nicorette gum (nicotine) helps to lessen craving.

• Antabuse (disulfiram) helps to prevent alcoholism relapse by creating unpleasant side effects if alcohol is used while it is being taken.

• Trexan (naltrexone) blocks all opiates while an addict is being treated with it. Thus, the addict will have no response to heroin if she or he happens to slip while in treatment.

• Finally, a number of amino acids are used individually or in combinations with each other to alleviate withdrawal and craving symptoms from addiction to various drugs. The theory is that these amino acids are used by the brain to make neurotransmitters that were depleted by the drug addiction. It is believed that the depletion in neurotransmitters is the cause of the withdrawal and craving. Common amino acids used for this purpose are Tyrosine, Taurine, Tryptophane, d,1-phenylalanine, lecithin and glutamine.

Medical intervention alone is rarely effective during the detoxification phase. Indeed, most programs forego medical treatment when the addict is not in any health or emotional danger from drug withdrawal. Intensive counseling, group work, and 12-step group participation have proven to be the most effective measures in engaging addicts into a recovery process and should be the main focus of all phases of treatment despite the many medical innovations being developed.

"I relied on the pills to keep clean, but I kept having relapses. They ain't Jack and the Beanstalk magic beans. And besides, they don't give you enough. They help you feel better but they don't cure you…not even close." Heroin addict in Phase 2 of treatment

Initial Abstinence

Once the addicts have been detoxified, their body chemistry must be given the opportunity to regain its balance. Continued abstinence during this phase is best promoted by addressing both the continuous craving for drugs and the problems in their lives which may put them at risk for relapse.

Anticraving medications such as those used during the detoxification phase can be continued during this phase when more traditional approaches like "voluntary isolation" (staying away from slippery places like bars, slippery people like co-users, and slippery things like drug paraphernalia), counseling, group and 12-step meetings are ineffective in controlling the episodic drug hunger during this phase.

Environmental "triggers" or "cues" often precipitate drug cravings. Addicts must learn to recognize their triggers which can be anything from drug odors to even hearing a song about drugs. They must then be prepared with a strategy to prevent themselves from using. It is important to note that drug craving is a true psychological response which is manifested by actual body changes of increased heart rate and blood pressure, sweating, specific electrical changes in the skin, and even an immediate drop of 2 degrees or more in body temperature.

Deconditioning techniques, stress reduction exercises, expressing one's feelings, and long walks or cold showers are all strategies used by addicts to dissipate the craving response when it arises.

As described in Chapter 3, Dr. Anna Rose Childress's Desensitization Program retrains brain cells to not react when confronted by an environmental cue. The procedure involves exposing an addict to progressively stronger environmental cues over 40 to 50 sessions in a controlled setting.

This technique gradually decreases response to the cues until there are no physiologic signs of a craving response even when the addict is exposed to heavy triggers. Every time an addict refrains from using while craving a drug, it lessens the response to the next trigger experience.

> *"I did it myself. Every day I would take out my Librium pills and look at them, touch them and even smell them. Then, I would put them back in the bottle because I knew I couldn't ever use them again. After a while, I lost interest in them altogether."* Recovering British Librium addict

In addition, medical approaches like Antabuse for alcoholism, naltrexone for opiates/opioids, and various amino acids like tyrosine or d, l-phenylalanine for many of the drug addictions have been used to support the work of the self-help groups by suppressing or reversing the pleasurable effects of drugs or decreasing the drug craving, all of which help encourage the addict to stay clean.

Recently, a benzodiazepine antagonist, Mazicon (flumazenil) injection has been approved for the treatment of benzodiazepine overdose. Further development of this drug and the research into a cocaine and a true alcohol antagonist may lead to treatments for these addictions in the same manner that naltrexone is effective in preventing readdiction to opiates.

Initial abstinence is also the phase during which an addict starts to put her or his life back in order from all the things she or he neglected to take care of while a practicing addict. A comprehensive analysis of an addict's medical health, psychiatric status, social problems, and environmental needs must be conducted and a plan developed to address all issues presented.

> *"I thought getting sober would take care of my problems ...that it was the alcohol that caused my messed up marriage, and so on. Drinking was just a symptom of how screwed up I was. Sober, I still had the same problems. I just became a sober, screwed up dry drunk." Recovering alcoholic*

Most importantly, addicts need to build a support system that will give continuing advice, help, and information when the user returns to job and home and is subject to all the pressures and temptations that made drug abuse begin. The support groups and 12-step programs like A.A. (Alcoholics Anonymous), N.A. (Narcotics Anonymous), C.A. (Cocaine Anonymous), and others are essential to maintaining a clean, sober, drug-free lifestyle. Involvement in group therapy and continued recovery counseling have been demonstrated to have the most positive treatment outcomes during the initial abstinence phase.

Long-Term Sobriety

The pivotal component of this phase occurs when an addict finally admits and accepts her or his addiction and surrenders to the long-term, one-day-at-a-time treatment process.

Continued participation in group, family, and 12-step programs are the key to maintaining long-term abstinence from drugs. The addict must accept that addiction is chronic, progressive, incurable, and potentially fatal and that relapse is always possible.

> *"We always say, 'I know that I have another relapse in me. I don't know if I have another sobriety in me.'" 7-year member of Alcoholics Anonymous*

It is also vital for the recovering addict to accept that her or his condition is "chemical dependency" or "drug compulsivity" and not just that of alcoholism, or cocainism, or opioidism. Individuals who manifest addiction to a particular drug such as cocaine, are well advised to abstain from the use of all psychoactive substances, including and especially alcohol. Even a seemingly benign flirtation with marijuana will probably lead to drug hunger and relapse. It is a common clinical observation that compulsive drug abusers often switch intoxicants only to find the symptoms of addiction resurfacing through another addictive agent or behavior. Drug switching is not an acceptable form of recovery-oriented treatment.

"I went from the weed to the alcohol to whatever else I could get my hands on until I got to cocaine. It escalated. And even with the cocaine, when I didn't have that, I went back to marijuana, "black beauties," Valium, and Darvon. I could have been compulsive about water. In fact, I became compulsive about food then and gained 70 pounds." Crack user

Recovery

Treatment and a continued focus on abstinence and/or sobriety are not enough to assure recovery and a quality lifestyle. Recovering addicts also need to restructure their lives and find things they enjoy doing that give them satisfaction, that give them the natural highs instead of the artificial highs they came to seek through drugs. Without this, one may have sobriety but will not have recovery. This integral phase of treatment has been validated experimentally by Dr. Vaillant, 1983. He indicates four components necessary to change an ingrained habit of alcohol dependence. In our model, the generic term "drug" is substituted for Vaillant's specific reference to alcohol:

1. Offering the client or patient a nonchemical substitute dependency for the drug such as exercise;

2. Reminding her or him ritually that even one episode of drug use can lead to pain and relapse;

3. Repairing the social, emotional and medical damage done;

4. Restoring self-esteem.

Continued and lifelong participation in the fellowship of 12-step programs along with the concerted effort to seek out natural, healthy, non-drug, rewarding experiences is the formula that most recovering addicts have found to be successful in achieving their treatment goals.

"I tell my clients that if they can't find something that is natural and healthy which gives them the high and the satisfaction that they got from drugs, then they won't have recovery. They won't have a quality life." Treatment consultant

Ethnic and Cultural Sensitivity

Cultural competency in treatment is another key element for successful outcomes. Programs which focus their development on a specific target population and provide culturally relevant prevention, intervention and treatment services have demonstrated the ability to attract, bond, and shepherd addicts into a recovery process much better than a general program with no specific focus. Models for such an approach have been developed for different ethnic, age, class, and professional target populations.

Treatment Works

Over the past quarter century, many innovations have been developed to treat chemical dependency, resulting in an increase in the effectiveness of treatment and appreciation that treatment works! Addicts can and do, enter recovery lifestyles which are much more rewarding than their previous lives. The earlier that an addict recognizes, accepts and surrenders to the treatment process, the better the outcome. The recovering community now represents a significant portion of the populations of most cities in the United States. This community offers practicing addicts hope that they, too, can change their lives should they choose to enter treatment.

"I'm not the same person that I was when I entered this fellowship. Through my recovery and the 12-steps, I have found meaning and purpose in my life. It feels especially good with my kids because they know that I'm here for them. There's no catchup anymore. I keep my promises. The challenge of a sober parent is keeping promises." Recovering speed addict

OTHER BEHAVIORS (Codependency, Enabling, and Adult Children of Alcoholics)

"Even though it was my dad that drank until he got sick, doing the intervention was harder for me than for him. I knew he denied his drinking. I didn't realize that I did too even though I didn't drink myself, and that

I had almost as many problems as he did." 31-year old adult child of an alcoholic (ACoA)

Current treatment focuses not only on the addicts themselves, but on their families as well. The use of drugs or alcohol impacts everyone in close contact with the heavy user. Recognized as addictive dysfunctional behaviors in the non-using family members are the conditions of

• codependency,

• enabling, and

• adult children or children of addicts.

Codependency

As addicts are dependent upon a substance, codependents are dependent on the addicts to fulfill some need of their own. For example, a wife may be dependent on her husband maintaining his addiction in order to hold power over the relationship. As long as he's addicted, she has an excuse for her own shortcomings and problems.

Enabling

When a family becomes dependent upon the addiction of a family member, there is a strong tendency to avoid confrontation on the addictive behavior and a subconscious effort to perpetuate the addiction, often led by a person who benefits greatly from that addiction, the "chief enabler."

Children of Addicts (ACoA)

Children of addicts take on predictable behavioral roles within the family which "co" the addiction and which continue on into their adult personalities. In addict families, the roles taken on by the children are usually one or more of the following:

1. Model child-high achievers: overly responsible and chief enablers of addicted parents by taking over their roles and responsibilities.

2. Problem child: experiences continual, multiple personal problems and often manifests early drug or alcohol addiction. They demand and get most of what attention is left from parents and siblings.

3. Lost Child: they are the withdrawn, "spaced-out" children, disconnected from the life and emotions around them. Often avoiding any emotionally confronting issues, they are unable to form close friendships or intimate bonds with others.

4. The mascot child or family clown: they use another avoidance strategy which is to make everything trivial by minimizing all serious issues. They are well liked and easy to befriend but are usually superficial in all relationships, even those with their own family members.

Effective treatment addresses addiction as a treatable and preventable FAMILY DISEASE. By the end of the 1980's, there was thorough recognition of the impact that addiction has on the entire family system. In the 90's, increased treatment strategies focus on the addict's family and programs which directly address ACoA and codependency. These programs have had a dramatic impact on making recovery a reality to more and more people in treatment.

The following are the 12-steps of Alcoholics Anonymous, the most successful recovery program for people who have lost control of their drinking. It was founded in 1935 by Bill Wilson and Dr. Bob Smith, both alcoholics, who found they could help themselves recover by helping others to recover. The program is successful because it suggests that a change in the way one lives, not just putting the cork in the bottle, is necessary for recovery. Alcoholics Anonymous and its offshoots—Narcotics Anonymous, Al-Anon, etc.—are spiritual programs not detoxification programs.

Step One
"We admitted we were powerless over alcohol—that our lives had become unmanageable."

Step Two
"Came to believe that a Power greater than ourselves could restore us to sanity."

Step Three
"Made a decision to turn our will and our lives over to the care of God <u>as we understand Him.</u>"

Step Four
"Made a searching and fearless moral inventory of ourselves."

Step Five
"Admitted to God, to ourselves, and to another human being the exact nature of our wrongs."

Step Six
"Were entirely ready to have God remove all these defects of character."

Step Seven
"Humbly asked Him to remove our shortcomings."

Step Eight
"Made a list of all persons we had harmed, and became willing to make amends to them all."

Step Nine
"Made direct amends to such people wherever possible, except when to do so would injure them or others."

Step Ten
"Continued to take personal inventory and when we were wrong promptly admitted it."

Step Eleven
"Sought through prayer and meditation to improve our conscious contact with God <u>as we understood Him</u>, praying only for knowledge of His will for us and the power to carry that out."

Step Twelve
"Having had a spiritual awakening as the result of these steps, we tried to carry this message to alcoholics, and to practice these principles in all our affairs."

Because many people dislike the spiritual references in A.A. writings and philosophy, a secular version of the program and the 12-steps has been formed.

REVIEW

FROM EXPERIMENTATION TO COMPULSION INTO TREATMENT

1. There are many theories of addiction. They can be divided into three main models: the addictive disease model; the behavioral/environmental model; and the academic model.

2. The addictive disease model states that addiction is an incurable yet treatable disease that is a consequence of genetic deficiencies in neurotransmitters and brain hormones.

3. The behavioral/environmental model states that environmental and developmental influences, such as stress, can result in changes in brain hormones leading people to seek and use drugs.

4. The academic model states that actual physiological changes of the body, due to excessive drug use, lead to addiction.

5. In the behavioral/environmental model, there are multiple levels of drug use: experimental; social/recreational; habitual; abuse; addiction.

6. The reality of drug abuse combines the three theories of heredity, environment, and psychoactive drugs, together, are what determine the level of addiction.

7. The compulsion curve states that we are all born with a certain sensitivity to drugs and that some are more sensitive than others. Users who are sensitive can fall into addiction very quickly, while those with low sensitivity will have to use a lot to fall into addictive patterns.

8. The hardest part of treatment is to get drug abusers or addicts to recognize their problem.

9. The four keys to a treatment program are detoxification, initial abstinence, long-term abstinence, and sustained recovery. This means getting the drug out of the system; counseling and group interaction to promote the initial abstinence; long-term participation in a group, individual, or family program to foster long-term abstinence; and developing a new set of emotions and feelings in addition to finding alternate natural highs to sustain the recovery.

10. Addicts need to find things that give them the same pleasure they initially sought from drugs. They need a natural high.

QUESTIONS

1. What causes addiction according to the academic model of addiction?

2. Describe the body changes which occur with the academic model of addiction.

3. What causes addiction according to the addictive disease model?

4. List five characteristics of addictive disease.

5. What causes addiction according to the behavioral/environmental model?

6. What are the five levels of drug use according to the behavioral/environmental model?

7. What are the three factors that determine addiction?

8. According to the compulsion curve, what is inherited sensitivity?

9. According to the compulsion curve, what moves a person along the compulsion curve from low sensitivity to high sensitivity?

10. How does the compulsion curve slope differ at the low sensitivity end as compared to the high sensitivity end?

11. What is the most difficult thing to overcome when treating addiction?

12. Why are drugs used during drug detoxification treatment?

13. What are the four parts of most drug treatment programs?

14. Once addicted, why can't the treated addict return to social or recreational use of the drug?

15. Why is habituation considered the dividing line between casual drug using behaviors and intensive drug misuse?

16. What is sensitization or imprinting and what role does it play in addiction relapse?

17. List three types of 12-step peer recovery programs.

18. How does Clonidine help treat the opiate/opioid addict?

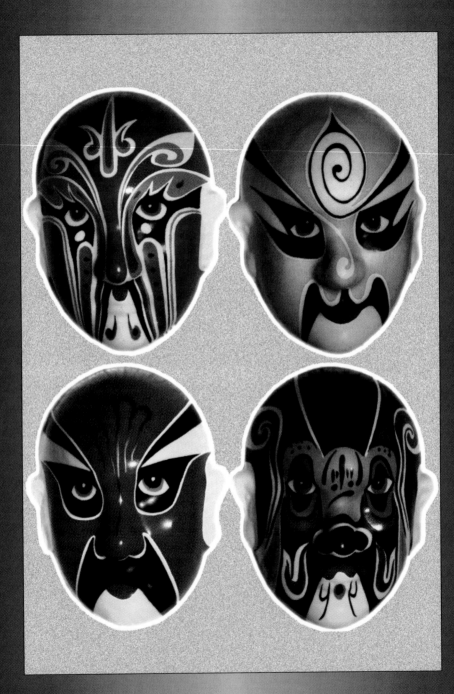

CHAPTER 12

DUAL DIAGNOSIS

OR MICA
(Mentally Ill Chemical Abuser)

1990

A-2 Wednesday, November 21, 1990 ★ ★ ★

Drug, alcohol abusers likelier to suffer mental ills, study says

By Alison Bass

1990
Obsessive-Compulsives

Psychiatric Drug Called Just a Start

By Charles Petit
Chronicle Science Writer

1991

Depression Stigma Keeps Many From Treatment

Sufferers urged not to blame themselves

By Clarence Johnson
Chronicle Staff Writer

DEFINING DUAL DIAGNOSIS

Although the field of dual diagnosis is new, the importance of the concepts presented in this chapter cannot be emphasized enough. The interconnection between mental illness and drug addiction is so profound that understanding this link gives one an extraordinary insight into the functioning of the human mind at all levels particularly when mental illness and/or addiction are involved. This chapter further helps one integrate the theories of addiction presented in Chapter 5 and 11.

A steadily growing number of chemically dependent individuals are under treatment with the condition known as "dual diagnosis." This condition is usually defined as a person having both a substance abuse problem and a diagnosable, significant, psychiatric problem.

The term dual diagnosis is more common in the chemical dependency treatment community. The term MICA (mentally ill chemical abuser) is more widely used in the mental health treatment community. Other terms like comorbidity and double trouble have also been used to refer to this condition.

"After more than 30 years of use, when I gave up the codeine and the Valium in treatment, I started to remember the pain. You know, the first thing that flashed through my mind was my uncle's face, when he was hurting me real bad, when I was 10. I hadn't remembered it for 32 years." 45-year-old woman with major depression

"This previous client is a case where the diagnosis should be written in invisible ink because so much is being revealed as she gets clearer and clearer. We've had major depression at different times, and there may be an underlying personality disorder, but we also have some post-traumatic shock syndrome too in the sense that she is discovering as she is getting clean and sober, an incest background and severe physical abuse from many

persons which she was not even aware of while when she was using. She wasn't just anesthetizing her feelings. She didn't even recognize the beatings as beatings." Dual-diagnosis counselor

The psychiatric disorders most often seen in dual diagnosis in combination with drug abuse are

• Major depression;

• Schizophrenia (thought disorder);

• Manic-depression (bipolar) disorder, or a combination of these.

Many treatment professionals also include other mental problems in their definition of dual diagnosis:

• Anxiety disorders, i.e. panic disorders, obsessive compulsive disorders, post-traumatic stress syndromes;

• Organic disorders;

• Developmental disorders;

• Somatoform disorders;

• Rage disorders;

and a few others such as sexual dysfunction and eating disorders. (Most of these disorders will be defined later.)

What this means is that a cocaine user might also have schizophrenia, even when not using drugs. An alcoholic might also have severe depression which persists even when the user is detoxified.

"I have this illness, mental illness, with manic-depression, and when I take the alcohol, my functioning isn't as clear cut, not as sharp as say the average person that isn't suffering any mental problems."
Client with dual diagnosis

It's important to distinguish between having symptoms and having a major psychiatric disorder. Everyone feels blue and sad sometimes. Everyone has the capacity for grief and loneliness, but this does not mean that a person is medically depressed, requiring medication or psychiatric treatment. It's really a question of severity and continuity.

THE DUALLY DIAGNOSED INDIVIDUAL

Depending on which drug is used and how it is used, psychoactive substances can create four types of dually diagnosed patients.

One kind of dual diagnosis involves the person who had a clearly defined mental illness and then got into drugs, for example the teen with major depression who discovers amphetamines.

"My mom asked my little brother if he thought I'd been depressed a lot in my life, and he said I'd been depressed ever since he could remember. The speed got me out of it except when I was coming down." *16-year-old boy*

Another kind of dual diagnosis associated with the use of psychoactive drugs occurs when there might have been an underlying psychiatric problem that wasn't fully developed as yet. There was no clear-cut depression nor clear-cut schizophrenia before taking drugs, but there were some unusual thought patterns that the person was experiencing which were not significant enough to be recognized as a mental illness. When that person started to use psychoactive drugs, the effects of those substances uncovered the underlying mental disturbance which had not yet surfaced.

"I think it was about six years ago when I had a suspicion of being a manic depressive, but I was so drunk and I really didn't know what was wrong with me. And when I quit using drugs, I just felt horrible, even worse than I had before, like I was dying." *38-year-old client*

The third way that dual diagnosis occurs is when the drug itself or withdrawal from the drug causes a transient depression, temporary psychosis, or another apparent mental illness. The imbalance in the brain chemistry in this type of dual diagnosis is usually temporary, and the mental illness will disappear within a few months to a year of abstinence. This is not a true dual diagnosis but only a temporary condition resulting from the toxic emotional effects of the drug.

"This speed run's only been 13 days, but I get these sores and I get paranoid and real crazy. After I come down it'll be weird. It will take weeks to get back into shape. And all that other crap will disappear." 43-year-old "speed freak"

The fourth kind of dual diagnosis happens when there wasn't a preexisting problem, but as a result of years of use or some extreme reaction to the drug, the user develops a chronic psychiatric problem because the toxic effects of the drug permanently imbalance the brain chemistry.

"My initial flip-out was in 1986 after snorting crank for six weeks straight, about a half gram a day. Three weeks later I had my first manic episode. Later they put me on Haldol and then Lithium. I have three diagnoses: amphetamine psychosis, psychotic depressive, and manic depressive." 28-year-old client

MAKING THE DIAGNOSIS

When assessing mental illness in a substance abuser, a general rule used by both mental health and substance abuse treatment professionals is that the initial diagnosis should be tentative.

"The doctor told me that a person who drank 25 years like me would probably take a year to clear. That was one reason that I never figured out that I was manic-depressive. I didn't notice it. I figured I was depressed because I was drunk all the time." 35-year-old man

The prevalence of dual diagnosis depends on when the diagnosis is made.

Since many mental symptoms are a temporary result of drug toxicity or drug withdrawal, an early diagnosis may merely be drug toxicity rather than dual diagnosis. Thus the prudent chemical dependency clinician treats all dangerous symptoms but holds off making a psychiatric diagnosis until the addict has had time to get sober and out of a drug intoxication or drug withdrawal state.

Other factors include

- The expertise of the clinician doing the diagnosis;

- The definition of "psychiatric disorder" that is used;

- The perspective of the assessment team (whether from the mental health or the chemical dependency treatment community);

- The population studied; the prevalence of dual diagnosis in a homeless drug-abusing population is greater than that seen in a group of school teachers.

INCREASE IN DUAL DIAGNOSIS

In a study by the National Institute of Mental Health in 1990, 53% of drug abusers and 37% of alcohol abusers had, in addition to their drug problem, at least one serious mental illness. Conversely, 29% of all mentally ill people had a problem with either alcohol or drug abuse.

The overlap is even greater with certain mental disorders. Sixty-one percent of people with manic-depressive illness and 47 percent of people with schizophrenia also had a problem with substance abuse. The drug of choice also matters. Seventy-six percent of cocaine abusers had a diagnosable mental disorder compared with 50% of marijuana abusers. Many were self-medicating their psychiatric disorder with street drugs.

"I believe I had depression all along, even before I started using, and so, through alcohol, marijuana, and even heroin, I was treating that depression."
Dual diagnosis client

Finally, the prevalence of a psychiatric illness, an addictive disorder, or dual diagnosis in prison populations was a remarkable 81%.

There are several possible reasons why the estimates on the number of dually diagnosed clients are dramatically higher than those made during the 1960's and 1970's.

The diminishing number of in-patient mental health facilities (Fig. 12-1) due to a reliance on prescribed medications such as antidepressants or antipsychotics and the increased reliance on outpatient mental health facilities have forced an increasing number of people with psychiatric disorders to deal with their problems on an out-patient basis or on their own.

Detached from the structure and intense professional supervision of hospital care, poor control of their prescribed medication and aggravation of mental problems are more likely to lead the client to turn to street drugs for help. Many people with mental disorders self-medicate with alcohol,

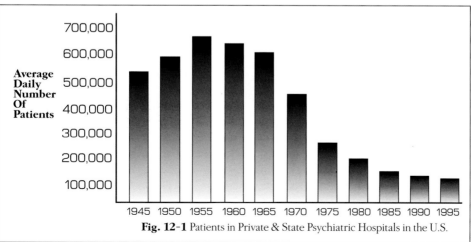

Fig. 12-1 Patients in Private & State Psychiatric Hospitals in the U.S.

heroin, amphetamines, or dozens of other drugs in an attempt to control their symptoms. For these and other reasons including the cutting of mental health budgets, the incidence of dual diagnosis among compulsive drugs users and particularly among the homeless remains extremely high.

> *"I had used heroin to control my depression as a mood stabilizer, and so withdrawing from it caused an even worse depression. When I came out of the sort of fog from the first five days of not having it, I felt better, but, the pink cloud feeling vanished quite quickly and was replaced with the usual depression that I was used to."* Patient in a half-way house

The growth of licensed professionals working in the field of chemical dependency treatment has resulted in a greater recognition and documentation of dual diagnosis. The increased abuse of cocaine and amphetamines has also increased the problem of dual diagnosis. A larger number of substance abusers means that more of them will also be dually diagnosed. Also, since stimulants are more toxic to brain chemistry than most substances, those with fragile brain chemistry are more likely to be pushed over the edge into chronic neurochemical imbalance and mental illness.

Finally, "managed care" and "diagnosis-related group" (DRG) payment for treatment services usually provide more financial incentives for the treatment of multiple medical and psychiatric problems than for just addiction treatment. This can pressure some clinicians to over-diagnose MICA.

UNDERSTANDING THE DUALLY DIAGNOSED PERSON

Understanding of the problem of the client with both a mental health problem and a drug problem is a new challenge for both drug treatment and mental health professionals.

> *"When I went into the hospital, I would tell them I had a problem, that I was on Valium and codeine. The first thing they would then give me was a shot of Valium. When I told them that Valium addiction was one of my problems, a doctor even told me, 'Go home and withdraw.'"* 40-year-old dually diagnosed woman

In the past, inability to treat a person who manifested both a drug and a mental problem, combined with an outright refusal to develop treatment strategies for the dually diagnosed client, resulted in inappropriate and oft-times dangerous interactions with those clients. They were often shuffled aimlessly back and forth between the mental health care system and the chemical dependency system without receiving treatment. Even though there's been an increase in facilities that address the "dually diagnosed client," inappropriate care is still the rule rather than the exception. Budget considerations and lack of expertise or resources have much to do with this problem.

Substance abuse treatment facilities do not want these patients because they see them as too crazy and too disruptive, and in many cases, too inattentive in group therapy, which is most often employed as the core of treatment. Psychiatric treatment centers also avoid these patients because they're perceived as disruptive and always relapsing. Their relapse and abuse of drugs and alcohol are not tolerated by psychiatric facilities which discharge patients routinely for relapse.

CHEMICAL DEPENDENCY TREATMENT COMMUNITY VS. THE MENTAL HEALTH TREATMENT COMMUNITY

The following list contains eleven differences between the mental health treatment community and the chemical dependency treatment community. These differences help one understand why good treatment for the dually diagnosed client has proved to be so difficult to obtain.

1. Mental health (MH) says, "Control the underlying psychiatric problem, and then the drug abuse will disappear." Chemical dependency (CD) says, "Get the patient clean and sober, and the mental health problems will resolve themselves. While these statements are true in many cases, there is still a third to a half of each group where concurrent treatment of both the addiction and the underlying mental problems is required.

2. In the MH system, limited recovery from one's problems is more readily acceptable than in CD programs where most believe that lifetime abstinence and recovery are possible.

"I've been to this one treatment facility three different times and each time I have been here I have benefited mentally. I have been in the mental health system for 30 years. I'm 52 years old and ever since I've been little, I've been exposed to alcohol." Woman with alcohol problem and manic-depression

3. Male dual diagnosis clients are more reluctant to seek help from the MH system than from CD treatment programs. This is probably because of the involuntary treatment aspects and the stigma of mental illness. Clients and their families hope that the problem is addiction from which they can more fully recover than they can from mental illness.

"I tell members of my family that I'm in a half-way house for drug addiction as opposed to mental health because it seems with drug addiction, I can get better but with mental health, people see it as a chronic, long-term problem. There's a stigma." 19-year-old dually diagnosed client with major depression

With women, the opposite is often the case. They experience more stigma about being an addict. They usually enter the MH system.

4. MH relies on medication to help the client function whereas CD programs promote a drug-free philosophy.

> *"I refused to take any psychiatric medication for a long time. I thought you had to be really crazy to take it, and I thought that this was a big conflict which would limit my recovery. If I take medication, I'm a drug addict. But I'm glad I'm taking it now. I'm able to sleep, and think."* 35-year-old client

5. MH uses case management, shepherding the client from one service to another, while in CD programs, self-reliance is emphasized. Doing too much for the client in CD programs is viewed as co-dependency.

6. MH has a supportive philosophy while many CD programs use confrontation techniques. A major conflict occurs when a patient is not responding to the substance abuse treatment and yet has a severe psychiatric disorder or is HIV infected. One can't use the same threshold of bad behavior to terminate that patient from treatment as one would with just an addiction disorder. A CD clinic will try to achieve a compromise between mental health and substance abuse treatment approaches, so that they put up with more drug using behavior when a patient also has a psychiatric disorder or HIV infection. It's difficult to medically discharge a patient being treated for MH or HIV when they relapse into drug addiction.

7. The MH system shares information while the CD field practices strict confidentiality.

8. In MH, most of the treatment team is composed of professionals: social workers, psychiatrists, psychologists, and the like. In CD programs, recovering addicts and professionals often work together. (In 1940, in the United states, there were just 9,000 psychiatrists, social workers, and psychologists. Now there are more than 100,000 psychologists, 60,000 psychiatrists, and probably 150,000 social workers, not to mention those in allied mental health professions.)

9. MH relies heavily on scientific diagnosis and prognosis of an illness and is more process oriented. CD programs rely heavily on the spiritual side of recovery and are more outcome oriented than process oriented. (Process oriented means that there is a rigid set of procedures which will be implemented at specific times during the course of treatment to achieve positive benefits for the patient.) These fine distinctions are often lost on the client.

> *"All I can tell someone is, 'I have a problem. I don't know which way you're going to deal with it or tackle it, but I have a problem, and I can't function, and I need help."* Dual diagnosis patient

10. MH pays a lot of attention to the idea of preventing the client from getting worse, while CD programs have more of a tendency to allow people to hit bottom, in order to break through the denial of addiction. In MH, if people are do-

ing badly, they are usually admitted to a more intense treatment facility. In CD, if people are doing badly (i.e., using), they are often kicked out to hit bottom. With the dually diagnosed client, it's inappropriate and dangerous to allow clients to bottom out.

11. In MH, patient education and training are nonstructured and individualized, while in CD programs they are more standardized, concentrating on information about the drugs themselves, the progression of addiction, and the twelve-step process.

From the perspective of the MH treatment community, dual diagnosis represents an almost insurmountable challenge to the clinical expertise of the staff of CD programs, their assessment skills, and even their underlying concept of recovery or sobriety. It is difficult to differentiate an underlying psychiatric illness from a drug-induced toxic psychosis or a post-addiction reactive depression. Too often, a diagnosis of mental illness is made too early in the treatment or assessment process, resulting in CD staff inappropriately referring patients who are having drug reactions to the mental health programs who, most often, then reject these individuals because of their drug abuse problem.

CD programs often lack or resist developing the expertise needed to diagnose and treat mental health problems. Fiscal and other limited resource problems prevent the expansion of their services to meet the needs of dually diagnosed clients,

creating a tendency to establish mental health problems as an exclusionary criteria for treatment admission or continued treatment in many CD programs. Even CD programs with expertise in this area sometimes mistake success in prematurely treating psychiatric drug reaction symptoms as proof that there is an underlying psychiatric diagnosis. This results in an early and inappropriate referral to MH services when the real problem is addiction, not dual diagnosis.

RECOMMENDATIONS

The dually diagnosed patient must be treated for both disorders and is best treated in a single program when appropriate resources are available.

CD programs need to establish linkages with MH service providers and vice versa, such that they can work together in providing the client with their combined treatment expertise. Each needs to recognize that mental health and substance abuse treatment are both long-term propositions, and therefore they need to establish long-range services to address the problem of dual diagnosis.

Triple Diagnosis

Triple diagnosis is the added condition of HIV disease in the dually diagnosed client. Persons with AIDS, an AIDS-related condition, an HIV positive blood test, or persons who are a partner of someone with AIDS require additional expertise and specific services to effectively address their chemical dependency.

As the epidemic has progressed out of strictly gay and intravenous drug-using populations and into the cocaine-using heterosexual population, triple diagnosis will strain health department resources and further complicate treatment.

Multiple Diagnoses

As the chemical dependency treatment community becomes more aware of other simultaneous disorders which complicate the treatment of addiction, it must be willing to accept new challenges such as:

- Multiple drug (polydrug) addiction,

- Chronic pain in the chemically dependent individual,

- Other medical disorders such as epilepsy, diabetes, sickle cell disease, and even sexual dysfunction.

These problems require the development of future drug programs which should be holistic, use several techniques and philosophies of treatment, and be multi-disciplinary to meet the challenge of the evolving, complicated, clinical needs of the chemically dependent patient.

The following sections will examine the different kinds of psychiatric disorders; discuss the relationship between heredity, environment, and psychoactive drugs in regards to mental illness and drug addiction; then examine the various treatments available for the mentally ill substance abusing patient, particularly the psychotropic medications used in therapy.

PSYCHIATRIC DISORDERS

A neurotic is the person who builds a castle in the air. A psychotic is the person who lives in it. And a psychiatrist is the person who collects the rent. —Anonymous

Although there are hundreds of mental illnesses as classified by the mental health community, we will describe the ones most often associated with dual diagnosis.

PRINCIPAL DUAL DIAGNOSIS DISORDERS

Schizophrenia

Schizophrenia is a thought disorder, believed to be mostly inherited, characterized by hallucinations (false visual, auditory, or tactile sensations and perceptions), delusions (false beliefs) and poor association of ideas, an inappropriate affect (an illogical emotional response to any situation), autistic symptoms (a pronounced detachment from reality), ambivalence (difficulty in making even the simplest decisions), poor job performance, strained social relations, and impaired ability to care for oneself.

The signs have to be present for at least 6 months for the diagnosis to be made.

"I was hearing voices, and the voices wouldn't go away, and they followed me wherever I went. I got into creating scenarios as to who they were and what they were doing." 28-year-old man with schizophrenia

Schizophrenia usually strikes individuals in their late teens to early adulthood and is usually with them for life. Occasionally there's spontaneous remission. It is extremely destructive to those with the illness and to the friends and families around them.

When diagnosing schizophrenia, clinicians determine what drugs are being used by the patient. If they don't, they will end up with a false or incomplete diagnosis. They accomplish this by taking a thorough medical history or by using urinalysis. Unfortunately, a large percentage of drug or alcohol problems are missed by clinicians.

Several abused drugs mimic schizophrenia and psychosis, producing symptoms which can be easily misdiagnosed. Cocaine and amphetamines, especially when used to excess, will cause a toxic psychosis almost indistinguishable from a true paranoid psychosis. Steroids can also cause a psychosis. Drug induced paranoia can be indistinguishable from true paranoia. Most drugs but particularly the uppers, LSD, MDMA (ecstasy), and even marijuana can cause paranoia.

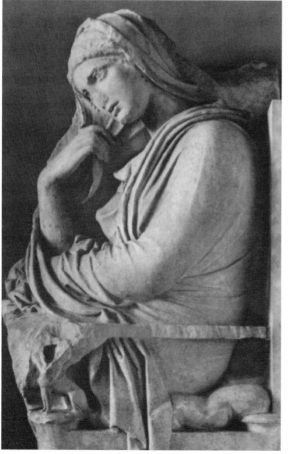

This Greek marble gravestone of a mourning woman from 400 B.C. is a reminder that mental illness was recognized throughout history. Hippocrates, the father of medicine, wrote about mental illness, particularly depression and anxiety (Metropolitan Museum of Art, New York).

The psychedelics such as LSD, PCP, peyote, and psilocybin are meant to disassociate users from their surroundings, so all-arounder abuse can also be mistaken for a thought disorder. Also, withdrawal from downers can be mistaken for a thought disorder because of extreme agitation. Many of the psychiatric symptoms will usually disappear upon treatment and detoxification.

Major depression

A major depression is likely to be experienced by 1 in 10 persons during their lifetime. It is characterized by:

- Depressed mood;

- Diminished interest and pleasure in most activities;

- Disturbances of sleep patterns and appetite;

- Decreased ability to concentrate;

- Feelings of worthlessness;

- Suicidal thoughts.

All of these symptoms persist without any life situation to provoke them. For example, a patient with major depression may win a lot of money in a lottery and respond to it by being melancholy or depressed.

For the diagnosis to be made accurately, these feelings have to occur every day, most of the day, for at least two weeks running. Organic causes such as an illness or drug abuse are ruled out as are natural reactions to the death of a loved one, separation, or a strained relationship.

"The depression just came when it wanted to come. I just sat there and thought about something, and I got depressed. The anger came because every male that has ever been in my life has beaten me or used me, you know, mentally and physically ... not sexually thank goodness." Severely depressed 17-year-old

The withdrawal symptoms which occur with most stimulant addictions (cocaine or amphetamine) and the "come down" or resolution phase of a psychedelic (LSD, "ecstasy") result in temporary depression which is almost indistinguishable from that of major depression.

Bipolar affective disorder (manic depression)

This illness is characterized by alternating periods of depression, normalcy, and mania. The depression is described above and is as severe as any depression seen in psychiatry. If untreated, many bipolar patients commit suicide.

The mania, on the other hand, is characterized by a persistently elevated, expansive, and irritated mood,

- Inflated self esteem or grandiosity;

- Decreased need for sleep;

- More talkative than usual or pressure to keep talking;

- Flight of ideas;

- Distractibility;

- Increase in goal-directed

activity or psychomotor agitation;

• Excessive involvement in pleasurable activities that have a high potential for painful consequences (i.e., drug abuse, gambling, or inappropriate sexual advances).

These mood disturbances are severe enough to cause marked impairment in job, social activities, and relationships.

"The manic feeling is a real feeling of elation and euphoria. There's also that grinding, angry sort of ... I don't really get angry and violent ...well, I did in jail, but I don't really want to hurt anybody or anything. And as far as being depressed goes, I can say I've only been depressed about three times, once to the point of being suicidal." 30-year-old man with a bipolar illness (manic-depression)

Bipolar affective disorder usually begins in a person's twenties and affects men and women equally. Many researchers believe this disease is genetic.

Toxic effects of stimulants or psychedelic abuse will often resemble a bipolar disorder. Users experience swings from mania to depression depending upon the phase of the drug's action, the surroundings, and their own subconscious feelings and beliefs.

OTHER PSYCHIATRIC DISORDERS

Anxiety disorders

These are the most common psychiatric disturbance seen in medical offices. There are eight classifications of anxiety disorders:

1. Panic disorder with and without agoraphobia (fear of open spaces);

"I'd be waiting for my prescription at a drugstore, and someone would just look at me, and all of a sudden, my whole body just went inside itself and I started shaking. My heart was racing. I couldn't say anything. I crossed my arms in front of me, and I was just in total panic. I couldn't move. All I did was shake inside like I was terrified. And my mind kept saying there's nothing to be scared of, but I couldn't control it. I had no idea what really triggered it. My husband would come up and hold me and sit there and say, "breathe!" And after a couple of minutes I would be alright and I would use one of my pills for anxiety, Lorazepam, a benzodiazepine. I think that my use of cocaine over a period of several years messed up my neurochemistry, particularly my adrenalin system. Then, I was always afraid of being someplace where I would have an attack and not be able to get help." 42-year old woman with a panic disorder

2. Agoraphobia without history of panic disorder (a generalized fear of open spaces);

3. Social phobia (fear of being seen by others to act in a humiliating or embarrassing way such as eating in public);

4. Simple phobia (irrational fear of a specific thing or place);

5. Obsessive-compulsive disorder (uncontrollable, intrusive thoughts and irresistible, often distressing actions such as cutting one's hair);

> *"I had a number of obsessions. The obvious one right now is my hair. I cut my hair obsessively in a crew cut, constantly, by my own hand. The thought would just come into my mind. It was something I didn't really have control over. I would smoke marijuana almost as compulsively as I cut my hair."* Patient with an obsessive-compulsive disorder.

6. Post-traumatic stress disorder (persistent reexperiencing of the full memory of a stressful event outside usual human experience, i.e. combat, molestation, car crash). It's usually triggered by an environmental stimulus, i.e. a car backfires and the combat veteran's mind relives the stress and memory of combat. This disorder can last a lifetime and be very disabling.

> *"I broke down after about six months over in Vietnam, and I was in charge of a gun crew. And when I broke down, seeing the deaths and all the abuse over there, some people's lives were lost.*

> *I'm responsible and it hurts. When I was med-evacked back to the States, I immediately jumped into alcohol and heroin."* 42-year-old Vietnam veteran with post-traumatic stress syndrome.

7. Generalized anxiety disorder (unrealistic worry about several life situations that lasts for 6 months or more);

8. Other anxiety disorders.

Sometimes it's extremely difficult to differentiate the anxiety disorders. Many are defined more by symptoms than by specific names. Some of the more common symptoms in anxiety disorders are shortness of breath, muscle tension, restlessness, stomach irritation, sweating, palpitations, restlessness, hyper-vigilance, difficulty concentrating, and excessive worry. Often anxiety and depression are mixed together. Some physicians think that many anxiety disorders are really an outgrowth of depression.

Toxic effects of stimulant drugs and withdrawal from opiates, sedatives, and alcohol (downers) also cause symptoms similar to those described in anxiety disorders and can be easily misdiagnosed as such.

Organic mental disorders

These are problems of brain dysfunction brought on by physical changes in the brain caused by aging, miscellaneous diseases, injury to the brain, or psychoactive drug toxicities. Alzheimer's disease, where older people gradually lose the mental ability to care for themselves, is one example of an organic mental disorder.

Developmental disorders

These include mental retardation, eating disorders, gender identity disorders, attention deficit disorders, autism, speech disorders, disruptive behavior disorders, etc.

Somatoform disorders

These disorders have physical symptoms without a known or discoverable physical cause and are likely to be psychologically caused, i.e., hypochondria (abnormal anxiety over one's health accompanied by imaginary symptoms of illnesses).

The passive-aggressive personality disorder, the anti-social personality disorder, and the borderline personality disorder

These disorders are characterized by inflexible behavioral patterns that lead to substantial distress or functional impairment. Most of these personalities "act out," that is, exhibit behavioral patterns that have an angry, hostile tone that violate social conventions and that result in negative consequences. Anger is key to all three of these personalities as well as chronic feelings of unhappiness and alienation from others, conflicts with authority, and family discord. This personality frequently coexists with substance abuse and is particularly hard to treat because of the "acting out," which is usually relapsing to drug use or creating a major disruption to their treatment.

HEREDITY, ENVIRONMENT, PSYCHOACTIVE DRUGS

It is important to notice the similarity between the psychiatric disorders and the direct effects or withdrawal effects of psychoactive drugs. For example, cocaine intoxication often results in behaviors identical to those of mania, anxiety, and paranoid schizophrenia.

The depressed mood, lack of interest in surroundings, and excess sleep, characteristic of a major depression, are quite like the direct effects of downers such as heroin, alcohol, and Xanax.

Cocaine and amphetamine withdrawal often look like a major depression. And, the short duration of action of the stronger stimulants, with their sudden ups and downs, mimic a bipolar illness that includes manic delusions and then depression.

Drug effects along with their withdrawal effects are so similar to the symptoms of mental illnesses that research strongly suggests similar areas of the brain and brain chemistry are involved. In fact, to properly understand dual diagnosis, it is crucial that one understand this relationship between brain chemistry and how a person acts.

NEUROCHEMICAL BALANCE

The three main factors that affect the central nervous system's balance and therefore a human being's susceptibility to addiction or mental illness, are heredity, environment, and psychoactive drugs.

Heredity

Heredity not only influences our looks but also gives us our neurochemical starting point. It might endow us with an excess of dopamine making us susceptible to schizophrenia; or it might impair our production of epinephrine making us more susceptible to depression. It might give us a nerve network that remembers theories better than facts making it easier for us indulge ourselves in flights of fancy.

Environment

Environment, particularly emotional and physical stresses of childhood, then moderates or distorts the neurochemistry that we're born with. It can create extra synapses between nerve cells or even block nerve pathways. For example, the neuro changes that were caused by fear can then make us more susceptible to new fears.

Psychoactive Drugs

Street drugs such as cocaine, heroin and marijuana (usually taken to get high) disrupt brain chemistry directly to make one more susceptible to either addiction or to mental illness.

It is hard to pinpoint altered brain chemistry, in and of itself, as the direct cause of these problems. The cause is, most often, the relationship between how people grow up, what they learn in life, how they react to their environment, what they do to themselves physically, how they develop their spirituality and their emotions that govern what they become; but certain patterns in their neurochemistry can exaggerate, diminish, or distort these influences.

Heredity and Mental Balance

How does heredity affect our mental health? Research has already shown a close link between heredity and schizophrenia, manic-depression, depression, and even anxiety. For example, the risk of a child developing schizophrenia is somewhere between 1/2 to one percent if the child has no close-order relatives with schizophrenia. On the other hand, if the child has a parent who has schizophrenia, the risk jumps to about sixteen percent.

"My great uncle's got schizophrenia and my nephew's got schizophrenia." 28-year old man with schizophrenia

"In my family, my mom, my aunt, and my grandmother were diagnosed as manic depressive. It runs in the family." 16-year-old boy

In addition, heredity affects susceptibility to drug addiction. Many studies have shown that if one parent is alcoholic, the child is 34% more likely to be an alcoholic than children of non-alcoholics. If both parents are alcoholic, the child is

400% more likely to be alcoholic. Finally, if the child is a male with a father and grandfather who are alcoholic, that child is 900% more likely to develop alcoholism.

> *"My dad was a raging alcoholic, so I was afraid to take a drink until I was 27. I blacked out that first time. It took 14 more years and a rotting liver to get me into treatment."* 41-year-old woman

Heredity creates this susceptibility to mental illness and drug addiction because each person is born with a different balance of neurotransmitters and "brain wiring" so some people can react to the environment and to psychoactive drugs in unique ways that trigger these hidden irregularities.

Environment and Mental Balance

The second major factor that affects our mental balance, environment, includes emotional influences, i.e. excitement, stress, anger, and ridicule. It also includes physical influences, i.e., physical contact including caressing as well as abuse, diet, exercise, and sexual contact (wanted and unwanted).

> *"My parents had a troubled marriage, and they'd fight and argue and my mother would be beaten. I think maybe some of the rage and some of the anger manifested itself into my schizophrenia or just triggered it."* 28-year-old man

The neurochemistry of persons subject to extreme stress can be disrupted and unbalanced to a point that their reactions to normal situations are different than most people's. Such persons usually become unable to handle stressful situations without running away or falling apart. The stressors they respond to don't have to be dramatic. They can merely be normal family expectations. For such persons, mother saying "It's eleven o'clock, I wish you'd get out of bed," can lead to extreme anger which further disrupts their neurotransmitters and therefore their thought processes and therefore their behavior.

> *"After my schizophrenia became really prominent, I noticed that little things, like on-the-job stress level, would get to me, and I'd have to quit and move on because it would trigger all sorts of problems."* 28-year-old client

> *"My dad beat my mom when he was under the influence of alcohol. He was an alcoholic. He also beat my older sister and me. When he came home I was always running and hiding. A few years after he left the family I was molested. I was screwed up but when I went into the service, I found that the marijuana and the heroin I abused in 'Nam kept my emotions under control."* Vietnam veteran

Well over 50% of the young adults who are psychotic and dually diagnosed experienced at least one form of abuse when they were children, and the rate is much greater in women than in men. Likewise, a very high percent (75% or greater) of women addicts have suffered incest, molestation, or physical abuse as a child or an adult.

> *"When I got addicted to the cocaine it was because I was being battered, and I used that to hide. When I left the cocaine, I used the drinking to hide. When I left the drinking, the cigarettes kicked in. When I left the cigarettes, I began to over-eat. It was like I had to fill up that hole with something."*
> 25-year-old woman

Notice that physical and mental abuse can lead to mental problems as well as drug problems.

....

This illustration ("The Extraction of the Stone of Madness") by Pieter Bruegal, the Elder, a satire of ways to treat mental illness, shows that even 300 years ago, people thought that mental illness was caused by something physical inside the brain. Compare this to the modern view of many clinicians that mental illness can be treated by changing the neurochemistry inside the brain, through psychotropic medication.

Psychoactive Drugs and Mental Balance

Along with heredity and environment, the third factor that can affect our mental balance, psychoactive drugs, deplete, increase, mimic, or otherwise disrupt the neurochemistry of the brain. This disruption of brain chemistry can lead to drug addiction, mental illness, or both.

If any nervous system receives enough psychoactive drugs, it will eventually develop mental problems, but it is the predisposed brain that is more likely to have a prolonged and permanent problem once exposed to drugs of abuse. The brain that is not predisposed is the one most likely to clear after abstinence.

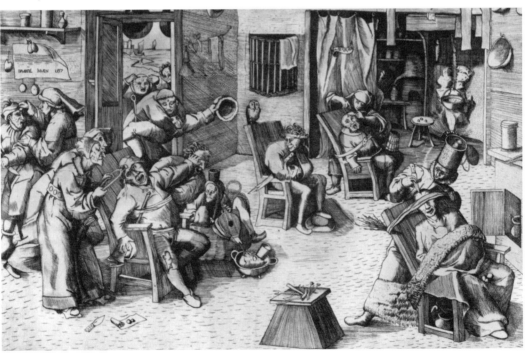

"Apparently, through three generations of my family and our alcohol drinking or smoking opium, I inherited a tendency to manic-depression that won't awaken under just alcohol abuse, so it took another drug stimulus that was a little bit out of range of a Northern European family to bring out my illness, and that was marijuana."
45-year-old man

Every time something enters the brain that is psychoactive, it changes the equilibrium, and the brain has to adjust to the presence of that substance. When exposure to that drug has ended, the brain does not always return to its original baseline. Those with susceptibility towards addiction or mental illness will then become ill.

TREATMENT

The close association of unbalanced brain chemistry with the disruptive effects of heredity, environment, and psychoactive drugs suggests that treatment of mental illness and/or addiction should be directed towards rebalancing the brain chemistry.

REBALANCING BRAIN CHEMISTRY

Heredity and Treatment

As of yet, we cannot alter a person's genetic code. We can't change a person with an alcoholic marker gene which signals a susceptibility to alcoholism, or alter a teenager with a mother and grandmother who have schizo-

phrenia. We can only alert some people that they are more at risk for a certain mental illness or drug addiction. (Even then, the research on identifying marker genes and knowing exactly what they mean is in its infancy. The Human Genome Project to identify all human genes is a step in that direction.)

Environment and Treatment

If we can't correct heredity, we can, however, attempt to correct the environment. It is possible to suggest a change in the environment itself. Also, through external treatment, we can attempt to correct some of the damage done by the environment.

If people change where and how they live, they can avoid those stressors and environmental cues which keep them in a state of turmoil, continually unbalance their neurochemistry, and make them more likely to abuse drugs and intensify their mental illness. For example, to help restore a sane way of living they can leave an abusive relationship, avoid their drug-using associates, get enough sleep, avoid situations that make them angry, seek out new friends in self-help groups to avoid isolation, or make sure they get good nutrition.

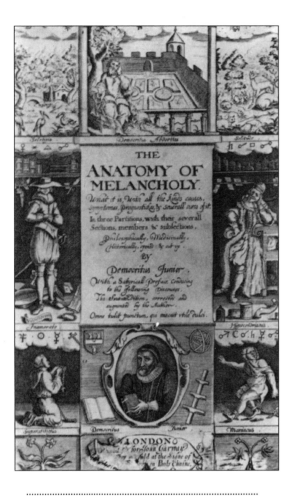

The Anatomy of Melancholy (1660), by Robert Burton, is a book about depression which shows that most civilizations were aware of mental illness and wrote about ways to treat it. This book even examines the benefits of confessing grief to a friend (National Library of Medicine, Bethesda, Maryland).

"I didn't really think that I was a mentally ill person. I thought, 'Well, I'm a drug addict and I'm an alcoholic and if I don't drink and I don't use, then it should just be a simple matter of just changing my entire life'...and I felt a little bit overwhelmed."
35-year-old man

But, hard as it might be, changing one's external environment is much easier than changing one's brain chemistry through manipulation of thoughts, feelings, or emotions.

Psychotherapy

Look into the depths of your own soul and learn first to know yourself, then you will understand why this illness was bound to come upon you and perhaps you will thenceforth avoid falling ill.
—Sigmund Freud, 1924

Psychotherapy, which was originated by Dr. Sigmund Freud in the late 1800's, is a way of helping the dually diagnosed patient. It helps clients explore their past to enable them to neutralize the emotional and neurochemical imbalance caused by the traumas and stresses of childhood, for example, by remembering sexual abuse that happened when they were a young child.

Individual or group therapy can be effective but, by necessity, it has to be a long-term project (even a lifetime project) to be truly effective in changing individuals or at least minimizing the damage they do to themselves.

"I go to Emotions Anonymous. I go there and it helps because I became a drug addict by not being able to deal with my emotions and my feelings." 25-year-old client

Psychoactive Drugs and Treatment

Finally, psychoactive drugs themselves can be used to treat mental illness. This form of treatment is attempted by both psychiatrists and by patients themselves who may self-medicate their condition with the use of abused drugs. Of course there are dangers in self-medication. The uncontrolled use of street drugs such as cocaine or some prescription medications like Ritalin can distort one's neurochemistry and magnify or trigger mental problems.

"I took both alcohol and lithium for my manic depression. The difference is that one is faster working. The alcohol works quickly, the lithium takes time to get there. But the alcohol caused other problems in my life in addition to my depression. I think I'll stick with the lithium." 50-year-old woman

But, there is an ever-expanding group of drugs called psychotropic medications (i.e., antidepressants, antipsychotics, antianxiety drugs) that are prescribed by physicians to try to counteract neurochemical imbalance caused by mental illness or addiction whcih help the dually diagnosed client/patient to recover or at least lead a non-destructive life. (We will examine the various psychotropic medications in detail later.)

The following table (Fig. 12-2) is a compilation of what we have been covering in these pages regarding the relationship between brain chemistry, drug addiction, and mental illness. In figure 12-2, Column 1 lists the neurotransmitters (the brain's messengers), Column 2 describes the natural regulatory function of the neurotransmitters, and then in Column 3, lists the street drugs that strongly affect them. Column 4 describes the mental illnesses associated with the disrupted neurotransmitters, and Column 5 lists drugs used to correct the disruption.

When studying the table, notice how many different neurotransmitters are affected by a single street drug, especially cocaine or alcohol; also notice the physical and mental traits that are affected by a neurotransmitter and how a street drug affects those functions.

Fig. 12-2 THE RELATIONSHIP BETWEEN NEUROTRANSMITTERS, THEIR FUNCTIONS, STREET DRUGS, MENTAL ILLNESS, AND PSYCHOTROPIC MEDICATIONS

COLUMN 1 Neurotransmitter	COLUMN 2 Some Major Functions	COLUMN 3 Street Drugs Which Disrupt the Neurotransmitter	COLUMN 4 Associated Mental Illnesses	COLUMN 5 Medications Used to Rebalance Neurotransmitters
Serotonin	Mood stability, appetite, sleep-control, sexual-activity aggression, self-esteem	Alcohol, nicotine, amphetamine, cocaine, PCP, LSD, MDMA (ecstasy)	Anxiety, depression manic depression obsessive/compulsive disorder	BuSpar, tricyclic antidepressant, lithium, MAO inhibitors, Prozac, Zoloft, tryptophan, Ritanserin, Anafranil, Paxil
Dopamine	Muscle tone/control, motor behavior, energy, reward mechanism, attention span, pleasure, emotional stability	Cocaine, nicotine, PCP amphetamine, caffeine, LSD, Ritalin, marijuana, alcohol, opiates	Schizophrenia Parkinson's disease	Lithium, MAO inhibitors, phenothiazine antipsychotics thiazine antipsychotics, tyrosine, taurine
Norepinephrine and epinephrine	Energy, motivation, eating, attention span, pleasure muscle tone, stimulation heart rate, blood pressure, dilation of bronchi, assertiveness, alertness, confidence	Cocaine, nicotine, amphetamine, caffeine, all stimulants, PCP, marijuana	Depression, manic depression, anxiety, and panic disorders, narcolepsy, sleep problems, attention deficit disorder	Tricyclic antidepressants, Lithium, MAO inhibitors, phenothiazine, antipsychotics, prescription amphetamines, Ritalin, clonidine, barbiturates, benzodiazepines, beta blockers (Propranelol), tyrosine, d,l phenyllalanine
Acetylcholine	Memory, learning, muscular reflexes, aggression, attention, blood pressure, heart rate, sexual behavior, mental acuity, sleep, muscle control	Marijuana, nicotine, alcohol, cocaine, PCP, amphetamine, LSD	Alzheimer's disease schizophrenia, tremors	Phenothiazine antipsychotics, Artane, Cogentin, lecitin, choline
GABA (gamma aminobutyric acid)	Inhibitor of many neurotransmitters, muscle relaxant, control of aggression, arousal	Alcohol, marijuana, barbiturates, PCP, benzodiazepines	Anxiety and sleep disorders	Benzodiazepines, glutamine
Endorphin, enkephalin	Pain control, reward mechanism, stress control (physical and emotional)	Heroin, other opiates, PCP, marijuana, alcohol, anabolic steroids	Schizophrenia, depression	Methadone, LAAM, Trexan, buprenorphine, d,l phenylalanine
Cortisone, corticotropin	Immune system, healing, stress	Heroin, anabolic steroids, cocaine	Schizophrenia, depression, insomnia, anxiety	Corticosteroids (Prednisone, cortisone), ACTH
Histamine	Regulator of emotional behavior, sleep, inflammation of tissues, stomach acid secretion, allergic response	Antihistamines, opiates	Depressive illness	Antihistamines, tricyclic antidepressants

PROBLEMS OF TREATMENT

There are several problems in the treatment of the dually-diagnosed client. The stigma of mental illness keeps many from seeking help, admitting to their illness, or even talking about it with family, friends, therapists, and groups.

Starting Treatment

With many dually diagnosed clients it is hard to know where to start treatment. Do you start treating the mental illness or the addiction or do you treat them simultaneously right from the beginning?

"I think that I start where the pain is. One patient, for example couldn't talk about his marijuana use without talking about how depressed and suicidal he was. We addressed the pain, the pain being his massive depression, and then we enabled him, by doing that, to back off his marijuana use. In the case of another patient, she was in such a massively tormented state in terms of anxiety, panic, fear, and depression behind her use of benzodiazepines and codeine that we had to start detoxing immediately, and we had to explain to her that we would be looking at the depression and the anxiety and probably medicating them as we detoxed her off her primary drugs of abuse."
Chemical dependency treatment counselor

A suicidal situation obviously needs to be attended to regardless of the cause. Similarly, if patients are dangerous, homicidal, or aggressive in some dangerous fashion, they have to be managed, often in a psychiatric facility. When these presentations are less malignant and less dangerous to self or others, then the treatment facility generally says, "What does it take to manage them?" And the first rule of thumb is, the patient has to be somewhat cooperative and manageable, so detoxification is usually the first step.

Impaired Cognition

Unfortunately, many clinicians involved in treatment believe that once dually diagnosed individuals put down the booze or drugs, they should be able to engage in treatment, but that's not always the case. In a screening exam at a Veteran's Hospital on neurocognitive function (ability to understand), they found that approximately 50% of the patients were mildly to severely impaired.

For the treatment provider what this means is the patient can repeat things, but the information and therapy don't sink in. It takes from two weeks to six months after detoxification for reasoning, memory, and thinking to come back to a point where the dually diagnosed individual can begin to engage in treatment. Treatment has to be tailored to the person's ability to process the information that the doctor or staff is providing.

Developmental Arrest

Drug abuse and mental illness often cause a pause in emotional development. Take the case of a young man in his late teens or early 20's who's full grown and pretty bright, but has been using drugs since the age of 11 or 12, and has also had emotional and mental problems. This type of patient comes to treatment with all kinds of problems, and one of the worst is that he's had a developmental arrest at the point where most people begin to work through issues and stresses in their lives. Most people mature through all the struggles and go on to become adults. But, if they've been using drugs and not having any feelings, and not having to go through that process, they still experience the emotions that they began to cut off five or six years ago.

"It's all those issues as a child that I seemed to take into my adulthood, and they come out. I'd get my buttons pressed. Someone gets me a little pissed off. You know, I really thought when I came into recovery, I wouldn't be angry anymore. Well, it took me almost three years here to realize that anger's a legitimate feeling. It's how I deal with it today and how I used to deal with it. That's what I'm learning about."
30-year-old dually diagnosed client

What happens is that many dually diagnosed clients have the character traits that are normal in children or adolescents but abnormal in adults, thus making treatment extremely difficult. Dr. Bert Pepper, a psychiatrist who treats young, dually diagnosed clients, lists eleven of these characteristics.

1. They have a low frustration tolerance.

2. They can't work persistently for a goal without constant encouragement and guidance partially because of the low frustration tolerance.

3. They lie to avoid punishment.

4. They have mixed feelings about independence and dependence, and then feeling hostile about dependency they test limits.

5. They test limits constantly because they haven't learned them yet or have rejected them.

6. Their feelings are expressed as behaviors; they cry, run away, and hit rather than talk, reason, explain, or apologize.

7. They have a shallow labile affect which means a shallowness of mood. Give kids a toy, they laugh; take it away, they cry.

8. They have a fear of being rejected. Extreme rejection sensitivity can even be expressed as paranoid schizophrenia.

9. Some live in the present only, but most of the older teens or young adults live in the past. Most dually diagnosed clients have no hope for the future, possibly because they remember the past too well or have trouble thinking.

10. Denial is a common characteristic in young children. One is

a refusal to deal with unpleasant but necessary duties. Another is an unwillingness to stop something that's pleasurable, like kids playing roughhouse until one gets hurt badly.

11. A feeling that "Either you're for me or against me," a black and white approach to every judgment in life, no modulation.

These characteristics are also very common in those being treated for chemical dependency alone.

What these characteristics suggest is that any treatment program has to be highly structured. What the client needs to do is learn all those behaviors, ideas, and emotions that were not learned before because of the drugs, the mental illness, or the turmoil of growing up.

These difficulties are all chronic or even life-long problems which cannot be treated with short-term therapy. These are problems of living, of living sober and of living with the symptoms of the mental illness. The best treatment has to be in the inpatient sector because it requires a great deal of monitoring and continuity over a fairly long period of time, but unfortunately, resources (financial and professional) for that type of inpatient care do not usually exist.

PSYCHIATRIC MEDICATIONS

Psychopharmacology

The field of medicine that specializes in the use of medications to help correct or help control mental illnesses is called psychopharmacology. The scope of this branch of medicine has grown rapidly in the last 10 years producing dozens of new medications and a new approach to mental illness.

Quite often the dual diagnosis patient does need medication for the psychiatric disorder; tricyclic antidepressants for endogenous depression; lithium for a manic-depressive disorder; anti-psychotic medication for a thought disorder. These medications have to be handled in a very carefully planned fashion because the individual has difficulty handling drugs. The clinician has to make sure the medication used for the psychiatric problem does not aggravate or complicate the substance abuse problem.

Medications are used on a short-term, medium-term, or even lifetime basis to try to rebalance the brain chemistry that has become unbalanced either through hereditary anomalies, environmental stress, and/or the use of psychoactive drugs. They are used in conjunction with individual or group therapy and with lifestyle changes.

One of the biggest debates in treatment centers is about the level of medication that should be used. Some clinicians look at psychotropic medications as a last resort. Others feel that they should be the first step in treatment. However, there is no question that judicious use of many medications has freed many people suffering from mental illness from a life of misery.

Pharmacology

The various psychiatric medications currently in use affect the manner in which neurotransmitters work in a variety of ways:

- They can increase or inhibit the release of neurotransmitters and even block the receptor sites (phenothiazines);

- They can block the reuptake of neurotransmitters by the sending neuron thus increasing the amount of neurotransmitter available in the synaptic gap. Prozac and Zoloft work this way on serotonin;

- They can speed up or inhibit the metabolism of the neurotransmitter (Nardil and MAO inhibitors);

- They can enhance the effect of existing neurotransmitters (benzodiazepines such as Valium).

Besides manipulating brain chemistry, some of the drugs act directly to control symptoms. Drugs such as beta blockers (propranolol) calm the sympathetic nervous system which controls heart rate, blood pressure, and other functions which can go out of control in a panic attack, or drug withdrawal state. They also calm the brain.

One problem with these medications (psychotropic medications) is that often, it's very hard to design a drug that will only work on a certain neurotransmitter in a certain way. There are always side effects, and since each patient and each illness is different, constant monitoring of each patient's reaction to the drug and the dosage is an absolute necessity. A careful explanation of the drug and a specific plan of use is necessary.

"The medication that we are thinking about giving you in this treatment program is really designed to correct some of the damage that you did to your body and to your mind with the drugs, or damage that had been happening as a result of some emotional or psychological problem. It does not mean you're sick; it does not mean you're defective; it does not mean you're weak. It just means that your biochemistry has somehow got out of balance, and the medications that we're recommending and especially the antidepressant medications are to rebalance those chemicals and bring you to a point where you can fully and effectively function and then begin to work on your other problems."
Stanley Yantis, M.D., Psychiatrist to a dually diagnosed client

Psychiatric Medications versus Street Drugs

One of the advantages of these medications over street drugs is that generally, except for the benzodiazepines and stimulants, they are not addicting. Psychiatric medications cause problems for the dually diagnosed client because he or she has been taught to stay away from all drugs during recovery.

Patients, when they are out on the street, feel a great deal of control over which drugs they ingest, inject, or otherwise self-adminis-ter. Patients, when they come to a doctor for treatment, which might include medications, have often expressed the feeling that they are not in control anymore of what is being given them. Thus, they are more apt to rely on street drugs rather than on psychiatric medications for relief of their emo-tional problems.

"Before I came to the clinic, I thought that using anti-depressants was taboo. I wanted to use street drugs but not any of these clinical ones. There's a stigma to it."
35-year-old client with depression and a problem with marijuana

OPTIONAL SECTION

This next section which classi-fies and discusses the specific drugs is rather technical and may be used as a reference source.

Just a few of the dozens of psychiatric medica-tions that are available to treat mental illness.

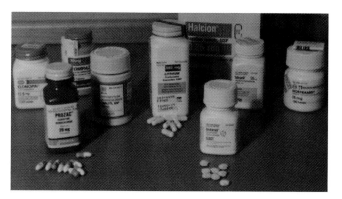

CLASSIFICATION OF PSYCHIATRIC MEDICATIONS

Some of the major groups of psy-chotropic medications are tricyclic antidepressants, MAO inhibitors, serotonin reuptake inhibitors, an-tipsychotics, anxiolytics (antianx-iety), lithium, beta-blockers, and sleeping pills.

We will discuss the drugs under the heading of the mental illness that they are generally used to treat (see Fig. 12-3). There is some overlap, for example, where a drug used for depression such as Prozac is also used to treat obsessive-com-pulsive disorder, or an anti-de-pressant is also used for manic-depression.

DRUGS TO TREAT DEPRESSION

Many in the psychiatric field feel that depression causes and in turn is caused by an abnormality of the neurotransmitters norepinephrine (adrenalin) and serotonin, plus a few other neurotransmitters. Antidepressants are meant to in-crease the amount of serotonin or norepinephrine available to the brain to correct this imbalance.

Tricyclic antidepressants

Tricyclic antidepressants such as Tofranil (imipramine) and Norpramine (desipramine) are thought to block reabsorption of these neurotransmitters by the sending neuron and so increase the activity of those biochemicals. This in turn forces the synthesis of more receptor sites for these neurochemicals. This seems to be the reason for the lag time in effecting a change in the patient. The patient might take 2 to 6 weeks to respond to the drug.

The tricyclics are very effective on patients with acute symptoms of depression. People without depression do not get a lift from taking a tricyclic-antidepressant as they do with a stimulant. In fact, they get drowsy from taking it.

"The antidepressants did not get me high as far as what I could feel, like feeling drunk or stoned. You don't get that sensation. The high I got is more like a lift, a mood lift. It's the difference between being lethargic and sad, or active and happy." 35-year-old man with depression and marijuana problem

The tricyclic antidepressants, available mainly as pills, can be dangerous if too many are taken, so careful monitoring of not only compliance by the patient with prescribed dosage but also constant feedback to the clinician about the effects and side effects are also necessary. Major side effects are dry mouth, blurred vision, inhibited urination, hypotension, and sleepiness.

"I went off anti-depressants. And after a month or six weeks, I began getting depressed again, but I had to be convinced that I was depressed again. And they said, 'You really should go back on medication,' and I didn't want to admit that I didn't want to be on medication. I wanted to exist without it." 35-year-old patient with major depression

These drugs are also dangerous to the heart, especially if they are taken with abused stimulants, depressants, or alcohol. Patients must abstain from abusing drugs while being treated with tricyclic antidepressants.

Monoamine Oxidase Inhibitors

MAO inhibitors such as Nardil (phenelzine), Parnate (tranyl-cypromine), and Marplan (isocarboxazid) are also used to treat depression. These very strong drugs work by blocking an enzyme which metabolizes neurotransmitters including norepinephrine and serotonin. This, in essence, raises the level of these neurotransmitters. Unfortunately, MAO inhibitors have several potentially dangerous side effects, so care and close monitoring are necessary in their use. They do give fairly quick relief from a major depression and panic disorder, but the user has to be on a special diet and remain aware of the possibility of high blood pressure, headaches, and several other side effects. Combined use of MAO inhibitors with abused stimulants, depressants, and alcohol can be fatal.

Newer Antidepressants

The newer antidepressants such as Prozac, Desyrel, Paxil, Zoloft, Welbutrin, and Xanax work through a variety of mechanisms.

Prozac (chemical name, fluoxetine)

The most popular of the new antidepressants, Prozac, has received a large amount of publicity both pro and con since its release in 1988. It seems quite effective in the treatment of depression with fewer side effects than tricyclic antidepressants or the MAO inhibitors. It is also used to treat obsessive-compulsive disorders and panic disorder.

Prozac is classified as a serotonin reuptake inhibitor because it increases the amount of serotonin available to the nervous system. The amount needed to be effective varies widely from patient to patient and has to be adjusted. It generally takes 2 to 4 weeks for the full effect to be felt. The side effects are usually insomnia, nausea, diarrhea, headache, and nervousness. Most of the side effects are mild and will go away in a few weeks.

Xanax

Xanax (alprazolam), a benziodiazepine sedative-hypnotic, though not labeled as a treatment for depression, has been used clinically by several doctors to control mild depression or mixed depression and anxiety, but if the patient also has a drug problem, benzodiazepines are only recommended for detoxification or immediate relief.

Stimulants

In the past, amphetamine or amphetamine congeners such as Dexedrine, Biphetamine, Desoxyn, Ritalin, and Cylert were used to treat depression. They work by increasing the amount of norepinephrine and epinephrine in the central nervous system. They were mood elevators when used in moderation, but the problem was that since tolerance develops rapidly, and the mood lift proved to be too alluring, misuse and addiction developed fairly rapidly with the drugs. The overuse led to various physical and mental problems such as agitation, aggression, paranoia, and psychosis. Ritalin is occasionally prescribed for elderly patients with depression and for young patient's with attention-deficit disorder. But for a dually diagnosed client, these drugs should be used with utmost caution.

Drugs Used to Treat Bipolar Disorders (manic depression)

Antidepressants, such as the tricyclics or, recently, Welbutrin (bupropion) or Prozac, are used to initially treat severe depression in the bipolar patient and an antipsychotic such as Thorazine or Haldol is used to initially treat a severe manic phase, but the main drug used for the treatment of manic-depression over the last 30 years is lithium.

Lithium

Lithium is started concurrently with an antidepressant or an antipsychotic. Lithium is a long-term medication used for years, even a lifetime. Clinicians are careful when making the diagnosis since the patient might be in the manic phase which resembles schizophrenia or the depressive phase which resembles unipolar depression. A bad diagnosis can be dangerous since long-term treatment of these other conditions is quite different.

Lithium doesn't really prevent a person from having moods. The patients still have high and low swings. What it does is dampen them. The high swings aren't as high and the depressions aren't as low, and it helps the bipolar patient to function. About 80% of bipolar patients respond to lithium. Symptoms begin to change within 10 to 15 days after starting the drug.

> *"The way manic depression works, at least for me, the medicine can control about twenty percent of it. The other 80 % is you. You have to learn how to control your moods with your mind, because the medication is only a small part." 40-year old with bipolar disorder*

Others

Tegretol (carbamazepine) is used in patients who do not respond to lithium alone. It seems to help patients who have more rapid "cycling" of their highs and lows.

Depakene (valproic acid) is used if the bipolar patient fails to respond to lithium and Tegretol. Its use with the bipolar patient is still limited to cases resistant to other medications.

Drugs Used to Treat Schizophrenia (antipsychotics)

In the early 50's a new class of drugs, phenothiazines were found to be effective in controlling the symptoms of schizophrenia. Some of the drugs such as Thorazine, Mellaril, Proloxin, and Compazine were initially referred to as major tranquilizers. More recently, non-phenothiazines like Haldol, Loxitane, and Moban have been developed. They act like phenothiazines and have similar side effects.

Researchers found that one of the major causes of schizophrenia is an excess of dopamine, a condition that is usually inherited. Most of the antipsychotic medications work by blockading the dopamine receptors in the brain, thereby inhibiting the effects of the excess dopamine. Generally, antipsychotic drugs do work, but they do not cure schizophrenia, and they can also cause serious side effects. The difference in side effects is the main difference between many of the drugs.

The main side effects of antipsychotics usually have to do with the decrease in dopamine in the system. From Fig. 12-2, you can see that dopamine controls muscle tone and motor behavior. By decreasing the dopamine, symptoms such as tics, jumpiness, and inability to sit still are common. Parkinsonian syndrome (mainly a tremor but also loss of facial expression, and slowed movements, etc), akathisia (agitation, jumpiness—exhibited by

75% of patients), akinesia (temporary loss of movement and apathy), and even the more serious tardive dyskenesia (involuntary movements of the jaws, head, neck, trunk and extremities). Often, a drug is given to block these side effects; Cogentin, Artane, Kemadrin, or even Benadryl.

Patients on antipsychotics can seem drugged, but for people suffering from schizophrenia who are agitated or violent, the sedating effect is very useful. These drugs are dangerous when used as a sleeping pill by patients who do not have schizophrenia or are not violent and agitated. The drugs can actually cause symptoms of mental illness in patients who are not schizophrenic. They also have severe side effects.

Antipsychotic drugs in general are also classified as high potency (Haldol, Stelazine, Prolixin, Trilafon, Navane) and low potency (Thorazine, Mellaril, Loxitane, Moban).

In an emergency situation, patients are generally started on a high-potency antipsychotic. They are given the drugs for several weeks to obtain a full response. If there is no response, either the dose can be raised or another drug tried. Most clinicians prefer to use low doses of these medications. The low-potency antipsychotics are used when patients also have problems sleeping. Manic patients are candidates for low-potency antipsychotic use.

Since antipsychotics are so potent, attempts are made to stop or decrease the dose of these medications as soon as possible, i.e. when the symptoms subside. This philosophy is particularly important in treating elderly patients.

Recently, atypical antipsychotic drugs have been developed. Clozaril (clozapine) is effective in the 30% of patients who do not respond to standard antipsychotic drug therapy. Unfortunately, weekly blood tests are necessary to monitor the side effects of Clozaril which make its use very expensive.

Patients who have been dually diagnosed with schizophrenia often use heroin and other opiates to control their symptoms. Alcohol, other sedative-hypnotics, and even marijuana or inhalants are used as well. Since all of these street drugs have dangerous toxic effects when combined with antipsychotic drugs, patients are exhorted to cease using them while under psychiatric treatment.

Drugs for Anxiety Disorders

For generalized anxiety disorder, as well as some of the other anxiety disorders, the benzodiazepines are widely used. The most commonly used are Xanax, Valium, Librium, and Tranxene. Developed in the early 60's, the benzodiazepines were considered safe substitutes for barbiturates, and the meprobamates (Miltown, Equanil). They act very quickly, particularly Valium. The calming effects are apparent within 30 minutes. Some of the benzodiazepines are long-acting (Valium,

Librium, Tranxene, Klonopin, Centrax) and some are short-acting (Halcion, Ativan, Restoril). The main problem with these drugs is that they are habit forming and do have withdrawal symptoms, so they are almost always avoided with the dually diagnosed patient for whom they can retrigger drug abuse. If the drug must be used, dosages are kept as low as possible, and the patient is monitored for addiction or relapse.

Buspirone (BuSpar) is the only other drug labeled for generalized anxiety disorder. It is a serotonin modulator and will block the transmission of excess serotonin which is considered to be one of the causes of the symptoms of many forms of anxiety. It also mimics serotonin, so it can also substitute for low levels of serotonin, a feature used by some doctors to use the drug for depression. It takes several weeks to work and is not nearly as dramatic, initially, as the benzodiazepines, so many patients are reluctant to use it. Its advantage, however, is that side effects are minimal and it is definitely not habit forming.

Drugs for Obsessive-Compulsive Disorder

For the obsessive-compulsive disorder almost every drug has been used, usually with relatively poor results. Anafranil (clomipramine) has recently been used with reasonable results. It is a serotonin reuptake inhibitor like Zoloft and Prozac.

Drugs for Panic Disorder

Several drugs are used to control panic disorder (as opposed to panic attacks). Panic attacks occur in someone who has panic disorder, in those on a bad LSD trip, someone having an extreme reaction to a stimulant, a heart patient experiencing tachycardia, reaction to various medications, and so forth. Panic disorder consists of multiple panic attacks accompanied by fear and anxiety about having more panic attacks. Situations where a panic attack might occur and they would be without help are also avoided. It is sometimes difficult to distinguish between a panic attack and a panic disorder.

Beta blockers such as propranolol (Inderal), and atenolol (Tenomin), and a dozen others, block beta receptors in cardiac muscles and bronchial and vascular smooth muscles. This helps calm the symptoms of a panic attack such as rapid heart rates, hypertension, and difficulty breathing because it blocks excess muscular activity in the vascular system and lungs. Beta blockers also have a calming effect on the brain which is helpful in treating panic disorders. It takes about one hour for the medicine to work, so many people with a panic disorder or social phobia will take a dose one hour before entering a stressful situation.

FIG. 12-3 MEDICATIONS USED TO HANDLE PSYCHIATRIC PROBLEMS

MAJOR DEPRESSION
Tricyclic antidepressants: imipramine (Tofranil, Janimine), desipramine (Norpramin, Pertofrane), amitriptyline (Elavil, Endep) nortriptyline (Pamelor), Doxepin (Sinequan, Adapin), trimipramine (Surmontil), protriptyline (Vivactil), maprotiline (Ludiomil)
Monamine Oxidase Inhibitors: phenelzine (Nardil), tranylcypromine (Parnate), isocarbox-azid (Marplan), pargyline (Eutonyl), belegiline (formerly Deprenyl) (Eldepryl)
New Antidepressants: fluoxetine (Prozac), trazodone (Desyrel), amoxapine (Asendin), al-prazolam (benzodiazepine-Xanax), bupropion (Welbutrin), sertraline (Zoloft), Ritanserin, paroxetine (Paxil)
Stimulants used as antidepressants: Amphetamines (Dexedrine, Biphetamine, Desoxyn), methylphenidate (Ritalin), pemoline (Cylert)

BIPOLAR AFFECTIVE DISORDER—(MANIC DEPRESSION)
Lithium (Eskalith, Lithobid)
Others: carbamazepine (Tegretol), valproic acid (Depakene), clonazepam (Klonopin)

SCHIZOPHRENIA (antipsychotics)
halperidol (Haldol), thiothixene (Navane), loxapine (Loxitane), molindone (Moban, Lidone), clozapine (Clozaril), pimozide (Orap), chlorprothixene (taractan)
Phenothiazines: trifluoperazine (Stelazine), fluphenazine (Proloxin, Permitil), perphenazine (Trilafon), chlorpromazine (Thorazine), thioridazine (Mellaril), mesoridazine (Serentil), tri-flupromazine (Vesprin), acetophenazine (Tindal), piperacetazine (Quide)

GENERALIZED ANXIETY DISORDER
Benzodiazepines: Short acting: alprazolam (Xanax), oxazepam (Serax), lorazepam (Ativan), triazolam (Halcion), temazepam (Restoril)
Long acting: diazepam (Valium), chlordiazepoxide (Librium), clorazepate (Tranxene), clon-azepam (Klonopin), prazepam (Centrax), halazepam (Paxipam)
Non-benzodiazepines: buspirone (BuSpar)

OBSESSIVE-COMPULSIVE DISORDER (OCD)
Clomipramine (Anafranil), sertraline (Zoloft), fluoxetine (Prozac)

PANIC DISORDER
First-line drugs: Imipramine (Tofranil), desipramine (Norpramin or Pertofrane), alprazolam (Xanax)
Second-line drugs: phenelzine (Nardil), tranycypromine (Parnate), clonazepam (Klonopin)
Beta blockers: propranolol (Inderal), atenolol (Tenormin)

SOCIAL-PHOBIA
Beta-blockers: propranolol (Inderal), atenolol (Tenormin)
MAO inhibitors: phenelzine (Nardil)

POST-TRAUMATIC STRESS SYNDROME
First-line drugs: benzodiazepines and sedatives as in treatment of generalized anxiety disorder
Second-line drugs: antipsychotics as in the treatment of schizophrenia

SLEEPING DISORDER
Sleeping pills: flurazepam (Dalmane), triazolam (Halcion), temazepam (Restoril)

REVIEW

DUAL DIAGNOSIS

1. Dual diagnosis is defined as a condition in which a person has both a substance abuse problem and a diagnosable, significant, psychiatric problem.

2. The three main psychiatric disorders used to define dual diagnosis are schizophrenia (a thought disorder), major depression (a mood disorder), and bipolar disorder (manic-depression).

3. Other mental illnesses used by some to define dual diagnosis include anxiety disorders such as panic disorder, phobias, obsessive-compulsive disorder, generalized anxiety disorder, post-traumatic stress syndrome; organic disorders; developmental disorders; somatoform disorders; and other personality disorders.

4. The use of abusable drugs can aggravate an existing mental disorder or create a new one.

5. A psychiatric diagnosis should always be conditional since abusable drugs can directly mimic symptoms of a mental illness. Withdrawal symptoms can also mimic the symptoms of some mental illnesses.

6. Four main differences between the mental health (MH) treatment community and the Chemical Dependency (CD) treatment community are

a. MH says, control the psychiatric problem and the drug abuse will disappear. CD says, get the patient clean and sober and the mental health problem will disappear.

b. In MH, limited recovery is more acceptable whereas in CD, most believe that lifetime abstinence is possible.

c. MH often uses psychiatric drugs to treat the dual diagnosis patient whereas CD promotes a drug free philosophy.

d. MH has a supportive philosophy whereas CD uses a confrontive philosophy.

7. Health professionals combine the two philosophies of treatment to develop programs that treat both illnesses (mental illness and addiction) of the dually diagnosed individual.

8. Triple diagnosis is the coexistence of a mental health problem, a drug addiction, and an HIV diagnosis.

9. The three factors that determine the mental health of individuals and their susceptibility to addiction are heredity, environment, and psychoactive drugs.

10. Each of the above factors manipulates brain chemistry, so one of the goals of treatment is to rebalance brain chemistry.

11. Treatment programs for the dually diagnosed individual should address both the mental illness and the addiction.

12. Treatment for dual diagnosis can be done through psychotherapy, counseling, the group process, and/or with psychiatric medications.

13. The major classes of psychiatric drugs are antidepressants, MAO inhibitors, antipsychotics, antianxiety drugs, Lithium, and Beta-blockers.

Optional

14. Drugs used to treat depression are tricyclic antidepressants, MAO inhibitors, amphetamines, and newer antidepressants such as Prozac and Zoloft.

15. Some of the drugs used to treat schizophrenia are the phenothiazines such as fluphenazine (Prolixin) and chlorpromazine (Thorazine); halperidol (Haldol); clozapine (Clozaril, etc).

16. The principal drugs used to treat anxiety are the benzodiazepines such as Valium, and Xanax and the non-benzodiazepine BuSpar (buspirone).

17. The main drug used to treat a bipolar disorder is lithium.

QUESTIONS

1. Define dual diagnosis.

2. Name the three mental illnesses that are usually present in a dually diagnosed client.

3. Name three other mental illnesses that are also found in dually diagnosed clients.

4. Name two of the four ways psychoactive drugs can produce a dually diagnosed individual.

5. Give two examples of psychoactive drugs mimicking a mental illness.

6. Name four differences between the mental health treatment community and the chemical dependency treatment community.

7. Compare recovery as defined by the mental health treatment community and the chemical dependency treatment community.

8. Define triple diagnosis and multiple diagnosis.

9. What is the difference between depression and bipolar illness?

10. Name four kinds of anxiety illnesses.

11. What are the three main factors that affect our mental condition?

12. What are three approaches to treating mental illness?

Optional

13. Name three different classes of drugs used to treat depression.

14. What is the main drug used to treat manic-depression?

15. Name the two classes of drugs used to treat anxiety.

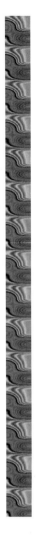

CONCLUSION

The search to understand drug use and addiction in humans has led researchers to two profound conclusions. One is that psychoactive drugs can only produce effects that already exist within us. That is, psychoactive drugs merely mimic, disrupt, or interfere with existing neurotranmsitters of the central nervous system and in that manner, create those feelings, emotions, highs, and relief from distress we try to get from drugs. And further, it means we already have the capacity to experience these highs or relieve our pain naturally, without the use of psychoactive drugs.

One can think of neurotransmitters as the body's scorekeepers. They keep track of our pleasure, satisfaction, elation, and pain and let us know when we are going in the right direction. The other amazing feature of our neurotransmitters is that we can control them through complex intellectual, emotional, physical, spiritual, artistic and even social endeavors. For instance, why else would we feel a surge of pleasure by solving a math equation or figuring out how to put the Christmas bike together.

The other conclusion is that the need to alter our state of consciousness is inherent in our makeup, even when we are in neurochemical balance. Humans seem to have a need to continually change the way they view, feel, and interact with the world around them as a way to seek pleasure or possibly to search for some idea or feeling beyond themselves.

The problem with using drugs to try to change consciousness and experience feelings such as pleasure, love, desire, accomplishment, elation, awe, and even fear, or avoid feelings like anxiety, pain, depression, and again, fear, is that the body has an inborn, relentless drive to remain in equilibrium.

What this means is that when drugs are taken to alter the neurotransmitters in order to create or avoid these feelings, the body senses that these are foreign, toxic substances, and through the mechanism of tolerance, it tries to adapt to, or neutralize, metabolize, and eliminate these chemicals. So, more drugs are needed to try to recapture or avoid those feelings.

And as use escalates, physical and mental side effects start to take their toll on the user's health and neurochemical balance, and it becomes harder and harder to duplicate that high, or relieve that pain. DRUGS ARE INHERENTLY SELF-LIMITING. Additionally, the continued use of the drug further alters the neurochemistry until a dependence on that drug develops. The user even forgets how to achieve many of the feelings without drugs.

Natural highs and techniques, on the other hand, are not self-limiting, have no side-effects, intensify with time, and can last for months, even years. We remain healthy because this is the way we were meant to blend with the world around us; this is the way we were meant to keep score with life.

What we are saying is that everyone needs to explore their natural states of consciousness and learn to seek and engage in daily activities which can produce the natural highs (or control the distress and pain), that some seek through drugs.

These natural highs can be physical, simple, and sometimes as brief as walking on a spring morning, playing a pick-up game of basketball in the school yard, eating a scrumptious dinner, or wearing a really comfortable shirt.

They can be more intellectual, complex, and longer lasting like getting an "A" on an exam one really studied for, planning a surprise party for a spouse's birthday, or performing a nice piece of carpentry on a house-building job.

They can involve more complex emotional relationships with people such as working well with a friend on a term project, sharing ideas, feelings, and thoughts with a brother or sister, or being willing to accept a spouse's faults and get on with your lives.

They can involve artistic achievements; painting, dancing, acting, or writing.

They can involve social and emotional commitments that span years; making sure your parents or your children are cared for, becoming accomplished at your job no matter what it is, being a support and friend to your neighbors, or remaining true to your promises

even when difficult.

Finally, they can span a lifetime, most often involving a daily dedication and adherence to a way of life, a morality, a spirituality, or a religious belief.

We're not saying that natural highs are all as easy to achieve as a swim at the beach. Many of them take time, a maturity, and a long-term commitment to see it through, but the results are equally rewarding. Which drug induced high compares in satisfaction and longevity with learning how to make peace with a parent you feared. We're also not saying that drugs are evil or bad in and of themselves. It is the way they are used that makes them that way. Some can be used in a rational, limited manner or in a compulsive, destructive way. The final decision is up to us.

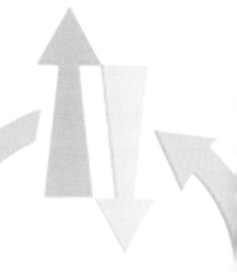

SELECTED BIBLIOGRAPHY

Besides the many interviews of drug abusers, former drug abusers, and health care professionals, we have consulted hundreds of articles, books, pamphlets, and studies. The follow list includes those we found most valuable.

Abadinsky, Howard. Drug Abuse: An Introduction. Chicago: Nelson-Hall, 1989.

American Psychiatric Association: Diagnostic and Statistical Manual of Mental Disorders, Third Edition, Revised. Washington, DC, American Psychiatric Association, 1987.

Banks, Dr. Robert, Jr., editor. Substance Abuse in Sport: The Realities. Dubuque, Iowa: The United States Sports Academy/Kendall/Hunt Publishing Company, 1990.

Briggs, et. a., Drugs in Pregnancy and Lactation. Baltimore, MD: Williams and Wilkins, 1986.

Carroll, Charles R. Drugs in Modern Society. Third Edition. Madison, WI: Brown & Benchmark. 1993.

Cohen, Sydney. The Chemical Mind: The Neurochemistry of Addictive Disorders. Minneapolis, MN: CompCare Publishers, 1988.

Davis, Kenneth, Howard Klar, and Joseph T. Coyle. Foundations of Psychiatry. Philadelphia: Harcourt Brace Jovanovich, Inc., 1991.

Department of Health and Human Services, Office of Inspector General. Adolescent Steroid Use. 1991.

Evans, Katie and J. Michael Sullivan. Dual Diagnosis: Counseling the Mentally Ill Substance Abuser. New York: The Guilford Press. 1990.

Fleming, Michael F. and Kristen Lawton Barry. Addictive Disorders. St. Louis: Mosby Year Book. 1992.

Gorman, Jack. M., M.D. The Essential Guide to Psychiatric Drugs. New York: St. Martin Press. 1990.

Leccese, Arthur P., Ph.D. Drugs and Society: Behavioral Medicines and Abusable Drugs. Englewood Cliffs, NJ: Prentice Hall, 1991.

Lowinson, Joyce H., M.D. et. al. Substance Abuse: A Comprehensive Textbook. Second Edition. Baltimore: Williams & Wilkins, 1992.

Miller, Norman S. Comprehensive Handbook of Drug and Alcohol Addiction. New York: Marcel Dekker, Inc., 1991.

Mottram, D.R. Drugs in Sport. Champaign, IL: Human Kinetics Books, 1988.

O'Brien, Robert, Sidney Cohen, M.D., et. al. The Encyclopedia of Drug Abuse. Second Edition. New York: Facts on File, 1992.

Physician's Drug Handbook. 5th Edition. Springhouse, PA: Springhouse Corporation, 1993.

Schultes, Richard Evans and Albert Hofmann. Plants of the Gods. Rochester, VT: Healing Arts Press, 1992.

Seymour, Richard B. & Smith, David E. Drugfree: A Unique, Positive Approach to Staying Off Alcohol and Other Drugs. New York: Harrington, 1987. Available from Haight-Ashbury Publications, 409 Clayton St., San Francisco, CA 94117.

The Guide to Psychoactive Drugs. New York, Harrington, 1987. Also available from Haight-Ashbury Publications.

Silver, Gary & Michael Aldrich. The Dope Chronicles: 1850-1950. San Francisco, CA: Harper and Row Publishers, 1979.

Snyder, Solomon H. Drugs and the Brain. New York: Scientific American Library, 1986.

Stafford, Peter. Psychedelics Encyclopedia. Third Expanded Edition. Berkeley, CA: Ronin Publishing, Inc. 1992.

Tricker, Ray and David L. Cook. Athletes at Risk: Drugs and Sport. Dubuque, IA. Wm. C. Brown Publishers, 1990.

U.S. Department of Health and Human Services. Alcohol and Health. Seventh Special Report to the U.S. Congress. Rockville, MD: U.S.Department of Health and Human Services, 1990.

Drug Use Among American High School Seniors, College Students and Young Adults, 1975-1990. Rockville, MD: U.S. Department of Health and Human Services [NIDA], 1991.

National Household Survey on Drug Abuse: Population Estimates 1992. Rockville, MD: U.S. Department of Health and Human Services, 1992.

U.S. Government. Abuse of Steroids in Amateur and Professional Athletics. (Hearing before the Subcommittee on Crime of the Committee on the Judiciary, House of Representatives, March 22, 1990.)

Wadler, Gary I. and Brian Hainline, M.D. Drugs and the Athlete. Philadelphia: F.A. Davis Company, 1989.

Weil, Andrew, M.D. and Winifred Rosen. From Chocolate to Morphine: Everything You Need to Know About Mind-Altering Drugs. Boston/New York: Houghton Mifflin Company, 1993.

Yesalis, Charles E. ScD. Editor. Anabolic Steroids in Sport and Exercise. Champaign, IL: Human Kinetics Publishers, Inc. 1993.

Zerkin, Leif & Jeffrey H. Novey, Editors. Journal of Psychoactive Drugs, 1967-1993. Available through Haight-Ashbury Publications, 409 Clayton Street, San Francisco, CA, 94117.

INDEX

A